MW00634620

ARCHITECT
OF
AESTHETICS

JOSEPH MURCI

DISCLAIMER: The information in this book is given to provide helpful information to the reader regarding the subjects discussed. This book is not meant to be used, nor should it be used, to diagnose or treat any medical condition. It is the sole responsibility of the reader to do their own research and use their own judgment before applying any of the methods or advice given in this book. Every reader should consult their physician before embarking on any training or nutritional program or advice as outlined here to ensure their safety and well-being. The publisher and author are not responsible for any specific health or allergy needs that may require medical supervision and are not liable for any damages or negative consequences to any person reading or following the information provided in this book. References are provided for informational purposes only and do not in any way constitute endorsement of any people, brands, institutions, or other sources.

COPYRIGHT 2017. JOSEPH MURCI. ALL RIGHTS RESERVED. No portion of this book may be displayed, copied, shared, or recreated under any means without explicit written consent by the author.

www.JOSEPHMURCI.com

Cover art: Garry Nguyen
ISBN: 978-0-692-93514-9

TABLE OF CONTENTS

THE 10 LAWS OF THE ARCHITECT OF AESTHETICS

MAXIMS OF AESTHETICS

REFERENCES

☾

PROLOGUE

GROWING UP, I WAS A BIT DIFFERENT than most
kids. Whereas the other kids were outside playing, I was
inside exploring a world of imagination and discovery. I was
an obsessive reader. I had a passion for art and drawing. My young
mind churned as I peered through my thick glasses to devise the
most magnificent structures I could muster with building blocks to
showcase in my room atop the shelf.

"That little boy is going to be a great scientist or architect
someday," people would say.

Being as I was, I didn't grow up with many friends. Who could
relate to me then?

I was shy, overweight, and shut out from hanging out with the
other kids. I was picked on, made fun of, and oftentimes found
myself sitting by myself in the lunchroom. Alone facing the silence

in a noisy room full of people. I didn't go to parties. I didn't go on dates. Most nights it was just me and my thoughts.

One day, I decided that I would make a change. I decided that I would stop feeling sorry for myself and living beneath my potential. I decided that I wanted more out of life, and it was *MY job* to go and get it.

See, my family comes from the poorest roots you can imagine. From trailer parks and the projects, my mother and father joined the military, said goodbye to their old lives, and crossed oceans and language barriers in pursuit of a better future than being broke, dead, or in prison. We never had much, but we what we *did have* was hard work and determination.

And I was going to use mine.

So one day, I told my dad I wanted to train and join in on his morning military routine. We were up before dawn running the streets while the rest of the world tossed and turned in their sheets. Bitter cold or blazing hot. It didn't matter. 3 miles of running followed by a circuit of calisthenics was my daily breakfast.

I'd be lying to you if I said it was easy. Most days my little legs wanted to give up. But my dad would always tell me:

> *"It's all in your head. You have to be motivated!*
> *You need to pick a point and say 'I'm going to*
> *reach it!'. Then you set another. And then before*
> *you know it, you'll be home."*

So I stuck to it. I pushed through. I toughed it out every morning there in the icy darkness when all I could see was my breath and the vision I had. And for the first time, I began to see my body change.

I looked in the mirror and saw the metamorphosis taking place before my very eyes. It was my first taste of training and I was hungry for more. So I started lifting on the old weight bench at home every night after school. I couldn't wait for the final bell to ring so that I could hop on the bus home and go train.

I began to fine tune my nutrition and devour any information I could to become better. I would plan, plot, and experiment with programs and ideas in a little notebook I carried with me everywhere. I was diligent and dedicated. I was lured in by desire but fell in love with the process.

...and the results poured in. I forged my body. Day in and day out. Rep by rep. Set by set. And as I did, my mind grew. I became stronger inside and out. I cultivated that part of me I never even knew I had.

As time went along, I progressed further and further in and out of the weight room. By the hands of fate, I went through many other major things as time went by that have molded me, changed my look on life, and made me into who I am today writing these words to you. I learned that LIFE is a gym. And no matter how hard it hit or how far I strayed, the weights were still right there waiting for me.

The problems I used to have back then are gone. When it came to attention and friends, I didn't have any. Now the problem is having too many. I went from having low self-esteem to paving the way to chase my dream. I was just a little boy who was looked down upon and wanted to change his life. And now everyone looks up to *me* and asks *me* for advice. I can't thank you enough.

And that's why I am here writing this for you all. For you to be the best *you* can be and live life to *your fullest potential*. It is my firm, unshakeable belief that *each and every one of you is special* and has something great to offer the world, and I'm going to take you there. One way or another. YOU. WILL. BE. GREAT.

Today, I don't design buildings nor do I run laboratory experiments. But as turns out, I did grow up to use my fascination of the world and love for discovery to build my dreams and a better life for myself and others. I did make it home. I did become an architect.

AN ARCHITECT of AESTHETICS.

FOR THE FUTURE KINGS AND QUEENS

For once you have tasted flight, you will walk the earth with your eyes turned skywards,
for there you have been, and there you will long to return.

Leonardo da Vinci

PART I: AESTHETIC FOUNDATIONS

1

THE START OF A
JOURNEY

Let him that would move the world first move himself.
Socrates

SET OF WEIGHTS AND A VISION. That's how it all began. It's been over 10 years since I hit my first set on the rusty old home weight bench with a mix of anger and excitement pulsing through my veins, and since then I've racked up knowledge and real-world experience through countless trial and error, extensive research on all things fitness and life, and reflections upon it all day in and day out in a quest for the best.

It's my passion, it changed my life, and it's all jam packed right here into this very book. Right here is the book I wish I had when I started out. Right here is what every soul who dreams of taking their body to its fullest needs to read. Everything you need to achieve your dreams and dominate. All yours. Use it well.

Dear reader, I don't you know you. And I likely never will.

But what I DO know *beyond a shadow of a doubt* is that within each and every one of you lies the potential for GREATNESS. Within you lies a WARRIOR. A FIGHTER. A CHAMPION. A HERO.

A work of art.

And it's my job to bring it out of you.

- Together, we will lift you to the heights you were destined to reach.
- Together, we will transform your life. Together, we will break boundaries and build empires.

...and it all starts with one building: the body.

Are you up for the task?

This journey isn't for everyone. But if you have what it takes, I can promise you that you will never be the same.

Let's kick things off by running through the benefits of the process of transforming the body through the weights and nutrition.

There's way more to lifting than meets *the eye*.

AESTHETICS

AESTHETICS. The fitness world is buzzing with this word like a bumblebee on cocaine, pre-workout, and lightning bolts from Zeus, and it's the ultimate prize sought after by lifters around the world. There's no surprise that physique is currency and will get you far in this world, and these juicy benefits of getting aesthetic on their *own* are enough to send most chasing gains to get aesthetic, but few know what it actually means.

Far from just a word to torment small children at spelling bees, Aesthetics are the branch of philosophy dealing with the principles of art and beauty. In other words: What looks good and why? And it goes way back.

For over 2500 years, philosophers from Plato to prom queens have debated just exactly what it is that makes things aesthetically pleasing, and for over 2500 years, no one seems to know for sure.

Many have argued that aesthetics are objective. Others shrug their shoulders and say that beauty is in the eye of the beholder.

What's the truth?

I'll break things down and give you the real deal right here in this book to take your physique to its aesthetic peaks.

THE AESTHETIC PHYSIQUE

We see beauty everywhere, but nowhere is this more evident than in the body and all that it's capable of.

In the notebook of the celebrated Renaissance polymath, Leonardo da Vinci, there is a drawing known as the Vitruvian Man. This drawing depicts a man in two extended positions enclosed by a square and a circle that demonstrates the ideal human proportion in all of its glory.

In that one little drawing, you see purpose, order, beauty, and harmony expressed through the human form. Incredible.

From Leonardo's sketch to the classical Greek sculptures to modern-day fitness icons and elite level athletes, it's impossible to evade the shell-shocking sensation of awe provoked by the simultaneous, paradoxical display of power and grace that the human body is capable of.

The body is a moving, moldable masterpiece that can be sculpted with attention to proportion, balance, and symmetry, and best of all? YOU are both the sculptor and the sculpted.

THE BENEFITS

People say looks don't matter. I say they're crazy. With one simple look at someone, you can tell a lot about who they are underneath and what they're made of.

There's much more to a person than their looks, but looks are the first thing people see and have extremely powerful effects out there in the world. First impressions last a lifetime. An aesthetic physique generates:

- ❧ SOCIAL PROOF
- ❧ RESPECT
- ❧ POWER
- ❧ INCREASED ATTRACTION
- ❧ BOOSTED SELF CONFIDENCE
- ❧ ENHANCED APPEARANCE

With an aesthetic physique, when you walk into a room, it's all eyes on you. Without speaking a word, you have already spoken volumes. People see the dedication and mental strength written all over you. There's a mix of jealousy, wonder, and respect. This will supe up your power level everywhere you go. You set the tone, and you're the example for others. Don't abuse it.

An aesthetic physique is like a cheat code to life, but you didn't cheat for it. You *earned* it.

Because of that fact, the body is a work of art to take pride in. Any fool with money can go to the store and pick up a new pair of shoes, jacket, or wristwatch. But to have a powerful, chiseled physique? That's something money can never touch.

An aesthetic physique is a badge of honor and a testament to the rock-solid character and dues that its beholder has paid... in – and OUT – of the weight room.

There's a reason it's a rare treasure out there.

Getting there will require:

MENTAL FORTITUDE

An aesthetic physique doesn't come without a price.
To reach the pinnacles of physical development, you've got to put in the time and work required. Aesthetics require impetus, commitment, and determination.

To train your muscles is to train your mind. To become the master of anything, first you must master yourself, and the gym will take you there.

Breaking past your barriers and achieving a new personal best in the weight room, staying on point with your nutrition, showing up consistently and putting in the work. That's the grind you can't fake - only cultivate.

You will develop patience, learn the value of responsibility, discipline, consistency, and self-control on as personal a level as there can be. The body is the most intimate possession you have.

WHO IS IN CONTROL?

It will fight and strive for dominion over you. Will you let it?

NO.

You will learn that it is your MIND that controls your body – not the other way around.

When you are tired and push forward despite your body's every aversion to the contrary – it is because of your mind. When you are tempted and led astray but stay firm to your goal – it is because of your mind. When before you rests that heavy heap of iron that is determined to crush your spirit, it is your MIND that sends the signal to your body that you CAN and WILL move that weight. That you WILL overcome.

Struggle, pain, temptation. You will not run from them.
You will *welcome* them into your life and learn to love them as your own. That's how you'll grow in the gym. That's how you'll grow as a person. That's what weightlifting can provide that other pursuits can't touch.

By all means, play cool songs and paint pretty pictures, but when you want to see what a person is really made of, put their body to the test. Throw them in the iron jungle and see how they handle the heat.

Don't let appearances fool you. Lifting weights is a mental sport above all else. It's you vs. You. The weights are just keeping score. It's all in your hands.

The gym is just a rehearsal for life, and lifting weights will strengthen the mind in far more ways than you can imagine. The mind is the origin of all reality, and to fortify it will enable us to do great things...

MAXIM OF AESTHETICS: THE MIND IS THE STRONGEST MUSCLE YOU HAVE.

Let's utilize this potential.

UNLEASH THE BEAST

What do you hate?

What pisses you off?

What's got you stressed?

What scars do you carry inside?

You feel that sinister surge rise up within you? Good. You're human and it's a cold, cruel world out there. Let's use that.

Within us all dwells a beast. A beast of unimaginable power. A maniac. A monster. Raw, primitive, and merciless. We all have a dark side. And it must be trained and wielded wisely.

For the majority of the time, we've got to keep it locked up tight deep within the chambers of our psyche, but there are times in which we can let it loose and give it free reign to frolic in the fires of its frustrations, lusts, and fury.

Rather than let it burn a hole inside of us and destroy or lead us into vices in the external world to cover up the hurt, we can channel that power for good in the weight room.

We can convert the pain into GAIN. The negativity into POSITIVITY. The hardship into CHAMPIONSHIP.

When you put yourself under that bar & barrel through that gut-wrenching set, you unleash that brazen beast and incinerate all of your frustrations, worries, fears, problems, stress, and tension within.

For that one hour, they don't exist. All that exists is you and your mission.

You transform from a civilized soul into a rabid werewolf howling upon the sight of the milky full moon and run wild, attacking that workout with fervent force. You leave that gym feeling like a champion.

You leave that gym feeling like a brand new person. And in a way...you are. You are transforming your body, your soul, and your mind.

Release your demons. Use your nightmares to fuel your dreams. Turn the enemy into your extra edge. That's the way you put pain in its place.

VITALITY

Look down at your hand and move your fingers.

Watch as the bundle of bones, a highway of blood vessels, and a grid of nerves work in seamless synchronization to carry out whatever you command. Your whole body is a masterpiece. Even your eyes that read this are more sophisticated than anything mankind will ever make.

Your body is the bridge from the mental world into the physical world. The primary and most important function of the body is allowing us to live life how life should be lived. Full of health and energy.

Crack open any anatomy textbook and you will be overloaded with the magnificent, intricate structures of incredible sophistication present throughout our bodies - all at our service to use to live and move in the world.

Lifting weights delivers the ammunition to function and feel better inside and out, move better, generate proper posture, and ensure strong tissues, bones, and joints. You have the ability to renovate yourself inside and out to strengthen your body and live as it was designed to live.

If nothing else, this is the single most important function of training that should never be jeopardized or neglected – for life. When the body is healthy, strong, and functioning as it should be, the rest of our life can unfold.

THE TEMPLE

Imagine the sports car of your dreams. What would it be?

A cherry red roadster? A murdered-out Italian monster? A silky white, curvaceous angel that floats across the asphalt at blistering speeds? Picture it in vivid detail.

If I gave you the keys to that car of your dreams, what would you do with it?

- ~ You would put the best fuel into it.
- ~ You'd wash, wax, and polish it every day.
- ~ You'd make sure you keep up with the maintenance and the repair religiously.

...so why don't you do that with your own body?

- ~ Hit the gym.
- ~ Eat well.
- ~ Dress well.
- ~ Sleep well.
- ~ Sit up straight.
- ~ Walk tall and proud.

The #1 reason why we lift - *the biggest of them all* - is because building the body and the process of doing so is the highest expression of self-love there is. Your body is your temple, and you only get one. Be proud of who you are and treat it like it deserves to be treated - the very best. Build that temple. Decorate that temple. Care for that temple. Brick by brick. Day after day. Train hard. Dress for success. Eat the very best. And rest like royalty.

Never take it for granted. Never. The body is not your enemy. It is your ally and best friend. It will speak to you. Listen. It will handle whatever you throw at it because it's there for you. This is the true meaning of the architect of aesthetics. Building that temple. 'Til death do you part.

Someday, we will all be buried and ashes. But the spirit that made that temple a work of art will never die.

TRANSFORM YOUR ENTIRE LIFE

Embarking on the journey of physical training and all it entails will unlock a world of potential for your life.

Whether you are a raw beginner or have some experience under your belt already, continually expanding your knowledge and abilities in the world of training, nutrition, and recovery is an investment that will pay you handsome returns now and as long as you may live.

The person you were when you first opened this book is not the same that will leave it. I'll make a winner out of you.

No man has the right to be an amateur in the matter of physical training. It is a shame for a man to grow old without seeing the beauty and strength of which his body is capable.

Socrates

2

THE SUCCESS
EQUATION

SUCCESS. What does that mean to you? Your dream body. Your dream life. What would you do if you could do *anything* you desired? No limits. No judgment. NOTHING holding you back.

Can you see it? No. Scratch that. Don't just see it. *FEEL IT* deep within you. Every detail. All of it.

Got it? Sweet. Hold onto that. That's going to be your future.

MAXIM OF AESTHETICS: SUCCESS BEGINS WITHIN.
BEFORE YOU CAN BE IT, FIRST YOU MUST SEE IT.

It's more than a vision. *It's previewing reality.* And it's all up to you to make it happen now.

But far too few actually do it...we'll fix that.

THE 4 P'S OF SUCCESS

Is success some sort of mythical monster that hides in a secret part of the woods and only comes out on a full moon during the third Friday of October? Is it just a product of sheer luck and wishful thinking? Do you have to sacrifice your first born, drink the blood of a unicorn, or sell your soul? The answer is no. Success is ripe, real, and up for the taking.

When you dissect success across history and even in the modern day, you will discover that there are several commonalities present that took seemingly common individuals to great heights.

Time and time again, someone rises from the depths, beats adversity, and cements their legacy in time. The impossible is made possible. The unthinkable becomes reality. Against all odds, limits are broken and great things are done.

...will you do the same?

MAXIM OF AESTHETICS: LEARN FROM THE GREATS - BOTH IN THEIR VICTORY AND IN THEIR DEFEAT.

When you boil it all down, success is achieved by nailing 4 fundamental areas:

PERSON + PURSUIT + PROCESS + PURPOSE = SUCCESS

THIS is the formula for success. The only one you'll ever need.

If you wish to succeed in fitness and in life, you will do well to abide by it.

PERSON

14 billion years ago amidst a sea of darkness, the Universe exploded into existence from a single point smaller than the head of a pin needle that has culminated in the richness of life of you and I.

You and I. Human beings. Alive with infinity ahead of us in this great big world full of potential.

The beauty of being human resides in our ability to transform who we are inside and out.

Mentally. Physically. Spiritually.

You can become whatever you want to be. And for as far as we can see when we peer out into the far reaches of the vast Universe and the stars from which we were made, we are the only ones in existence who possess this gift.

...what are you going to do with it?

CAPTAIN OF YOUR SOUL

Your life is whatever you make of it.

The whole world will tell you what *they* want you to do. They'll tell you what you *should* do. They'll try to tell you what you *can* and *can't* do. Don't listen to them. It's not theirs to decide. It's yours.

You will sculpt your life and sculpt yourself based on your vision. You will become your own work of art. This is YOUR job, and your job alone. Embrace this fact and embrace this freedom.

From this point forward, you will stop looking at yourself like a victim of your situation and blaming others for your shortcomings. You will stop blaming society, your genetics, the government, your family, your friends, and whoever else you feel like is responsible for you not being where you want to be. No more. It's all on YOU. You're the captain of this ship, and heaven, earth, and the Seven Seas are all open for you to explore.

From this point forward, you will assume responsibility for your life and everything in it. Good or bad. It doesn't matter. It's all there to build you. It's all there for your glory. If you're not willing to accept your past, then you don't deserve to take credit for your future either. Own it. It'll make your story greater.

From this point forward, you will face the world with your inner strength as a person. Toss aside all of the masks and materials. Step out from your phantom fortress of status and fame. That's what cowards do. You must be great without them or you are nothing with them. It's all about you. Everything comes from within.

From this point forward, you will rely on yourself and yourself alone as the ruler of your reality. You were born alone, and you will die alone. Others can help you in your journey, but people come and go like the seasons, and at the end of the day when everything is said and done, you're all that you've got.

When that heavy bar is on the ground, who lifts it? When life knocks you down, who is it that stands up? When things get tough, who is it that refuses to give up?

You. And it's *your* job to make yourself into the best version of you that you can be. Only then will you truly succeed now and forever.

But where shall you start?

THE ORACLE

In Ancient Greece, travelers of all shapes and sizes came from far and wide to the Oracle at the Temple of Apollo in Delphi in search of answers.

Young and old. Rich and poor. Amongst them was even the Spartan King, Leonidas, before taking his fearless 300 Spartans into brutal battle against the monstrous military forces of Persia. It was revered - a sacred place. A place of wisdom and guidance.

Yet do you know what the wise elders had inscribed upon the entrance of this temple for all of the hopeful to see upon their arrival?

"GNOTHI SEAUTON."
"KNOW THYSELF."

You come seeking knowledge...You come seeking answers...You come seeking truth...

But first, KNOW THYSELF. *This* is the beginning of all knowledge.

MAXIM OF AESTHETICS: KNOW THYSELF. YOU ARE YOUR BIGGEST ALLY OR GREATEST FOE.

Who are you?

Not what society *thinks* you are. Not who you *pretend* to be. The true you. The you that only *you* can ever see.

- A human being. With heart and soul. Mind and body.
- A person. With a past that has brought you here to read this very sentence in one way or another.
- An individual. With thoughts, dreams, and beliefs. Character, values, and skills.

To know thyself is to know who you are deep down at your core.

What are you made of? Why do you do the things that you do? What are the thoughts in your head? What are your strengths and weaknesses?

Now get up and go look yourself in the mirror. Stare long and hard.

You see that? That's you TODAY. Focus on who you will BECOME tomorrow. Your past does not determine your future. YOU DO.

That vision of success. You can do that. I promise you. You've got to believe down to the deepest fiber of your being that you can do it.

That you WILL do it.

BUILD THE PERSON

Nothing comes into being without first passing through a PERSON. Great things happen because GREAT people do them. Therefore, *you must make yourself great.*

> YOUR MIND.
> YOUR BODY.
> YOUR CHARACTER.
> YOUR VALUES AND VIRTUES.

Work on these. Always and forever. You will never go wrong with investing in yourself, but you *will* go wrong by investing in everything else.

Break me down and bury me, and I will come back bigger and better than before. And you damn well better believe the same. Within you is infinite possibility. You have such power, and you don't even realize it.

But you will.

Become the best version of YOU that you can be, and the Kingdom will open its doors for you with submissive pleasure.

PURSUIT

An expert sniper is shown to be excellent by aiming at his target and hitting that bulls-eye.

YOU may be great, but where will you aim this greatness?

Where will you pour the most valuable things you have in life - your time, effort, and attention?

This is where you place *your life.* It will expand and expand. It will generate a mountain of compound interest over time that delivers a powerful payoff.

Every day when you wake up, you have a choice to make. What will you do with your day? This is your choice. And your will and choice are sacred. If you made the choice, you could do absolutely nothing at all until the day you withered away and died.

You are free. You always have been. You always will be.

So see to it that everything that you do in life is YOUR choice that brings value to you AND to others. This will make your life and the world at large a better place - just the way it should be.

Every thought. Every action. Every day. That's all you. Choose wisely.

THE MISGUIDED

Look at the world's definition of success and what they pursue. Money, fame, and material items. Look at why they do what they do. To conform to the norm. To cover themselves up with things that can never satisfy them or fill that empty hole within them.

Free by law, but slaves to themselves. We will do better.

Listen up and listen good. Nothing - *absolutely nothing* - could EVER make you more valuable as a human being than who YOU are within. The world is change, and you'll waste your whole life chasing external satisfaction with nothing to show for it but pain and lost time.

Your life is of infinite value. Don't trade it for society's opinion or something that comes with a warranty.

Your pursuit must be much more. Don't ask so little from life.

BE THE EAGLE

Think about what you love to do.

Think about that thing you'd dedicate yourself to for nothing in return. That thing that the mere thought of gives you that little leap of joy inside you. THAT'S what you need to pursue in life.

Pursue your passions. Pursue what moves you. Pursue what springs from within naturally. Pursue what you love where time stops, a week passes by in an instant, and the mere act itself paints the world in vibrant hues.

Don't waste a second of your life pursuing something that doesn't resonate deeply with you and bring you unconditional joy. Don't waste it chasing hollow dreams. All you'll get is struggle and disappointment.

When your pursuit is on point, life will come easy and struggle is a thing of the past.

Does an eagle struggle to fly? No. That's what eagles were BORN to do.

So escape from your cage of invisible bars. Get your feathers out of the mud and put yourself where YOU belong - high in the sky. Doing what *you* were born to do.

Afraid?

Have FAITH. Leap off of the cliff and you'll see your wings take you wherever you want to go.

MAXIM OF AESTHETICS: CHASE NOT MONEY NOR FAME. CHASE YOUR PASSION, AND ONLY THEN WILL THE WORLD REMEMBER YOUR NAME.

Here, our pursuit will be to tap into our fullest physical potential. To take the body to the heights and glory it was destined to reach. Bettering yourself - that's as noble a pursuit as you can get.

We will develop a love for the iron. We will find joy in the steps we take - no matter how small. Devising plans, plotting our progress, fine-tuning and refining. Growth. Advancement. Self-improvement. Conquest. This is our art. This is our joy. This is our pursuit.

PROCESS

Our process is the string of events that take our pursuit and transform it into the reality we wish to see. Rest assured, if there is something you wish to achieve, there exists a way to make that a reality. You just need to figure out *how*.

For anything you wish to achieve in life, you must ask yourself these questions:

I.   WHAT IS MY GOAL?
II. WHAT IS NECESSARY TO ACHIEVE THIS GOAL?
III. WHAT ARE THE CONSTRAINTS?
IV. HOW DOES THIS FIT THE BIGGER PICTURE?
V.   GIVEN THE ABOVE, WHAT IS THE BEST WAY TO CARRY THIS OUT?

This will create your process.

When you've got this figured out and set things in motion, success is inevitable. That's right. **INEVITABLE.** Rejoice. It's just a matter of time. It couldn't be any other way.

So don't sweat success. It's yours. It just likes to flirt and play hard to get.

Now what you'll need is the right knowledge and application.

KNOWLEDGE

The body is an incredibly complex work of art, but I will give you the fundamental knowledge and tools you need on training, nutrition, and much, much more to accomplish your goals with flying colors.

No bullshit. No new tricks. No magic bullets.

We will take the knowledge from scientific research and study of various fields and COMBINE that with first-hand, real world experience to create the optimal program. You can't stick to just one or the other. That's tunnel vision. When and where we need to, I will fill that in with educated decision making and time-crafted intuition to put you in your best firing position.

The fitness industry thrives on myths and loves to sell hype and lies, but *there is no magic bullet* - it's all about the *basics* and *who's pulling the trigger.* Aesthetics are all about CONSISTENCY.

Consistency. Showing up and putting in the work day in and day out. Nothing worthwhile in life comes without consistent effort. 1 step more. 10 steps more. Ever forward. JUST KEEP MOVING. Keep driving those legs 'til you're in the end-zone and living life at the after party.

THAT'S what separates the kings and queens from the common complainers. THAT'S the way you win. And that's where application comes in.

APPLICATION

A great person, a worthy pursuit, and the right knowledge are all stopped dead in their tracks by a faulty process. When we're met with failure, it's often the process – not the person. Application is critical. Remember Newton's Law:

An object in motion will stay in motion unless acted upon by an outside force.

Therefore, we will *remove* those outside forces so that you have an unobstructed path to pay-dirt for the winning touchdown. The only thing standing in your way is your own desire.

In the fitness world and society at large, people think more pain is more gain. They think success is all about sacrifice and working harder, and if you don't succeed, then you need to be more dedicated and disciplined. They may succeed for a little while, but it never lasts and they all burn out and fade away. Fuck all that.

You do not sacrifice. You will use your mind and assess all the valid requirements and constraints and when there's no way out, you make TRADEOFFS instead. Sacrifice is for victims. This is for your glory and you love it. Watch the words that come out of your mouth or run through your head. They matter.

Dedication and discipline are beautiful things, but only where they are necessary. Don't wear yourself down fighting battles that don't need to be fought. Do what you need to do and save your energy and attention for the important things so that you're fresh and always at your best.

THE BETTER WAY

Driven by the goal, we will take those requirements and constraints and weave them into a workable process that is best for YOU as an individual.

We will maximize the results through effectiveness and efficiency by choosing and using the right tools and eliminating wasted effort or second-class methods from the process.

We will devise the optimal workout program that takes all factors into account. You as a person. Your current level. Your life as a whole. What's best in theory is not always best in practice, and where I see fit, I will put my focus on YOUR success rather than the success of a concept. We must make your success F.A.T.E.

FUN. ACCESSIBLE. TIMELY. EASY.

Success has to be like a game. Moving forward has to be an available option at all times. It's got to be there whenever and not require you to sign away your entire life. It's got to be simple, easy, and flexible. How can you NOT succeed in a system like that?

Life is all about the journey, and THAT'S how you maximize the journey. We will do what we need to do and leave some space for life to shine through. Clean, simple, and efficient. We'll be flexible and adapt. We will achieve AND keep the results. We will...

BE LIKE WATER

We will be wise and choose the right, crystal clear stream to flow unobstructed, adjusting our path to whatever we're met with – just like water, the essence of life.

Water always maintains its fundamental properties, but it molds and bends to adjust to the things it encounters. When it's in a glass, it becomes the glass. When it's freezing out, it freezes. When it's hot, it evaporates. A river flows and winds around the stones and follows the current.

Flow. Adapt. Be like water. Unattached. Free. Keep flowing and crashing like a mighty waterfall. Unstoppable.

Success is built on the little things. Consistency. The never-ending successive victories. Step by step. Drop by drop.

What will keep that river flowing with peak force? For that, you need:

PURPOSE

In life, it's not so much what you do. It's *why you do it.*

It's not about what happens, but *how you view it.*

Life is all about PURPOSE. The purpose that drives you. The purpose that you see in yourself and the world around you. No matter where you are - like or dislike, you HAVE to find purpose in what you're doing or you'll never make it. You're what gives it life and value.

Strong purpose can move mountains. Purpose will give you one more rep when you didn't think you could move another inch. Purpose will turn the negative into positive. The difficult into doable. Purpose will push you to unparalleled heights and open up the doors for possibilities you never dreamed of when the only one on your side is the reflection staring back at you in the mirror.

Even if you're stuck with a poor pursuit or a poor process, purpose will step in and carry that load like a mighty ox.

Motivation is for amateurs. What you need is PURPOSE.

This purpose can come from many areas. Many are driven by a variety of external factors. Wanting to impress others, wanting to be respected, wanting to feel accepted. No. Not good enough. Most people don't even like or respect themselves, and the only opinion that ever matters is your own that comes straight from the heart.

The TRUE, long lasting embers of unstoppable drive must always come from within. It's got to quake your very existence. It's got to be bigger than you. It's got to give you chills just thinking about it.

WHAT IS YOUR PURPOSE FOR PICKING UP THE WEIGHTS?

Sit in silence with nothing but the trickle of thoughts that cascade through your mind. With your body, you can do great things, but the body is corruptible. There must be more.

M   U   R   C   I

WHAT DO YOU WANT OUT OF LIFE?

WHY?

What is it that gets you up in the morning? Your alarm? Or your insatiable hunger to be the best version of **You** that you can be and pursue your dreams?

Today is a good day, my friends. You are alive and well with breath in your lungs, and many cannot say the same.

- How will you use it?
- What difference will it make that you woke up today?
- What difference will it make that you were ever even BORN at all?

Today, tomorrow, or twenty years from now when the Grim Reaper comes knocking at your door, are you going to be filled with regret and remorse?

"I wish I..."

"If only I..."

No. Fuck that. You wish nothing.

You say "THIS IS WHAT I WANT!" and you go out there and YOU make it happen. It's YOUR life and no one is going to live it for you.

Get out there and take risks. Throw yourself into the fire. Dare the world to knock you down so you can get back up and show them all who they're dealing with.

As long as there's another ounce of life in you and you have your vision and your purpose, you WILL NOT give up!

Succeed or ~~fail~~ learn lessons to become even better, you will go to bed every night knowing you gave it your very best and lived today the way it deserves to be lived: to the absolute fullest.

An ironclad purpose - DESIRE planted at the very roots of your soul - will catapult you to heights you can't even conceive of should you water it and let it flourish. It will push you in your darkest times and deliver you unto the Light. Despite all the odds, a strong purpose will override it all.

Discover this purpose. You are not complete without it.

MAXIM OF AESTHETICS: A HUMAN BEING WITH NO PURPOSE IS A HUMAN BEING WITH NO PULSE.

With these 4 factors of success in your hands, a thousand armies couldn't break you. No trials or tribulations can shake you. This formula will make you.

Now let's go get it.

3

THE AESTHETIC
PHYSIQUE

I saw the angel in the marble and carved until I set him free.
Michelangelo

ICHELANGELO was a young Italian Renaissance artist full of promise. At the tender age of 26, he began his tremendous work on sculpting David, one of the most celebrated and recognizable works of art in history - a task that would take him over 2 long, obsessive years of concentrated, passionate work. When Michelangelo revealed the sculpture of David for its placement on the roof of the church for which it was destined, the City of Florence decided upon having it placed elsewhere, for it was simply too beautiful to stay up there so far from view.

Over 2000 years prior to Michelangelo in the southeast off the isles of Greece, the Trojan War kicked off as thousands of ships set sail to the wind en route to Troy after the beautiful Helen, wife of the king of Sparta, eloped with the Prince of Troy and was taken off to live there. Legendary warriors such as Ajax and Achilles fought their battles amongst legions of soldiers to win her back.

Human beauty.

There can be no doubts that the human form is capable of incredible beauty and has captivated and intoxicated us since we left our first footprints on the soft soil of Mother Earth. Even more apparent is our human ability to create beauty - and that is what we will do - in ourselves and in the world.

FACTORS OF THE AESTHETIC PHYSIQUE

Aesthetics deal with the principles of art and beauty, and our goal is an aesthetic physique. But what does that look like? You know it when you see it, but why? Is it just in the eyes of the beholder or is there a definitive standard?

All of the above.

The fields of philosophy, modern neuroscience [1,2,3,4], biology, practical experience, and much more offer insights that point towards several conclusions that have led me to determine that the maximally aesthetic physique must be:

I.   INTRINSICALLY VISUALLY APPEALING
II.   BIOLOGICALLY AGREEABLE
III.   CULTURALLY ACCEPTABLE
IV.   PERSONALLY LIKEABLE

To be a truly great artist, you must be a student of the senses and the mind, the body that sustains them, history and the times in which you live, and the hearts and souls of others.

The artist is not a mere man with paint and a chisel. He is wise in the ways of the world and life.

PERSONAL
FACTORS

CULTURAL
INFLUENCE

**AESTHETIC
PHYSIQUE**

PURE VISUAL
BEAUTY

BIOLOGICAL
BIAS

These factors exist along a continuum that feed into and support each other, and that's why the shape is rounded. Most people see one alone as the source of aesthetic appeal. That's not enough. They're ALL involved because they're all a part of who we are.

- The two bottom factors are the strongest, constant, and support the two that lie on top of them.
- The top two stem from the ones underneath and feed into each other. The experiences we have create the culture and the culture influences us in return. It's a two-way street.

Now let's look at each in further detail to peek under the hood and give you your aesthetic foundations.

PURE BEAUTY

All of the knowledge you have or *ever will have* of the world has come via your senses.

Everyone thinks of the sensory superstars like sight, sound, taste, smell, and touch, but you have more: the sense of reason and meaning (intellect), a moral sense, and a sense you use to relate with others to perceive and connect with their feelings and point of view. All of these allow you to make sense of the world and acquire knowledge of what's going on in it.

BEAUTY in its purest form is the perception of order in accordance with the framework of what is pleasing to those senses [5,6]. Each sense and each situation where it is employed has its own world of governing principles, and they often overlap because many senses are stimulated through one work.

BEAUTY THROUGH THE SENSES

CORPORAL		MENTAL	
THE BIG 5	INTELLECT	MORAL	RELATIONAL
Music Cuisine Art Texture Aroma	Math Science Philosophy Design/Intent	Law Virtue	Literature Movies Lyrics Interaction with others

For example, we find beauty in:

- The arrangement of color, shape, line, and proportion in art [1,2,3,5,7]
- The mixture of flavors, textures, temperatures, and aromas in cuisine
- The actions of a person in a particular situation [8,9,10,11]
- The mixture of words unfolding to produce poetry or the plot in a story [12]
- Notes, rhythm, harmony, tempo, panning, and sound selection to create a song [13,14,15]
- Numbers or premises arranged to produce mathematical or philosophical truth [16]

In each of these, the elements are arranged in *distinct* ways that create a favorable effect on that sense and produce pleasure in the mind. If they violate certain structures of that sense, it is noticeable immediately and disliked. Bright clashes of color, noisy music that's out of tune and off beat, an evil action, and so on.

☙ COMBINED EFFECT

When more than one sense perceives beauty, the aesthetic effect increases [17]. Live music with great lyrics and visuals are one easy example.

☙ PILLARS OF PURE BEAUTY

If an object is offensive to the senses, then its beauty disappears unless another one supports it like a building with many pillars. This is why ugly art can still be described as beautiful. It conveys a symbolic *meaning* from the artist that arouses that sense of beauty. The other sense picks up the slack.

...but why is it beautiful?

From processing fluency theory to divine creation, there are several theories as to *why* we perceive these things as beautiful to the sense alone, but we will not venture into them here. They do nothing to further or weaken our 4-pronged topic of discussion. Our focus will be more on the practical takeaways.

PURE AND PRACTICAL BEAUTY

Once you've got the pure beauty, you can add in the other factors from the 4-cornered shape and get *practical beauty*. This creates total aesthetics, or the aesthetic effect.

All sensory input have to be processed and passed through the filters of the mind to create the aesthetic effect:

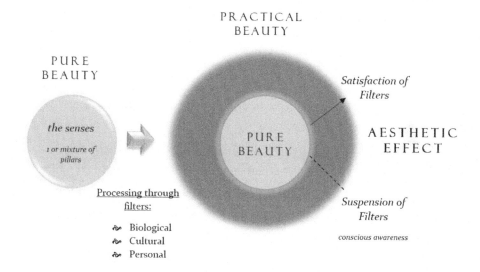

This my current model of aesthetics.

You take that nugget of pure beauty through one or a combination of many sensory stimuli and either satisfy the remaining 3 factors that we'll speak about next or figure out how to turn them off and focus on only that pure essence without judgment or bias, like a sliver being carved out of the fog to see straight within.

You can think of the large sphere of practical beauty as a mask or a fog around the pure beauty that alters the perception of the pure beauty inside. Sometimes, this is desirable and increases the aesthetic effect. Other times, it is not and destroys or distorts it completely.

Turning off the filters can be done through mental training and heightened perspective by mentally disconnecting from the picture, but you can only do this for yourself, so to appeal to the maximum amount of people, you'll need to satisfy the rest to achieve the maximum aesthetic effect.

OBJECTIVE BEAUTY?

Isn't beauty just in the eyes of the beholder?

With regards to pure beauty, beauty *is* objective. Pure beauty always exists. Whether *you* can see it or not is irrelevant. It's like a DVD. You need a working set of TV and speakers to watch it, but that beauty is still written into the disc waiting to be tapped into and experienced.

Practical beauty adds the individual and opinion into the equation and is what gets the results in the world as we as unique individuals add in our own element. To understand the difference between pure and practical beauty, you simply have to understand this:

*"This is pleasing to the eyes, but not to **me**."*

Now we'll look at the factors that create that practical beauty through morphing or masking perception. This is what gets real results we care about out there in the world. Let's get going by starting off with the biggest and most powerful, biological bias.

BIOLOGICAL BIAS

It's the middle of the night, and you're submersed in a deep sleep. The bed is soft and warm, and you don't have a care in the world.

Then out of nowhere, you're ripped from your sheets, kidnapped, and dropped in the middle of the jungle leaving everything you know and love behind. There is nothing and no one to save you. No food. No clothes. No water. No shelter. Nothing. How long would you make it?

Not long.

Today, we're surrounded by skyscrapers, technology and all of the luxuries and comfort of the modern world, but make no mistake - the world is a cruel, harsh place that'll eat you alive if you don't fight for what's yours. Survival is a very real issue out there in the wild.

BASIC NEEDS

Getting your basic needs covered is the prerequisite for anything else you do in life. The body needs to maintain homeostasis and acquire everything it needs for optimal function at all costs, so food, water, shelter, and so on are essential requirements for any living organism.

But we aren't alone in the world. There is safety and power in numbers, so over time societies formed to provide more resources and protection amongst the group. Because of this, from a basic, crude perspective, how others view you is important in ensuring that you've got what you need to survive in the wild world.

Nature, in all of Her wisdom, has given you a body that takes care of all of your vital functions on autopilot. Your heart beats, your internal processes carry on like clock-work, and your systematic levels are maintained very well within tight ranges.

But that only speaks for the *internal side* of things. You still have to satisfy your *external* requirements for life.

Therefore, She's even done the same for *your mind* to propel you towards satisfying those base requirements. Basic desires and strong emotions are tied to these requirements to influence behavior in such a way as to lock these down.

I've outlined the translation from basic survival needs into the base human desires below.

SURVIVAL NEEDS	BASE HUMAN DESIRES
Food	Pleasure
Water	Control
Shelter	Abundance
Protection	Power
Health	Security
Reproduction	Safety
	Importance
	Respect
	Ease
	Time (Speed, duration, etc.)
	Permanence
	Maximize benefit
	Reduce harm

As you can see, the items on the right side of the table are very closely linked to the basic needs on the left both from a fundamental and social perspective.

MENTAL FILTERS

Because of this reality, sensory input that activate that mental radar favorably are going to be seen in a more positive light than ones that don't. This forms the basis for biological bias.

Unfortunately, this same mental system makes the path to true success and happiness in life a tough one and opens the doors to all the pain, mediocrity, and suffering in the world, past and present.

In the table below, the factors that trigger biological bias are on the left, and their behavioral consequences can be found on the right.

BASE DESIRES	EGO OPERATING SYSTEM
Pleasure	Selfishness
Control	Binary Scales and Labeling
Abundance	Greed/Hedonism
Power	Jealousy
Security	Identification with the Self
Safety	Seeking of Meaning in External Things
Importance	Living in the Past/Future
Respect	Attention Seeking
Ease	Impulsiveness
Time (Speed, duration, etc.)	Irrationality
	Self-rationalization
Permanence	Reactive/Defensive
Maximize benefit	Attachment
Reduce harm	

Look familiar? The behavioral systems on the right form the basis of *the ego*, the irrational mental autopilot program associated with the identity of the self and securing the resources required for the survival of that self. It has to be understood and controlled. I will show you how to manage the mind in a later chapter.

IMPLICATIONS FOR AESTHETICS

How does this apply to an aesthetic physique? Easy.

- ❧ The body must be a symbol of health, energy, strength, and life because a part of the mind is built to identify benefit or harm in the world and others
- ❧ It must represent all of the top-notch factors of vitality for both men and women
- ❧ It must look natural [18-24]

Doing so subconsciously ups the aesthetic rating, attraction level, and social pull of the physique.

Many claim this is the origin of beauty itself, but even though our senses and survival benefit are *related*, this is not the end all be all and must take other filters into account as I've laid out [25].

❧ AVOIDANCE

Because of these considerations, physiques that are too frail, too muscular, too lean, fat, misshapen, disfigured, and things of that nature have the opposite effect on the viewer and trigger intrinsically negative responses by disturbing that mental filter.

There is much more to human beings than their physical side, and we are not limited to this obsolete knee-jerk response, but these are not desirable things to the subconscious mind, so ensuring a pleasant, healthy, balanced appearance is key for aesthetics.

CULTURAL INFLUENCE

Since the day you were born and even before, your mind has been morphed and molded by everything around you.

Everything your senses can touch has been processed and stored away in your mind like a gigantic supercomputer. This has created your standard for reality and lays down the brickwork of your mind. It's your reference point by which everything else is judged, and it creates the bricks that you'll use to build your thoughts and your life. All reality is the origin of thought.

This is what I call **Mental Input Material (MIM)**, and it covers everything from your surroundings to media to people. Want to live a better life and change your mind? Expose yourself to better input. Don't put your eyes, ears, and attention on anything less than the best that lifts you up and takes you places.

AESTHETIC ARCHETYPES

Because of this, your idea of aesthetics is going to be impacted in relation to everyone you've seen in life and the influence that this has had on you in defining the normal standard of beauty.

The cultural standards are heavily impacted by pure beauty and biology, and that's why they're seated atop the shape. These tastes and trends fade in and out or change over the course of history and across different modern cultures, but they're never enough to override the senses or biology completely.

Celebrities, actors, models, and artists have the most impact in the modern day. Everyone wants to look like them. Everyone wants their workouts and diets. They're at the forefront of attention and work to define that cultural standard. Not to mention, the social pull, resources, and status they have activate the biological bias and throws in a bunch of extra desire to get on their level in hopes you live just like them.

NOVELTY FACTORS

Because of the standard, you can separate yourself from it to draw more attention and intrigue. People love what is new and challenges their pre-existing concept of something. However, this must be done mildly. Going too far past the norm can have the opposite effect and be rejected by its stark differences.

Don't stray too far from the modern ideal. It makes the people uncomfortable.

PERSONAL

Finally, we turn our attention to the personal. We live life through our eyes and everything we've been through. Based on your perspective as a person, everything can change - for better or worse. This is the wildcard that brings a close to the aesthetic factors.

EXPERIENCE

One way or another, your past and personal experiences have led you here today and will influence the way you view things around you.

No matter how intrinsically beautiful or ugly something is, your unique experiences as a person can flip the tables and cause you to view it in a completely different light because of the emotion-laden memories or beliefs you hold.

These can be deceptive. They can have their origins in powerful past experiences that you've long forgotten and lay low in your subconscious. You don't know why you feel that way about a certain something, but you do. Look within. You'll find your answer.

MOOD

The personal effect also extends to the mood that the observer is in. A positive state of emotions will lead to a better perception, and vice versa for a negative state. For the optimal aesthetic, always aim to have the observer in a pleasant mood for maximal effect.

FACTOR TAKEAWAY

There is not much that can be done about this factor, but by looking at the big picture, you can certainly relate to your audience on a personal level through shared experiences that we all have been through. How can you connect with your viewer 1 on 1? What brings us all relief and joy? What struggles do we all face at some point or another?

These are the questions to ask.

FACTOR SUMMARY

When all four of those factors are in optimized and in play, they bring about a well-rounded note like the warm strum of a rich chord on a guitar.

Reflect upon how these factors drive the perception of human beauty around you - both throughout history and across modern civilization worldwide.

Also reflect upon how the violation of these factors are deemed undesirable by the majority. To understand this is to understand why aesthetics are a key component of bodybuilding, but the standards of competitive bodybuilding are not determinant of aesthetics.

IMPLICATIONS FOR OTHER AREAS

This discussion of aesthetic theory has been centered around maximizing the aesthetics of the physique, but these conclusions have very far reaching effects into the arts and product development. Each field is unique, but by optimizing these 4 areas, you will be able to produce better material for your target market.

WHY IT MATTERS

What's the meaning of all this talk on aesthetics?

They're so common that it's easy to take them for granted, but aesthetics are a fundamental component of our everyday life.

From the buildings we live in and places we want to go to the food we eat, music we listen to, and clothes we suit up in, aesthetics are always there guiding our decisions and enriching the world around us.

Art is our escape and speaks to us all on a deeper level. It has been an integral part of human culture for thousands of years, no matter which culture or age group you look at. It's the common language of who we are and represents a deeper part of us all.

HIGHEST EXPRESSION

Furthermore, creating beauty is the highest expression of humanity there is. Nowhere else can we express ourselves and utilize our intelligence, choice, and creativity like in the arts and our actions.

To see a musician lost in their performance, an artist absorbed in their work, or a writer flowing from the marks of their pen leaves such an impression on us that we can't do anything but sit back and admire.

To take the chaos of the world and ground it under your power.
To take the body and sculpt a physique.
To take a life and sculpt a legacy.

That's what makes us human.

4

ELEMENTS OF THE AESTHETIC PHYSIQUE

No one is an artist unless he carries his picture in his head before painting it and is sure of his method and composition.

Claude Monet

OW THAT YOU KNOW what goes into an aesthetic physique that creates the best effect on the viewer, we can look at *how* to make that happen.

We will be using that theoretical framework to fuel the organization of artistic elements to sculpt the physique.

The primary visual elements we have at our disposal to create an aesthetic physique are the same as any visual art:

- PROPORTION
- SYMMETRY
- FLOW: SHAPES, LINES, AND ARRANGEMENT
- DETAIL/DEFINITION
- COLOR

And finally, as any great artist, we will discuss the MEANING we wish to convey to the observer.

PROPORTION

Nothing requires the architect's care more than the due proportions of buildings.
Vitruvius

Proportion is the first and most important aspect of the aesthetic physique.

It deals with the relationship between the various sizes and lengths throughout the body. This applies to muscle groups, joints, and all of various areas of the body. Because it's associated with *relative differences* and not absolutes, proportion is a magic trick and a balancing act tightly wound into one.

To reach the pinnacles of aesthetics, you've got to spur the body into growth and get lean, but to do so recklessly without regard to proportion is a recipe for disaster.

It must be in the *right place* to the *right degree*.

Our goal is to highlight the important points for our cause and maintain a strong balance across the body. Not too much, nor too little. Harmonious balance.

MAXIM OF AESTHETICS: STRIVE FOR BALANCE ABOVE ALL... IN LIFTING AND IN LIFE.

GODS AND GODDESSES

Aesthetic proportion all starts at the waist.

The physique of a man and a woman are distinguished and drawn up by key defining characteristics that are centered around the waist and the proportions on either side of it.

Aesthetics will skyrocket by taking these natural characteristics and blowing them up through proportion [26]. You focus on the pure, unfiltered essence of masculinity and femininity and expand it to wow the observer and leave an impact.

You've got to hit a homerun here because this technique doesn't just stop at proportion. It applies to everything else and trickles into fashion, style, behavior, language, and body language as well. Take what the people want and crank it up.

    ⇛ MEN

For men, the name of the game is the Shoulder:Waist ratio - also known as the V-Taper.

Broad, booming shoulders seated atop a trim, chiseled waist is a symbol of masculinity as old as time itself. It's the mark of the leader. The alpha. The go-getter who can hold things down amidst a world of chaos. Women love it, and the guys respect it. It'll give you the look like you just jumped out of a comic book.

To do this, you'll need to work on wide, sweeping lats and boulder shoulders with leanness to create a slim waist and round out the cap of the deltoids through enhanced muscular separation. By default, this will also play into the appearance of the lower body.

❧ WOMEN

Goddesses in the making will look to hone their hourglass figure. That's the Shoulder:Waist:Hip ratio.

A tight, narrow waist, and wide, womanly hips alongside a gentle V-taper, full legs, and rounded glutes are the peak of femininity and beauty - amongst other things. This means women will need to focus on well-rounded leg days with special emphasis on the glutes and just enough upper body work to create that figure that allows the viewer to get lost in her calming curves and creates a seamless silhouette.

This, coupled with the Goldilocks level of leanness that's *just right*, will create a stunning physique fit for a goddess. Women hold their visual appeal without tremendous leanness much more than men.

In fact, this idealized standard has been in play for thousands of years dating back to some of the first art ever produced by humans. It has carried that tradition throughout history, and it's no coincidence why.

GOLDEN GUIDES?

For eons, architects, artists, and sculptors have carried out their work seeking the optimal proportion of ocular pleasure. Many have been said to use the Golden Ratio of 1:1.618 to arrange the elements of their work in such a way that is most beautiful to the human eye. Also known as the Divine Proportion, it lies mischievously hidden in plain view within marvels such as the Great Pyramids, The Parthenon, and the riches of the Renaissance as shown in the Mona Lisa and Michelangelo's David.

This ratio has been observed to ground beauty and design across the cosmos, nature, and even within the human body itself - from the outlay of a beautiful face and hand down to the very double helix of the DNA that serves as its architectural blueprint. In fact, its usage continues in modern times as many designers, photographers, and even surgeons utilize it in their disciplines to create their best work.

Some lifters have even dared to aspire to reach this numerical guideline to create the ideal physical proportions, as demonstrated by things such as the Adonis index. Yet this is solely **one** piece of the aesthetic puzzle of a human being as we have thoroughly proven thus far. Practical beauty is more than the purely visual standards.

Proportion can and *should* be manipulated beyond these numerical ideals to create compelling visuals. If you stick to numbers only, you're missing the jackpot. You want to push past proportion norms in key areas of the physique.

The mirror is our guide, so put away the tape measures.

WHOLE BODY PROPORTION

Once you've got your base frame by enhancing the masculine and feminine proportions, you've got to enhance the proportions of the rest of the body to match. This will convey strength and vitality as the muscles grow in size in response to the training to fit the enhanced gender proportions.

Consider these relationships, for example:

BOTTOMS UP	LOCALIZED	CROSS-BODY
Feet:Legs Legs:Waist Waist:Shoulders Shoulders:Arms Arms:Hands Shoulders:Head	Joints:Muscles Quads:Hamstrings Biceps:Triceps Traps:Shoulders Hips:Waist	Calves:Bis/Tris Upper body:Lower body Head:Body Hands and Feet: Body

And that's just the tip of the iceberg.

As you can see, the artistic appeal of the body is interconnected and tightly woven together. When you add to one, you have to consider another - and vice versa. All must be kept in balance.

This means you'll need a well-rounded training program to achieve the optimal aesthetic. No preferential treatment. No skipping leg days for guys, and no skipping upper body days for girls. You need the whole package.

SPOTLIGHT

Every show has its star.

To add extra flair to the physique, we can emphasize one area in particular to truly stand out, draw attention, and add our own personal touch and uniqueness to the body. Generics are forgotten. Spice things up and throw in a little novelty.

This is primarily accomplished through capitalizing on our genetic potential which you will learn more about in the next chapter.

Perhaps you have gifted quads. Perhaps your waist or hips are shaped magnificently aesthetically. Perhaps your biceps peak perfectly. The possibilities are endless, and each has their own that even when moderately developed will be a pleasing sight to behold, even if it slips a bit out of proportion.

Although most desirable, this special body part need not be a muscle group or other body part per se. The face, hair, or even elements of fashion can be used to bring about the same effect. The aim is to create a distinguishing feature of the body.

SYMMETRY

From the outspread wings of a mighty eagle soaring through the piercing blue skies of a sunny Spring afternoon to the structure of a delicate snowflake fluttering to the Earth on a serene Winter evening and much more, across nature we are met with mesmerizing symmetry.

Symmetry between two opposing sides is a pleasing sight to behold. It demonstrates order and unison. When one side is off balance, it throws off that ideal.

In the human body we also find symmetry in abundance.

Eyes and ears, hands and feet, legs and arms. Even mind and body. One side is matched and balanced by the other. We work as one whole functional unit - one day humanity will achieve the same.

Ensuring that the musculature of one side of the body does not become under or overly developed in relation to the other is critical for aesthetics and creating a balanced visual.

MAXIM OF AESTHETICS: TOO MUCH GIVEN TO ONE WILL CAUSE ALL TO TOPPLE.

In fashion and style, symmetry can be toyed with tastefully to create visual intrigue through patterns, colors, and accessories, but the body itself does not lend well to asymmetry. Bodily symmetry is a very important marker of health and attraction on a basic biological level.

It is instead the firm foundation for fashion and style to flourish upon.

FLOW

Geometry has stunned the human psyche through its sophisticated simplicity and bold beauty for thousands of years. Beauty is perhaps no more objective than in the proofs of mathematics and geometry. Many have gone so far as to call it the "language of God".

Look around you.

The world is built by the lines, shapes and angles of geometry, and the flow of a physique is created by the arrangement and the interplay of these various lines, shapes, and angles of the body created by the muscles, their layout, and posing. The eye is drawn to the dance of taut, uniform lines and smooth, wide curves.

Through this flow we find harmony and structure. This arrangement and movement of the various parts of the body will lead the eye like a composer leads the ear through his symphonies of strings.

From the stable base notes of the waist, the tension rises through the arcing ascent of the lats to be punctuated by the crisp crescendo of capped delts cascading off into muscled arms and the hands that built them.

CORE AREAS

When you consider the muscular arrangement of the body, there are 5 key areas that deserve special attention to create a visual balance across the frame. They are:

- ࢚ SHOULDERS
- ࢚ LATS
- ࢚ FOREARMS
- ࢚ GLUTES
- ࢚ CALVES

Based on their position on the body and across various angles and movements, these areas anchor the eye and create a harmonious, balanced visual.

Because of this, special attention must be given to ensure that these muscle groups stay in proportion are not underdeveloped. In fact, extra emphasis on these muscle groups will produce a favorable result in the aesthetics of the physique by virtue of their position and role in favorable proportions.

POSING AND BODY LANGUAGE

The body is a moving work of art, not a statue, and flow is also vitally important for posing and body language considerations.

We can continually change the arrangement of the body and the effect it creates on the observer by altering our posture or movements and creating a different work of art on the "canvas" of our physical space made up by the areas we can reach with outstretched arms and legs.

The same body put in different postures, movements, and positions will create two completely different effects [27-31]. You must be flowing, not rigid. You'll ruin all of your hard work if you don't get this down. You've got to exude grace and confidence.

Stand up tall, act big even if you're small, and be smooth and poised as if you created it all.

Hype up your masculinity or femininity and create an addictive aura.

The ties between motion and emotion are no etymological coincidence. The animation of the body will adjust the perception thereof, and **no** aesthetic physique is immune to the far-reaching effects that posture and posing imposes.

As we move our bodies, we move the souls of others.

DETAIL AND DEFINITION

Throughout history, some of the finest art that has ever graced the globe has been produced for temples and places of worship. From the intricate stone work and stained glass of the towering European cathedrals to the tiles and patterns of the mosques of the Middle East, we find breathtaking, dizzying detail. This same level of detail can be achieved in our Temple - the body - to display its structure in all of its glory.

Through patience and proper nutrition, the physique is chiseled out like marble and the details that have been carved in diligently within the confines of the iron dungeon are made visible by removing their subcutaneous cloak - just as a master sculptor removes the drapery from his creation to present it to the world.

Round, full muscle bellies are brought out in full view. Rippling striations formed by the sinewy spindles of forceful fibers are thrust to the forefront of attention as the muscle contracts and performs its duties under the command of its master.

A heightened degree of definition can lift a lackluster physique into unforseen heights by implementing a newfound layer of detail and accentuating the proportions of the body, although this degree must be tempered as not to submerge into the murky pools of excess created by the image of frail, sickly physique that is off-putting to the observer.

COLOR

For the final visual element, we turn our attention to color.

Few can deny the internal impact of a violet and amber sunset at dusk, the serenity of staring out into the bright blues of the salty oceans extending into the infinity of a pure blue sky, or the smorgasbord of bright colors scattered amongst a robust garden in full bloom.

Although outside of the realm of physical dimensions like proportion, definition, and flow, color still has a very large impact on aesthetics. Through the spin of the color wheel, we can select and coordinate colors to produce a stunning visual impact.

Every person has their unique set of skin tone, hair color, eye color, and so on. These are more or less fixed, but color has very far-reaching applications when you consider fashion and style.

Through different colors, patterns, graphics, and contrast, the body can be accentuated and added an additional layer of visual intrigue that creates a pleasant mystery [32-34], divides up space, and draws the eye, so this is an important factor for dressing the aesthetic physique.

MEANING

Lastly, a discussion of aesthetics would be hopelessly hollow without paying homage to the value that the observer places on the meaning and symbolism of the physique.

All art must be given the breath of life by its observer, and no work of art is complete until that observer adds their final personal stroke of symbolic meaning to finish the piece.

An aesthetic physique goes far beyond the effect of shape, line, and color. Through our strategic work with proportion, symmetry, flow, definition, and color, it is a walking display of beauty and several powerful truths of its beholder that amplify the visual effect for all with eyes to see it.

On a raw, primal level it demonstrates power, strength, and vitality. It inspires confidence, trust, and respect. It is a beacon of health and energy that all aspire to attain.

To see an awe-inspiring physique is to see diligence, dedication, and drive manifested in its physical form. The inner world is transmuted into external reality through the toils of time in the weight room and proper nutrition.

Because of innate biological considerations, we must never take our art to egotistical excess. Monstrous magnitudes of muscularity and the extreme limits of leanness left unchained will evoke knee-jerk emotions of repugnance and distaste that lose touch with the effervescent effect that an aesthetic physique will provide its viewer.

You want to look like gods and goddesses. Not the monsters they'd be fighting.

The true mark of an architect of aesthetics is to take his creation teetering on the cliff of the extreme so that it is on the cusp of impending doom before pulling it back under his wisdom and sagaciousness to the applause and relief of the audience suspended in terror.

STAND FOR MORE

Be a symbol that others can look up to. The meaning behind a work of art adds to the appeal of that work of art [35,36]. If you have a powerful back story or have made an incredible transformation, you will always win out against the natural. People can relate to you. They can feel your story and your journey. I didn't reveal my past in the prologue for no reason. I want you to feel what I went through and light the fire in you to show you that you can do this. We aren't so different. I may be teaching you, but we are in this together.

Don't despise your current situation or genetics; use them to your advantage.

Through your work in the weight room, you can be an inspiration to others and motivate millions to change their life for the better. That's worth it even by itself.

SUMMARY OF THE COMPONENTS OF AESTHETICS

Having discussed the factors in play that make a physique aesthetic, we have seen the variables in the play that dictate EXACTLY what it is that makes an aesthetic physique aesthetic.

- Well balanced cross-body proportions of heightened muscularity and leanness
- Emphasized proportions for the defining characteristics of men and women
- Specially developed body part to create uniqueness and visual intrigue
- Physical symmetry that can later be the stable base for artistic flare through fashion and style
- Accentuated muscular curves and line, shape, and angle of the body
- Proper arrangement of the visual elements through posture, posing, and body language
- Balanced frame markers of the deltoids, lats, forearms, glutes, and calves
- Increased muscular definition - not to excess
- Positive, profound meaning to the observer

Doing so will ensure that we not only appeal to the eye, but also the biological, cultural, and personal worlds of the observer that can view the physique as a symbol of beauty, power, life, health, respect, and even inspiration.

We can now turn our attention to what OUR role is in this. First, we must start with examining ourselves and the potential we have.

5

GENETICS AND AESTHETICS

Regard your soldiers as your children, and they will follow you into the deepest valleys;
look on them as your own beloved sons, and they will stand by you even unto death.
Sun Tzu

W E ARE MADE OF TRILLIONS OF CELLS, and together, they serve as our army that we as generals must determine how to deploy in battle most effectively based on their personality and characteristics.

Imprinted into every cell of your body is the biological blueprint of life, DNA.

A complex code more intricate and extensive than the most advanced computer programming conceivable to man lies in the bedrock of your very essence as a living human being. Those are your deoxyribonucleic assets that'll set the rough landscape for how you look and perform.

Our genetics will impact our journey, so here we'll look at what they do for us - both internally and visually.

INTERNAL FACTORS

Within the body there lies a myriad of things going on at a cellular level that very heavily impact the results we get from diet and training [1].

The main ones are our:

- METABOLISM [2,3]
- RESPONSIVENESS TO TRAINING [4]
- HORMONES [5]

These factors will vary from person to person, gender to gender, and age to age. For example:

- Some people can put on muscle faster than others - overall and within certain body parts.
- Some people put on a better proportion of muscle to fat when they're looking to gain muscle in a caloric surplus.
- Some people hold up better mentally or physically at lower body fats or during periods of dieting.

The examples are numerous of how two seemingly similar people can have vastly different internal worlds and responses to training and nutrition. These effects cannot be underestimated.

Nevertheless, outside of hopping on pharmaceuticals or jumping in a time machine and genetically engineering yourself, there's really not much you can do about these factors without meticulous manipulation for marginal gains, no matter what any guru magic has to say about it.

The best you can do is *flow with the current* and adapt to them.

Because of this, we won't dwell or spend much time on these factors. There is no sense in stressing over something you can't change, and a respectable physique can be built regardless of the genetic factors present that are far too often the scapegoat of poor progress.

The principles don't change, just your ROI. It's all about your strength and drive as a person.

VISUAL FACTORS

If you hear a voice within you say 'you cannot paint,' then by all means paint, and that voice will be silenced.
Vincent Van Gogh

When an artist sets out to do their work, they stare at a blank canvas and decide how to proceed from there. As an architect of aesthetics, we can look at the physical potential of a person and see how to move forward with regards to our training.

Just by looking at someone with zero formal training, you can get a solid understanding of how their journey will look based on their physical starting point. The main ones we will discuss are:

- HEIGHT
- BONE/JOINT STRUCTURE
- MUSCLE SHAPE/INSERTIONS

All of these play a role in how you'll look and what that means for your training and physical development based on the core components of aesthetics discussed earlier.

HEIGHT

Aesthetics are going to be impacted by your height and width -- your height and how densely you fill out your frame.

Tall, lanky individuals and short, stocky people are a stereotype for a reason. Having too much height without width and having too much width without height simply isn't as visually pleasing as a more favorable ratio. You must remain proportional to your overall height.

For this reason, taller individuals will have to work hard to ensure that they fill out their frame properly, and shorter individuals in pursuit of aesthetics must put aside their Napoleon syndrome and seek to use weights as the tool they are - not a status symbol. Ultimate size is not a good goal to have for aesthetics because growing as large as possible will do nothing for the size of your head (ego, perhaps) or hands and feet.

Height and length of limbs also plays a huge role in the mechanics of a lift, and for this reason, certain exercises may be better for some people than others. For example, taller, long limbed individuals tend to excel in pulling movements such as the deadlift or rows, and shorter individuals are better suited for pressing and squatting movements.

That means that those involved muscle groups will develop very well and extra care will have to be ensured to develop the rest accordingly.

BASE FRAME

The base skeletal structure has a large role in the perception of proportion. This is your default size of joints, shoulder width, waist, and hips primarily, amongst other things.

Due to the magical effect of proportions, smaller joints will create a more pronounced effect between the joint and the muscles on either side of it. Those with smaller joints can 'appear' bigger despite having the same muscular size simply by virtue of not having to grow as much to make the muscle groups pop.

If you're a guy with a narrow waist and wider shoulders or a girl with wide hips and a thin waist by default, you already have better natural proportions that'll only get better with proper training. This explains why some people who either don't lift or are new to training can look more aesthetic than those with more experience under their belt.

This is also why speaking of gains in terms of raw numbers like your weight, how much you squat, and size of your muscles is silly from an aesthetic standpoint. It simply doesn't tell the whole story.

Smaller frames and joints often lead to difficulties in pushing heavier weight and joint issues, but this is balanced by simply needing less growth to get a nice visual effect. Bigger joints call for bigger muscles to get the same visual effect, but they are better suited to move the heavier weight necessary to do this. And thus, balance is maintained in the Universe.

The role joints play in the picture also has big repercussions for choice in fashion. Making your joints wider is a big no-no if you want your aesthetics to extend past being naked. Slim fits are the way to go.

MUSCLE SHAPE/INSERTIONS

Joints aren't the only thing that have a most direct impact on the default visual appearance of the body. The *shape* of the muscle and *where* that muscle inserts on the joint also has much play in this.

The impact of muscle shapes and insertions can most readily be seen in muscles such as the biceps and calves. Having a calf muscle with a high insertion can make it difficult to "fill out" the calves properly and create a well-rounded leg. Having long biceps can make it harder to get a nice, round peak that pops.

Most related to many fitness goals, ab shape can vary a tremendous amount between people. No matter what you do, if your abs are asymmetrical, they will stay that way. If you only have a 6 pack, nothing will get you 8.

Training can only enlarge the muscle that is already there. No exercise will change your default muscle shape.

SUMMARY OF GENETIC FACTORS

By this point, you may be over-analyzing yourself and celebrating or pouting in the corner.

Genetic factors are extremely impactful, but they do not determine your success and will not negate the magic that consistent work in and out of the weight room can provide.

Even if you think that your genetics are poor, don't let your mentality be poor with it. How far will that get you?

Ten soldiers wisely led will beat a hundred without a head.
Euripides

THE FINAL COMPONENT

Hidden here for you to find, dear reader, is the final component of aesthetics - the weakness. All aesthetic masterpieces must have their weakness to be truly world class.

This weakness creates vulnerability that paradoxically elevates the beauty of the object in question by comparison. It creates contrast. It demonstrates your humanity. It makes you accessible and related. Utter perfection is unsettling. We like for things to be a little messed up - just like us.

The greatest leaders in history were not treated as gods amongst men for their power - but because despite their power, they fought on the frontlines and demonstrated their humanity.

You can search for perfection for a lifetime, but until you realize the beauty of the imperfection, you will never truly achieve what you set out for.

MAXIM OF AESTHETICS: BUILD UPON YOUR STRENGTHS AND WORK WITH YOUR WEAKNESSES. YOUR ONLY LIMITATIONS ARE THOSE YOU IMPOSE UPON YOURSELF.

There is only one of you out there, and it is YOUR mission to make yourself into the best human being you can be - no matter where you start or what you have to work with.

Every block of stone has a statue inside it and it is the task of the sculptor to discover it.
Michelangelo

6

THE BATTLE
STRATEGY

Study strategy over the years and achieve the spirit of the warrior. Today is victory over yourself of yesterday; tomorrow is your victory over lesser men.
Miyamoto Musashi

E'VE GOT THE VARIABLES OF SUCCESS, aesthetics, genetics, and the direction that that's pushing us towards now. In this chapter, we will look at the way we'll attack such a complex beast, the knowledge base driving our decision making, the key components of any program, sustainability, the importance of setting targets, and the time frames to wrap it all up. No matter what you do, this is a chapter you cannot miss.

POINTS ON THE MAP

We've got a lot on our plate to make you great. It's all good. We'll take things step by step. Here's how your journey through these pages is going to look:

GYM AND EQUIPMENT

First, we'll look at the gym and everything you need to get your solid workouts in. We'll go over what you need to look for in a gym, clothing and attire, gym accessories, and music to fuel your training sessions.

TRAINING

Training is what will slap size on that statue of yours.
We will talk about the principles of muscle growth and how to carry that process out to perfection through managing your workout intensity, volume, frequency, exercise selection, progression, periodization, and workout programming.

I'll also tell you exactly what you need to know about warm-ups, time off, and the role that cardio plays in getting your best results.

NUTRITION

Training is the trigger, but all the training in the world will go straight down the drain and take you with it if you don't get your nutrition dialed in.

In the nutritional part of the book, I will show you how to optimize your progress to maximize muscle gain, fat loss, and hit that cruise control for maintaining your physique by teaching you the ins and outs of calories, macronutrients, how to split your meals, which foods to eat, how to measure them, and supplements that can help you out on your journey.

RECOVERY AND REALIGNMENT

You'll be training hard, so you'll be resting hard to match.
In this section of the book, I'll give you all the tips and tricks to ensure that you are resting and repairing from your training sessions the right way, and we'll get you in proper alignment and posture so that you're moving and feeling your best to give it your all to your training.

PROGRESS

All this work will do you no good if you don't have a way to ensure progress. Here we'll discuss tracking your progress, plateaus, and common pitfalls for sustained progress by ensuring consistency, dealing with injury, and managing social issues.

MINDSET

The hardest battles aren't fought on the battlefield. They're fought within your own mind.

All the attention is given to the flashy superstars of muscle growth and nutrition, but not enough is given to the person inside who's making all of that happen and how they use their minds to view and live in the world. Not here. The biggest obstacle you have is yourself, so I'm going to give you the way to use your mind to its fullest potential to achieve your goals.

BONUS

You think I could leave you without giving you some know-how on how to present your best package to the world? Think again.

In the bonus section of the book, I'll give you tips to tune up your thread game and hit the streets with style no matter where you are to show off all that hard work you've put in.

I'll also give you pointers to bring up your body language to match that masterpiece you've made in the gym to maximize your results. It's not just about how you look, it's how you carry it in the world that makes a world of difference.

PHYSIQUE PHILOSOPHIES

These days, fitness is all the rage. Everyone is an expert, and there is an endless stream of fitness advice running rampant out there in the world. It's all over TV, magazines, and the Internet, and it's an information overload.

Some of it is decent. Most of it is terrible.

This is not a book to win the flashy workout or feel good contest for the masses. This is a book to take you to the pinnacles you deserve to reach.

Everyone out there has their own way of sculpting the body, but let's take a look at how *we're* going to approach the various areas vital to your success here:

EVIDENCE-BASED, BUT REALITY PLACED.

A good decision is based on knowledge and not on numbers.
Plato

The information and recommendations in this book are going to come from a combination of several areas. They all have their place, but none of them by themselves are the winning ticket. Let's take a look at each.

1. SCIENTIFIC RESEARCH

For most of the history of training, routines and rules were born from custom and tradition. Lifters in pursuit of aesthetics made their decisions based on 'feeling', what was popular at the time in the community, and whatever the most jacked folks were cranking out in the gym and spilling about their dietary habits in between sets.

This avenue of thought led to the infamous temple of 'bro-science' and brought birth to a plethora of myths around training, recovery, and nutrition that still circulate locker rooms worldwide.

In addition, the intense desire to achieve the pinnacles of health and aesthetic appeal has a long, fruitful history, and whenever there is demand, a businessman isn't far behind. As a result, supplement companies pushing product, magazines and shows from the TV to the internet channels looking to gain a wider audience, and even personal trainers have all jumped on the bandwagon to make fancy claims at the expense of others and bastardize the noble pursuit for fitness in hopes of gaining fame and making a quick buck.

Such a dynamic duo has proven to be quite a force to be reckoned with, but we're living in a great era because the shaky claims of bro-science and business scams are being combatted and replaced more and more by concrete scientific research.

In questions of science, the authority of a thousand is not worth the humble reasoning of a single individual.
Galileo Galilei

The scientific method allows you to draw conclusions about the nature of the physical world and the interactions of different variables by creating controlled experiments and observing the results. Through the work of researchers, we've been able to gain tremendous insight into the different mechanisms of muscle growth and nutrition, and every day more and more myths and commandments of bro-science that made fitness success a steep mountain to well-intentioned people are being slain.

Here we will use the latest and greatest scientific research and data to ground your processes and make better decisions to optimize your results.

NOT SO FAST

Nevertheless, scientific research is not the end all be all.

Factors such as study length, sample size, the studied population, and perfectly controlling every factor all play a role in determining the applicability and extent of their conclusions. This is especially true for lifting and nutrition where programs are built upon many variables, one variable often alters another, and *changes take time.*

In addition, research speaks *of averages*, but not everyone responds the same to certain methods, so there are outliers and different degrees that need to be taken into account before drawing definitive conclusions about every single individual. We've got to add other factors into the mix to create the best program for you.

2. PERSONAL EXPERIENCE

Science will tell you the cold, hard facts about physical systems, but it can't touch the subjective experience we all have. What works best in theory doesn't always work best in practice, and every program has to account for what it's like to go through it on a personal level.

I've been lifting for over 10 years, so you're getting the real deal right here. Before I run around recommending things to you, rest assured that I've been there done that.

I know what it's like to go through it all. Busting through a burning set of squats with over twice your weight on your back. Fighting through the trenches and temptations to get into shredded condition. Combining that with a social life. Taking the body to its peaks.

Because of that, I have knowledge from the first-person point of view. I know what you feel, how you feel, and what it's like to put these things in practice.

If I wouldn't do it, I'm not going to put you through it, so before anything gets to you, it's got to go by me first because I can relate. That's what makes a good coach great.

3. PRACTICAL EXPERIENCE

Lastly, we've got the real world out there to observe trends and see what works and what doesn't. This gave rise to the mighty temple of bro-science.

Today, bro-science is beaten and abused, but there's still a tremendous amount of value in seeing what works out there so long as you keep your mind right.

Science still has a lot of catching up to do, and if there's a lot of people out there doing something that's working, it warrants giving things a closer look.

As such, over the years I've stacked up the experience from those I've worked with, corroborated with many other physique architects and athletes, and studied the various practices past and present to gain clear-cut, tangible proof of the methods getting results out there to take the body to its peak.

A WINNING COMBINATION

If you want the best results out of your program, it's going to take a combination of all of these factors. They all have their pros and cons.

Think of it like this:

There's a big building and each one of those areas of science, personal experience, and practical experience is a room with one window in it. These rooms are all located on different sides of the building.

As such, they all have different views when they look out of that window. Sometimes, their field of vision overlaps and they see the same things, but because each one has a limited perspective, they've all got to spend time in each other's room to really see what's going on.

"But wait...there are 4 sides to a building and they only occupy 3 sides of it."

And that's <u>exactly</u> why you've got to stay humble.

We have to take the conclusions from *all* of these different areas and then apply critical thinking to pick the best option for you and your goals based on sound decision making.

They're nothing more than tools at our disposal to use for our artwork.

OPTIMAL FOR YOU

If you cracked open this book looking for the sorcerer's stone or a magical solution, I've got some bad news for you.

There is no best program. None. You will never find it.

There is only an optimal program for *you* based on *your current goals and level of development*. Every single person is different.

Nevertheless, the same principles still apply to the responses of the body to training and nutrition, and I've provided the framework to make adjustments as needed to optimize your program based on your results, so the content in this book will get you where you need to go when you put them into play. I've done that part for you.

Your job is to make sure that you make it happen, so for that, let's talk about some key components of application.

SUSTAINABILITY

The most fundamental component of any workout or nutrition program is **sustainability.**

The journey of achieving the ultimate physique is a long one with many twists, curves, and obstacles, so you need to design your program to weather the storm and take you to the promised-land.

Aesthetics aren't an overnight success. It's all about showing up and putting in the work day in and day out.

Therefore, when you're creating your programs, you've got to aim to get the results you want, stay healthy and injury free, enjoy the process, and allow for flexibility and freedom. For any protocol you're even thinking about going on, ask yourself this one extremely important question:

Am I cool with doing this for the rest of my life?

That simple question will set you straight. Any program you do needs to gear you up for success **now and forever.**

I know the industry will try to tell you that you can achieve mountains of muscle fast, get shredded in a week, or take this pill to become immortal and all powerful. I also know that a part of you wants to believe them. But these are nothing more than lies.

You may get results with such ridiculous protocols for a short amount of time, but you're going to hate it, and you'll lose all those gains when you drop out and can't keep up with it anymore. The body teaches us all a very valuable lesson:

GREAT THINGS TAKE TIME.

Always keep your eye on the prize in the horizon. There is absolutely nothing when it comes to building your physique that demands strict, aggressive methods that put you through hell.

People fail, damage themselves physically and mentally, and form a negative outlook on fitness by becoming too impatient or concerned with hunting mythical creatures rather than consistent, effective work. You've got to live and love that grind.

AESTHETIC SUCCESS

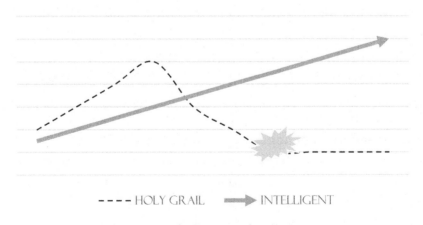

- - - - HOLY GRAIL ➡ INTELLIGENT

Nice results, but can you keep 'em?

We're playing long ball here. You've got to enjoy your journey of transforming yourself and keep that tip top physique for LIFE.

We're here to build statues, not sandcastles.

With these things in mind, the optimal program for you is going to come down to 3 fundamental factors:

THE 3PS OF A PHYSIQUE PROGRAM

To create any optimal program for you, it's going to come from maximizing the areas of:

- PHYSIOLOGY
- PSYCHOLOGY
- PRACTICALITY

The **physiology** we'll handle with the evidence-based approach we saw earlier. This is the backbone of the program and will ensure that you've got the right things going on within your body to achieve your goal. Whatever you do in your program has got to work and take you to that goal. Your program needs to follow sound principles, and everything you do has got to a have a rationale behind it that utilizes your resources most effectively.

The **psychology** is how you feel about your program. If you're not loving that journey of improving your physique and health, something is up. Cranking out your workouts, whipping up your meals, tracking progress and seeing those results pour in needs to light a fire in you. You've gotta love it. That's the only way you'll make it.

Practicality comes from making those other two factors fit in with your lifestyle. If I had all the resources in the world, I could take you to the level of Adonis or Aphrodite, but in the real world, you've got other obstacles to weave through. Sometimes, you've got to make tradeoffs, but most of the time, you just need to think through the principles and make the best call given all the factors laid out on the table. To help you do just that, let's look at setting up your targets.

FITNESS FRAMEWORKS

Everything in life has pros and cons, risk and reward, cost and benefit. Fitness is no different.

As you go along in your reading, I'll tell you everything you need to know about maximizing your physical potential based on those 3Ps, but there's one more thing you simply have to know: The law of diminishing returns and the importance of setting targets.

FITNESS RESULTS

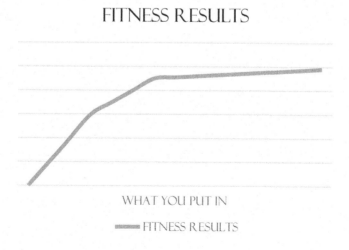

WHAT YOU PUT IN

━━━ FITNESS RESULTS

Get to know that chart very well. The more time, energy, and effort you put into your training and nutrition, the better the results you get will be, but that's not true into infinity. After a certain point, you're going to be putting in tons of effort just to get marginal gains. You can put in a certain amount of work to get the majority of your results, but to squeeze out that little bit extra, you've got to double it. Your job is to always understand where you're sitting on that curve and ask yourself:

Is this worth it to me?

Maybe it is. Maybe it isn't. I can't answer that for you. I can only give you the tools to your success. You've got to look at your life and make that call. Are you living life and enjoying that process? How are the other areas of your life integrating with your program?

To help you gain more clarity on this, let's take this one step further.

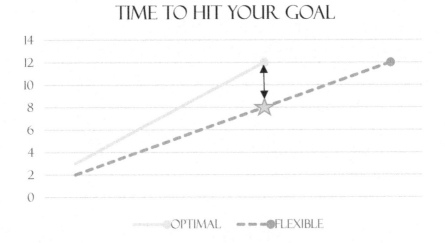

Let's say you were a perfect specimen and nailed everything day in day out like a machine. That'd be the top line.

On the bottom, you make that tradeoff between optimality and a more flexible approach. It takes you a little longer, but you enjoy the process more, and look at where you're at when the optimal approach hits its peak. Pretty damn good when you look at where you started.

Regardless of which you choose, the recommendations I give you will be based on the *optimal solution*, so you're going to need to assess the information I give you and set your levels based on that optimal target and how it pertains to your goals and lifestyle.

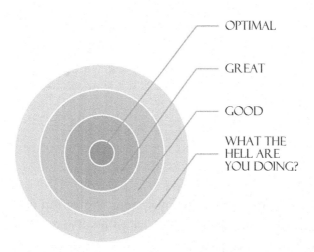

You don't have to stay seated on that bullseye, but by having that bullseye set, you know exactly what to aim for. And that makes the difference between putting points on the board or poking people's eyes out. You don't need perfection. You need **direction**.

Lastly, you need to understand that every day you have a dart to throw at that target.

The process of achieving your ultimate aesthetic physique is a long one, and your success is not an on or off switch. It's a bank account.

Today you may miss. Tomorrow you may hit it spot on. Some days you'll be closer than others. This is all normal. What you need to focus on is making sure that your plots stay consistent.

HITTING YOUR PROGRAM TARGETS

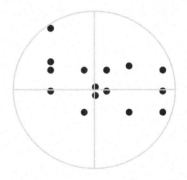

There will always be variation in any system. Perfection is a fairy tale and a moving target, and you'll drive yourself crazy like a cat chasing a laser on the wall. As soon as you pounce, it moves. So don't sweat it. A little high, a little low. But when you step back to see the clusters, you'll see you're heading where you need to go.

Set your targets, aim steady, and recalibrate your scope if you find you're falling shy too often. Improvement is a never-ending love affair.

SEAMLESS SYSTEM

Now let's wrap this all up. With the knowledge I'm going to dish out to you, you're going to need to create a system that works for you and allows you to keep going sustainably. For that, I'm hitting you with these 4S.

1. SUCCEED
2. SIMPLIFY
3. STANDARDIZE
4. SUSTAIN

If business is your thing, I'll throw in another S for you to replace that last one at no extra charge: Sell.

1. SUCCEED

Once you find that combination based on the information in this book that you enjoy, gets you the results you want, and fits in with your schedule and lifestyle, you've hit success.

Perfect. That's the first step.

2. SIMPLIFY

From there, you just have to simplify it and ask yourself what you can do to make it more refined and optimal for you.

I'll have you recording your progress over time, so when you look back, you can pinpoint what works, what doesn't, and what can improve or get cut altogether to get closer to that moving target of perfection.

3. STANDARDIZE

Next, you'll take that and create your standard. Your standard is that base template of effectiveness made up of your habits, routines, and core principles that deliver the goods.

Here are the standards that you will create for yourself as you go along. The particulars will depend based on you as an individual.

TENENTS OF FITNESS SUCCESS

TRAINING	NUTRITION	LIFESTYLE
Structured workout for your goals at least 3x/week Proper warmups Workout the entire body Focus on progression	Keep calories in check Adequate protein, EFA, hydration, and micronutrient intake Meal times and foods you enjoy	Proper sleep each and every night Active every day Minimize stress Mindfulness Mental Input Material (MIM) Posture, tissue quality, and movement quality

This right here is most of the battle. Once you've got this down pat, everything else is just minor details that can fluctuate and flutter all over the place depending on the circumstances. Success is simple. You just need to know what you're doing and lay it all out.

No matter what, you will maintain this standard. That'll lay your brickwork down and serve as your stable base.

This will eliminate your guess work and streamline your processes.

Should I go to the gym...?
Should I eat well today?
Should I go to bed on time tonight?

Those are questions that don't need to be asked. It's automatic. This underlies my simple philosophy:

Live clean so that you can get messy.

When you've got the basics of your fitness, finances, and life on point, you've got plenty of space for everything else. When you want to turn up, splurge, or relax, you've got the room.

That's how you flow like water. That's flexibility.

4.   SUSTAIN

Lastly, all there is left to do is keep it up. It'll become a part of you, and there will come a point in which you can't stay out of the gym or stop that fitness lifestyle.

Nevertheless, always keep your eyes and mind open and continually seek improvement in everything you do. There is no end to this. And you don't want one. Where's the fun in that?

That's how you succeed.

THE TIME FRAMES

You have taken the first step in coming here to drink from the cup of knowledge on training and nutrition, but perhaps you are feeling a bit antsy and impatient. The allure of changing your body and henceforth changing your life can be quite enticing. So, you may ask...

"When putting the principles in play properly, how long will it take for me to achieve my goal?"

All who embark on their physical journey come from a different starting point, and as noted, we all dispose of different genetic factors that mean that all take a different route in achieving their goal. Different routes and starting points, same direction. However, I bring good news:

Assuming an average starting point executed well:

- ❧ You will be above average and quite proud after 1.5 years.
- ❧ You will radically transform your physique within 3 years.
- ❧ After 5 years of consistent training, you will be near the upper levels for your body's capacity.

From here, the quest for further improvement is far from over, as you will continue to improve, learn, and refine your technique as time carries on, but these are rough guidelines as to what you can expect from putting the knowledge of training and nutrition I outline in this book into play.

7

THE 10 LAWS OF THE ARCHITECT OF AESTHETICS

*L*ASTLY, BEFORE YOU SET SAIL and disappear into the horizon in pursuit of gains and glory, there is one more thing that you must know.

Over the years in the pursuit of aesthetics and physical prowess, there have been many bloody battles that have stained the pure cloth of the noble desire of self-actualization. Many have risen to the occasion, and many have fallen and failed.

Divides have been established amongst the people, and those who seek their goals have been crushed amidst the confusion and tyranny that has been established.

Despite the madness, however, there is hope.

Passed down from generation to generation and guarded heavily amongst the wisest in the world are these golden nuggets of Ancient wisdom that I will bestow upon you:

THE 10 LAWS OF THE ARCHITECT OF AESTHETICS

It will take a wise person to obey these laws. Many are not up for the task and will break them in their own ignorance or at the expense of those they encounter.

You, future champion, are better than that, however.

Study these laws. Revisit them often. Let them guide you in your times of confusion. In training, in recovery, in nutrition - and for those with the eye to see, in life.

I.   HONOR YOUR GOAL

VICTORY results from driven FOCUS.

You must know EXACTLY what you want. Only THEN are you unstoppable in your pursuit.

Indecision and fickleness will lead to little more than defeat and time sifting through your fingers like grains of sand to be lost in the wind and never return.

When you're strong on both sides, you're weak on both sides. Pick your path and be congruent through and through.

II. THE BODY OPERATES ON A SPECTRUM

Right/Wrong. Good/Bad. Black/White. Effective/Worthless.

Abandon this foolish thinking.

There are only varying DEGREES. It is up to YOU to decide how far to go and when to pull back. The power lies in your hands.

Does that frighten you?

III. THE BODY ACTS IN PHASES

The body is not subject to rapid swings. Results don't flash and disappear like lightning in the sky. They are molded by time and persistence like a great canyon.

Time doesn't reset at midnight within the body, and it cares not whether it's Tuesday or Friday.

Time is a mental construct, and you will not be bound by it. You will plant yourself in the PRESENT and use time as a tool to devise your plans but nothing more. If you live in the past or future, you will never truly live at all.

Observe as the body follows its rhythm through time and remain patient. Work with it. Stay consistent. Patience is a virtue, and the best moves are the slow and strategic ones that turn the tide of war without anyone being the wiser.

Acting on impulse has led to few successes but thousands more destructive defeats.

IV. THERE ARE NO HARD RULES. ONLY TECHNIQUES AND TOOLS

Does an artist paint with one brush, one stroke, or one color alone? Or do they bring life to their work through various shades, styles, and colors?

We will adopt the position of an artist and use what best suits what we are trying to create with the things at our disposal.

Nevertheless...

MAXIM OF AESTHETICS: ALL IS VALID BUT NOT ALL IS VALUABLE.

When you internalize this, you will truly be free.

V. CONSIDER ALL OF THE VARIABLES ON HAND

Rarely are there isolated variables in the process of physical development. Everything is connected, and where you alter one, you alter another. Learn to measure your tradeoffs.

Hover above the situation unchained, seeing things for what they are in their entirety. Only then can you make the best decision.

VI. THE BODY IS MASTERFULLY BUILT TO SURVIVE AND ADAPT

The crux of physical development is knocking the body out of homeostasis to bring about some change. Overloading the muscle to spur growth. Creating a caloric deficit to drop body fat.

While we can do many things with our knowledge of the body to bring about good changes, let us recognize that we cannot outsmart Mother Nature through magic and manipulation. She's a much wiser vixen.

In regards to extreme actions and stubborn dogmas, a simple question sends silly ideas to the guillotine:

How does this make sense from a survival standpoint?

Rest in pieces.

VII. SIMPLICITY IS THE SOLUTION

The allure of fanciful techniques, concoctions, and programs is high.

You will be put to the test by distractions and terrific claims, but you must never lose sight of the basic principles.

A great tree must have its roots planted firmly within the soil. The seasons change and the leaves come and go, but true to its roots in the steady Earth the tree will remain.

VIII. MAKE GOLD OF WHAT IS GIVEN

The true mark of an architect of aesthetics lies in taking what he is presented with and turning it into a masterpiece. Every human being is presented with their own unique situation from their life to their body to their circumstances. We will work with this like alchemists.

Alchemy is the ancient science and philosophy of purifying and perfecting material items. The mortal into immortal. The base metals into GOLD. The architect of aesthetics is an alchemist applied to human form. You will take what you are given and make gold.

The things that you've been given aren't as important as what you can do with them. Let's see what you're made of.

IX. STAY HUMBLE

From the brisk breezes of Japan that tickle the pink rose blossoms in full bloom, the philosophy of kaizen has traveled and fluttered into our hands.

The philosophy of kaizen is the philosophy of continuous improvement. Every day, in any way, there lies some step to improve. Some way to progress. If you believe you can...

No matter how far we come, we will remain humble and open to new ideas, learning, and growth. No matter how far we come, we will remain innocent and ignorant like the child who has just stepped into the light for the first time from its cradle in the cave.

"I am wise for I know nothing." said Socrates. Are you much greater?

X. NEVER FORGET THE HUMAN BEING

We speak of taking to the body to its highest splendor, but let us never forget that animating and wielding that body is a PERSON.

A person with a past. A person with dreams. A person with interests, feelings, and a life outside of the walls of the weight room and the echoes of the iron.

The true architect of aesthetics recognizes that:

MAXIM OF AESTHETICS: FITNESS IS JUST THE MEDIUM - NOT THE MISSION.

You will place the success of the INDIVIDUAL over the success of the system. You will place LIFE above lifting.

You shall never forget the human being.

ONWARD TO OLYMPUS

With that, young architect, I roll up the scroll and pass it into your hands. Treasure it, and treat it well.

Are you ready?

At the flip of this page awaits a world before you that will change your life forever. If the time is right, drift off into the sparkling coast and relish your journey as you experience the new lands and adventures that await you beyond the horizon.

Go forth and build your temple. We shall reunite at Mount Olympus.

PART II: GYM AND EQUIPMENT

8

THE GYM

IN THE GOLDEN AGE OF AESTHETIC BODYBUILDING, Venice Beach, California was the mecca of muscle.

The atmosphere was electrified with enthusiasm and burning passion for the weights. The air was rich in the scent of the salty oceans blowing through the wind and the rusty iron being tossed around in the gym.

There was an almost magical quality about it that you just couldn't quite put your finger on, but you could somehow feel it grip the air like a humid cloak, and it was here that created the perfect training grounds for many a legendary physique that set the foundations for modern bodybuilding and continue to inspire us today and for generations to come.

Choosing your gym is a critical step on the path to constructing your physique. It is here where the work will take place that will sculpt your body, mind, and spirit. It is here where you will face your battles. It is here where you will conquer, test your limits, and grow.

FACTORS IN A GYM

There are several factors to take into consideration when it comes time to select your iron asylum. We need a place that can provide the proper tools we need to sculpt our physique and boost our spirits through an environment that is conducive to our success. Here we will look at equipment, facilities, the crowd, timing, logistics, the vibe, test drive, and price points before looking at the home gym alternative.

EQUIPMENT

First things first. We need to make sure the gym has the equipment you need to form your aesthetic workshop. Here's what to look for:

- Dumbbells up to 100lbs (standard preferred; adjustable will require set-up and clean-up time)
- Barbells (standard 45lbs)
- Benches (flat and adjustable)
- Power-racks
- Standard free weight plates (45, 25, 10, 5, and 2.5 pound)
- Cable station with attachments (single handle, rope, bar)
- Seated/standing calf raises machine (a leg press or loaded barbell will work here)
- Mirrors

At minimum, look for these fundamentals. More than one option for each is preferred and is a great luxury to have depending on the time you hit the gym and how big the crowd is.

For extra needs or due to your special requirements, other machines and set-ups are nice to have and can offer variety on top of the bare minimum. This includes cardio equipment, angled set-ups, specialty bars, and so forth.

Good news is most gyms these days have all of the above, so you've got your bases covered. Let's look at some more factors.

FACILITIES

Behind the necessary equipment, check to ensure that the facilities are spot on. The gym must be neat, orderly, and well-taken care of across all areas. This will tell you all you need to know about how important a pristine workout experience is to the staff.

Safety, maintenance, and cleanliness are important, and having to go on a scavenger hunt for equipment and weight plates is a waste and will murder your workout momentum.

Also ensure that it big & open with adequate space to move around in without having to adjust your position constantly to accommodate others. A designated warm-up area with smaller weights and foam rollers is a definite plus, and A/C units, heaters, and clean water are a definite must.

Other important points to make note of are the design and decoration. This can impact your mental state and make you feel fully in your element or out and place and unable to get in a good workout. The colors, posters on the wall, content playing on the TV, and other factors all add up to make a great place to train.

You'll be spending a lot of time here over the years, so make the right choice and don't sacrifice on service and your surroundings.

CROWD

Take a look around the gym and observe the clientele. What do you see?

MAXIM OF AESTHETICS: THE PEOPLE YOU SURROUND YOURSELF WITH ARE THE PREDICTORS OF YOUR SUCCESS.

Seek out gyms with a crowd that is hungry for success. They must have respect for each other and the gym. They must be passionate about pursuing progress. This energy is contagious and fuel you on a subconscious level. Seeing a bunch of zombies will do nothing but drag you down. You need people who not only lift weights but also lift YOU up. And you better be one of them.

If you're a lone wolf and the gym is your world away from the world, find the gyms and times where the gym is empty and let out your inner beast without distractions. The gym can be the best sanctuary there is. For that hour of the day, it's your sacred bubble. Guard it.

TIMING

Don't hit the gym when it's packed if you can help it.

Having to pull a number to wait in line for your next exercise is not an effective use of time, and we need unimpeded consistency and work flow to make gains.

If nothing else, structure your gym schedule and workouts around the herd. Monday is national chest day, so hit legs instead on that day. If the machines are all occupied, use the empty space between to knock out some dumbbell lunges. You get the idea.

LOGISTICS

Find a gym that's close to home, close to work, or both. Most gyms will allow membership across their network, and if they don't, negotiate.

You're more likely to go when it's close, and you'll waste less time in transit to and from the gym, so there's less of an investment in going which frees up your schedule more and takes the excuses out of the equation. A 1 hour workout is more than just 1 hour at first glance.

Of course, having a home gym is the most accessible gym there is, and you may choose to go this route either by personal preference or be forced due to the circumstances.

Because of the plus sides this has, I recommend that everyone have at minimum some basic equipment on hand.

VIBE

The factor that stands above all else is the atmosphere and vibe.

- When you walk through that door, do you feel inspired to go hard and pump some iron?
- Can you feel the energy floating through the air?
- How does the environment make you feel deep down?

This is the X Factor - a cocktail blend of numerous variables that can range from the lighting to the color scheme, to the clientele, to the layout, to the building itself.

The effect this has is different for everyone, but the important thing to take away here is that you must feel in harmony with your surroundings.

It's a bit hard to put your finger on, but when it's there, you know it. It'll light that fire in you.

TEST-DRIVE

Before committing to any gym, give it a test drive.

Most gyms will offer an introductory training pass for a period of time. Take advantage of this.

Go, get some workouts in, and judge the experience as if you were already a member. Get a tour of the facilities so you can get a feel of the place, and then make your decision.

CASH

Go for the best gym that you can afford in regards to what you will use it for and your personal taste based on the factors that we've gone over and will continue to discuss throughout the rest of the book.

Your choice in gym is just like any other buying decision, so use your good judgment - perhaps even more important considering you'll be spending several hours of your week here.

Quality rules all, and your home away from home is no place to cut corners.

HOME GYM

Getting a great workout in doesn't require a boat load of equipment. It's all about the basics.

With a few bits of equipment and a dash of creativity, you can create your own home gym and still get the gains you're after. It's never closed, there's no traffic, and you're free to do as you damn well please and train insane.

Even if you do have a gym membership, investing in some basic equipment for home is a fantastic idea. Life can be chaotic sometimes, and things come up. Being able to get a workout in at home can come quite in handy in a pinch.

At bare minimum, a bench, a set of adjustable dumbbells and some solid know-how can give you a productive full-body workout without the need for a gym. More can be useful and is dependent on its utility to you, so glance over at the required gym equipment and determine what - if any - is worth your while in accordance with the rest of the material presented in this book.

9

PROPER ATTIRE

HETHER OUT IN THE CITY STREETS taking care
of business, enjoying a night out with the entourage or a
sexy someone, making moves in your career, or crushing
iron at the gym:

D R E S S F O R S U C C E S S.

The way you portray yourself to the world and subconsciously to
yourself MATTERS and is an integral component of generating a
positive ecosystem of progress and abundance to send your life
hurtling with magnificent momentum towards your goals.

You need to care just as much about how you look for your workout
as you do for a first date. Actually, you better care *more*.

You need to treat *every workout* like a date with destiny. People
need to look at you and know that you're about your business and

aren't just there to "stay in shape" or catch up on the latest scores or useless drama.

In the gym, you won't be blazered up with crisp, colorful pocket squares and slick loafers or mini-skirts and high heels, nor will you be flashing the tight leotards and cutoffs of the 80s, but choosing the right threads will make a world of difference in how you feel and gear you up to get your work done the way you're supposed to.

CLOTHING GOALS

When it comes to workout attire you have these 3 priorities:

1. LOOK YOUR BEST

The gym is a place to build yourself up and hone your health, and the gym is a big room full of mirrors, so you're going to be seeing a lot of yourself. Take pride in your appearance and the work you're about to put in. Working out is not a chore. It's a CHOICE. Set the example for others, and respect your craft.

2. FEEL YOUR BEST

What you wear to the gym should be cool and comfortable. Avoid rough fabrics and constrictive clothing. It needs to feel right and be able to breathe a little as you power through the workout.

3. PERFORM YOUR BEST

Most importantly of all, you've got to be able to crank out the high performance required. That's why you're in there in the first place.

Eliminate any loose fabrics, accessories, or hair that can get caught or get in the way during your exercises or anywhere in between.

Let's look at some practical recommendations to hit all of those now.

CLOTHING CHOICE

For guys and girls, well-fitting athletic shorts or joggers/leggings and a snug T-shirt or tank top fits the bill like a charm.

This will make sure that your clothes are comfortable, don't interfere with your workouts or movements patterns, and give you that extra oomph of confidence as you see yourself putting in that work and building up your physique.

Color-wise, opt for vivid colors or patterns that contrast with the dull, lifeless colors of most gyms and their equipment. This is stimulating to the eye and speaks sparks of high energy. A bright shirt, shorts, or shoes all have that eye-catching effect that allows you to stand out from the background and enhance the workout experience.

❧ LAYER UP

Along with these recommendations, learn to dress in layers - especially as the cold months draw near. During warm-ups, you want the muscles and joints to be warm and fluid. As the workout progresses and your intensity increases, you can strip down like you've got daddy issues and continue to knock out your sets as the pump and heat gets to be too much.

In the hot months, some compression shorts or leggings will trap heat better without being overwhelming. This can lead to a better perceptual workout and potential tactile feedback for muscular contractions in the legs. Give it a shot.

FOOTWEAR

For lifting weights, get yourself a flexible, slim, flat-soled shoe with an excellent fit. The more minimal, the better.

Arch support and angles are great for lots of running, but in the gym, we want as close to a natural feel as possible while still providing protection and grip. Your feet are biomechanical masterpieces. Let them do their job.

This is especially important for leg exercises such as deadlifts, squats, and calf exercises, and if you've ever seen folks performing these lifts in Tarzan mode by going barefoot or in socks alone, this is why. It lets the foot do its work and places the weight more on the heels where it should be and enables better biomechanics on the lift.

SOCKS

As you'll see later in the book, leg days are coming hot off the grill with a nice few sets of Romanian Deadlifts. Due to the form on these, you may find yourself scraping up your shins as you keep the bar snug to your body. To get around this, you can opt for longer socks on these days. If not, some compression pants or leggings will do the job.

HATS

Fitted hats and baseball caps will cover up your savage hair that's sure to surface when you're training full blast. With the brim down and hat snug, you'll create that feeling of more isolation and seclusion from the outside world. It's a sign you're in your zone.

Throw your earbuds into the mix, and you're a force to be reckoned with. Just watch out for the tightness. You don't want to hamper blood flow and circulation. If there are marks, it's too tight.

Outside of fitteds or baseball caps, beanies, hairties, and headbands are A-ok.

ACCESSORIES

Accessories are the cornerstone of any great outfit, but in the gym, be a minimalist.

The max you can ever pull off is a sports watch to monitor your workout time and rest between sets, a bracelet that fits snug on the wrist, a chain or necklace that stays tucked and out of the way, or a pair of earrings.

Go for them all, or go for none. Your phone can serve as a stopwatch just as easily, but if you do this, throw it on airplane mode, do not disturb, or eliminate all lock screen notifications that'll distract you from the mission at hand. Your phone is for recording your progress, music, monitoring the time, and checking your form on occasion only. Tell your fan club or secret admirers to hit you up later. They'll still be there.

10

LIFTING ACCESSORIES

O N TOP OF THE GYM AND PROPER ATTIRE, there are some other things that are going to be useful for your workouts. This chapter is all about lifting accessories. We'll go over things to help you get a better grip on your training, belts, music, and gym bags to gear you up to get your best work done.

GLOVES, STRAPS, AND CHALK

Bars are made of metal. Hands sweat. Sweat + metal bars = slippery. Hold your applause.

Most bars have tread to help with grip, but when you're loading up like a shotgun to deadlift several plates, a slippery bar can cause you to fail the lift despite your ability to spank that weight like it colored on the wall. Gloves, Straps, and Chalk get around this issue.

GLOVES

Gloves are the most widespread and popular method of dealing with grip in the gym. Additionally, for businessmen, females, folks in the service or food industry, and anyone else, gloves can prevent those calluses from bursting like Mount Vesuvius on a set of raw deadlifts that'll leave your clients, cohorts, and customers running in fear.

Don't get thick, bulky gloves. This isn't a boxing match or handling ebola vials. Overly thick designed gloves will alter the natural feel of the hand gripping the bar and impede workout performance [1].

STAY STRAPPED

Straps are another common remedy for getting a grip on the weights. These are most relevant on exercises like rows and deadlifts where gravity is fighting against you from a superior position. If your arms or legs can move the weight but your grip strength is failing you, it would make sense to introduce some straps until you get things sorted out.

The objective is to train the targeted muscles, and when grip becomes a limiting factor for the targeted muscle group's progress, action needs to be taken until the weak point is fixed.

Straps can have their place, but using them in conjunction with getting your grip strength up is the better option. You want your forearms and grip to adapt. Use them sparingly on your heaviest sets or late in the workout when grip starts to tire out and slowly ween yourself off of them.

CHALK

Last but certainly not least in the grip department is chalk. Commercial gyms frown upon the white stuff because of the mess, but you can sneak in a bit as long as you don't go overboard trying to create a Christmas wonderland around the squat rack.

More serious athletic or powerlifting gyms will have chalk dishes readily available around workstations, and if not, you can always buy your own chalk to use. They typically come in plastic-wrapped bricks that you put in your own small plastic container for easy transport and to keep the mess under wraps.

Lord help you if you get stopped by the police with the bricks of the stuff in the passenger seat. Better act like you don't know me.

❧ NAILS

For the ladies out there, make sure that you keep an eye on your nail length. Long nails will interfere with your ability to grip the weights fully and properly, so tone down the claws. A little bit is fine and pleasantly feminine, but too much will detract from the workout.

BELTS

Outside of legitimate physical injury reasons, weight-lifting belts are more of a luxury than a necessity.

The idea behind belts is to increase intra-abdominal pressure and strengthen the core for the weight being lifted. This sounds logical and good on paper, but the problem with this is that it also affects the biomechanics of the lift unfavorably [2].

If you've never tried for yourself, the difference behind a belted squat and a non-belted squat is significant. Outside of heavy sets (5 reps and under), belts simply aren't necessary. Train without them from the start with solid form and your body will adapt accordingly as you progress.

The body works as a full functional unit. Build your natural belt. Your abs will develop.

WRAPS/SLEEVES

For joint and muscular support during their workouts, many people turn to wraps and sleeves. These offer compression and additional warmth to the area and can allow for a more stable structure that will support the demands of the workout.

Unless you have a specific chronic/ pre-existing injury or are moving heavy weights, these are more of a fashion statement than a requirement, and you should only look to use them if you truly need them.

If you do, you'll know. This should be done alongside a proper correctional routine, for most of these stem from underlying issues that must be addressed either through posture or movement patterns.

MUSIC

Music is a moral law. It gives soul to the universe, wings to the mind, flight to the imagination, and charm and gaiety to life and to everything.

Plato

There's nothing quite like grinding out your set when the beat drops and you're hit with that euphoric symphony of rhythm and energy.

There is a special species out there that prefers to lift in silence, but music is a must-have for any worthwhile workout. Time and time again, music has been shown to improve moods, performance, energy level, and reduce our perception of effort and fatigue [3-7]. Don't do without it.

CREATE PLAYLISTS

Take the time to craft your own playlists with your favorite music. You can get creative with this and create general mixed playlists, playlists by genre, or even playlists by workout day.

Heavy metal & hard rock can be just what the doctor ordered for leg day, whereas on upper body days you get more pumped with the bass-rich shockwaves of the 4 to the floor that some good EDM provides or the lyrical flames produced by your favorite rappers and the seismic undercurrent of 808s.

Something so simple as looking forward to lifting to your favorite new song can provide you with newfound energy and passion for your workouts. Utilize it. If you don't get chills, do better.

SEGMENT YOUR PLAYLIST

To take this even further, you can segment out your music selection based on workout phase.

For example, you play one type of music for your warmups, another for your heavy compound work, and yet another for your higher rep hypertrophy style work. The sky is the limit here. This can help for mentally segmenting your workout out.

ADJUST THE SET

For the workout itself, toggle the volume and song selection to correspond to your working sets, rest times, and workout portion.

- Warm ups get slower music at a lower volume
- More intense sets get louder volume with tremendous energy and impact
- Lighter work gets somewhere in the middle
- And rest times get something above warmups but less than a lighter set. They're there to keep the flow and momentum up while creating contrast between your working sets where you want to be fully amped.

This will take some trial and error to nail correctly, but once you DO get it, your workout will be like its own movie or symphony, complete with build ups, climaxes, and the like that transform the simple act of lifting weights into an event you can't wait to experience.

MUSIC EQUIPMENT

Invest in a great set of headphones or earbuds. Don't skimp on quality here. Training is a way of life, and when you're in the gym multiple times a week, there's zero sense in cutting yourself short over something that will radically alter your workout experience for the better.

Seek for a full range of frequencies, durability, and sweat resistance. You want solid, tight bass and crystal-clear highs. Proper volume output is a must.

Outside noise reduction is an excellent feature to look for as well. This can help towards creating your own little bubble and seclusion from the outside world.

MORE THAN SOUND

The proper length of wire here is also key. Too long and you may be getting it tangled, and too short will leave your full range of motion restricted as you crane your neck to accommodate the short length. A helpful tip is to tuck the wire underneath your shirt so that it doesn't get in the way of your movements. Better yet, go wireless.

Regardless of what you do, ensure you secure your device. A clip, strong case, arm band, or zippered pockets are all advisable here. Ever gone back for bench presses and had your phone fall out of your pocket or accidentally hit your phone with a dumbbell? Then you know what I'm talking about.

This will also keep it out of the way and prevent it from becoming a distraction. For example, when doing deadlifts with the phone in your pocket, you may be tempted to alter your movement pattern so that the bar doesn't drag on your thigh and bump into your device. Form is key, so never let the attire or equipment be the limiting factor.

GYM BAG

Every year, thousands of homes are torn and broken by the result of forgetting earbuds or pre-workouts after getting to the gym.

To make sure that you have all of your bases covered required for killer workout and don't suffer the same fate, pack a gym bag that contains everything you need beforehand and keep it handy.

A good gym bag should contain:

- Change of gym clothes and shoes
- Any lifting accessories
- Earbuds
- Portable charger
- Towel
- Hygiene products
- Water Bottle
- Any supplements or meals on the go*

By doing this, you'll always ensure that you have what you need when the time strikes to go hit the gym. Keep it locked and loaded at the house, at the office, in your car, or wherever you are to ensure that there are no excuses when it's go time.

*You'll see my thoughts about supplements and workout nutrition in the Nutrition Section of the book.

PART III: TRAINING

11

OBJECTIVE OF AESTHETIC TRAINING

HEN YOU STEP FOOT INTO THAT WEIGHT ROOM with desire in your eyes, what's your objective? A great plan for success *always* surges from a clearly defined and honored objective. On the battlefield, in business, and in the weight room: Know what you want and employ your efforts and resources mercilessly to make it happen. Leave *nothing* to chance.

MAXIM OF AESTHETICS: IF YOU FAIL TO PLAN, THEN YOU PLAN TO FAIL.

Which objective will we honor when we go head to head with the iron? Let's first determine our objective by deciding which of them are NOT for our goal:

- ❧ Our objective in the weight room is NOT to be the strongest and lift the most amount of weight at one time.
- ❧ Our objective in the weight room is NOT to have the longest, most intense workout possible and leave thrashed and beaten.
- ❧ Our objective in the weight room is NOT to burn a ton of calories and drop fat.
- ❧ Our objective in the weight room is NOT to look cool by doing fancy fruity exercises.
- ❧ Our objective in the weight room is NOT to enhance athletic performance.

Nope. Try again. That's not gonna cut it.

> The objective of weight training for our goals is to *stimulate the growth of muscle mass* to our frame in strategic locations to form a flowing, aesthetic physique.

PERIOD. We will apply laser-like focus to this objective. Forget the rest. It isn't our cause. Those extra results are purely secondary.

Everything else we talk about will be going to this goal, so it's important to get it right. This is the principle of **specificity.** Decide what you want. Then gear up to *go get it.*

BE SPECIFIC

Imagine that in front of you there is a series of buckets. Each one represents a particular muscle group or skillset that you want to develop.

Now let's say that I give you 20 marbles, and you have to place these marbles in the bucket you want to build the most. I'm magical, so once you make your decision on where to put the marbles, I snap my fingers and your body transforms to match the decisions you made on which buckets to put the marbles in.

Where would you put them?

This is how you need to create your training program. Those 20 marbles represent your time, energy, and recovery capacity. You only have so much to go around, so you MUST choose wisely how you're going to deposit those resources based on your goal.

*Our goal is muscle hypertrophy of specific areas to form an aesthetic physique, so where we put our resources absolutely **must** go towards that goal.*

- A girl with her eyes set on being a goddess is going to have a different program than a guy looking to compete in powerlifting.
- A guy on a quest for maximal aesthetics is going to have a different program from an athlete training for performance.

You can hit the gym for all sorts of reasons from injury rehab to health to size and strength, but not all paths lead to the same goal. This leads us to:

THE CRUCIAL QUESTION

If someone were to look at what you're doing in the gym and ask you why you're doing that particular exercise, that many sets, that rep range, that order, and any other variable in your training program or nutritional plan, your answer needs to be logical, solid, and support that goal that you've set out for yourself or else you're just screwing around and shooting in the dark.

Does that mean you can't do anything else ever? No. But you are *conscious* of that fact and *make that choice* despite knowing it isn't optimal. And that's cool. That choice may make the difference between enjoying your program more & giving it your very best or dropping out and not achieving your goal.

There's diminishing returns to all things fitness and nutrition, so that extra effort may not be worth it to you, but you at least have your TARGET firm and set. Even if you miss that bullseye, you're damn close and aiming in the right direction. Even if it takes you a bit longer, you'll still get there. That makes all the difference. Remember:

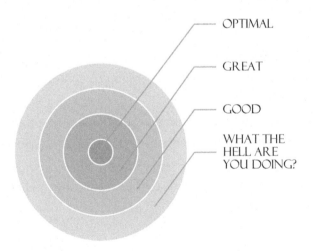

OPTIMAL

GREAT

GOOD

WHAT THE
HELL ARE
YOU DOING?

Building your physique isn't picking what you want on the menu at the restaurant or filling up your cart and clicking 'checkout' for some online shopping.

Building your physique means investing your valuable time and money, putting in work on intense workouts for years, pushing past your barriers, and dedicating yourself to the gym grind, so you better make the right decisions. How tragic it would be to go through all that and not even get what you want.

You don't pick your training 'just because' or 'I feel like'. You pick what you do because *this takes you closer to your goal.*

End of story.

MAXIM OF AESTHETICS: YOU MUST BE ABLE TO SATISFACTORILY JUSTIFY EVERYTHING IN YOUR WORKOUT, DIET PROGRAM, AND LIFE.

With that in mind, let's talk about some GAINS.

THE THREE AESTHETIC TRAINING MUST-HAVES:

When it comes to this goal of putting on muscle mass, we have three main priorities:

1. STIMULATE
- Provide the challenge and trigger for growth
- Balance Intensity, Volume, Frequency

2. RECOVER AND BUILD
- Recover from the training session through proper nutrition and rest
- Consider whole body and mental recovery

3. PROGRESSIVE OVERLOAD
- Improve and grow by increasing that stimulus over time until desired muscular levels are achieved

This is very cut, dry, and methodical. And that's the point. To dial up a great training program, you've got to take a scientific approach. You're a doctor prescribing a physique remedy. We will briefly talk about the basics of what each consists of and then lay out the training principles that will satisfy these requirements to build our routine.

1. PROVIDE THE OPTIMAL STIMULUS FOR GROWTH

Hypertrophy (the white-coat way of defining muscle growth) depends on overloading the muscle and is accomplished through several factors to varying degrees including mechanical tension, the metabolic stress, and the damage inflicted upon the muscle being worked [1], with mechanical tension being #1 and the biggest factor.

To keep things clean and crisp, in practical terms, every workout program is going to come down to a balance between *training intensity, workout volume, and workout frequency*:

FREQUENCY

OPTIMAL
TRAINING
ROUTINE

INTENSITY   VOLUME

These 3 factors are all very closely related, thus the equilateral triangle. Intensity and volume form the base of the program and are the most important by both *defining the adaptation* and the *magnitude of that adaptation*. Frequency has more of a connecting role and helps you to manage those two for optimal results.

INTENSITY can primarily be defined by weight, reps, proximity to failure, and rest times. There is a direct relationship amongst these factors. The type of exercises performed here also plays a role in determining the intensity of a workout.

VOLUME is king [2,3] and refers to the total amount of the work at that intensity being performed over a period of time (week/workout). In its simplest form it can be thought of as:

WEIGHT x REPS x SETS

This also called *total tonnage* or *workload*, and for ease of use it can often be used to refer to just the number of sets you're doing since a minimum intensity level of weight being used is often a given.

The weight will impact the reps you can perform as well as the number of sets you can reasonably do within the workout. Outside of the workout, this will impact our next factor of training: Frequency.

FREQUENCY deals with how often you're working out that particular muscle but also to a lesser extent - how often you're working out in general.

Making the best gains depends on spreading out your volume to allow for the best quality training you can do and ensuring that the muscle is being trained to maximize its growth cycles [4].

You must also ensure that frequency allows for total body performance to be on point, so living in the gym is not a good idea if you're truly serious about your training. Let your lust for the lifting regenerate. You'll get your best workouts and life balance that way.

T O T A L   V O L U M E

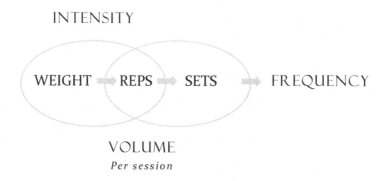

INTENSITY

WEIGHT ➡ REPS ➡ SETS ➡ FREQUENCY

VOLUME
Per session

When you factor in the frequency, you get TOTAL VOLUME. The *total volume* you do is the biggest determinant of growth [2,3].

GET THE BALANCE RIGHT

Any program worth its salt is going to find sound balance amongst these 3 factors. If it doesn't, run far, far away. Because of this, many programs work, but not all programs *are optimal* or optimal for *you*.

For example:

- You can go all out but volume and frequency will suffer.
- You can go very frequently but not with a lot of volume or intensity.
- You can do a lot of volume but intensity will be lacking and frequency won't be very high.
- If you go high on none of them, you won't grow well at all.
- And lastly, if you go high on all of them, you will be visited by the ghost of death and dragged into the Shadow Realm.

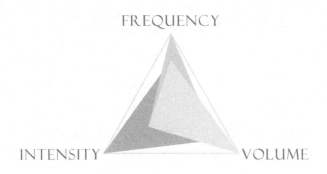

FREQUENCY

INTENSITY   VOLUME

None of these factors in isolation is the answer, and the most you can really ever push is 2 of these factors before you completely wreck yourself. It takes a charming cocktail of these factors to achieve optimal hypertrophy.

For example, to achieve the best growth, you can't just release the Kraken to crush a 1RM (1 rep max) and call it a day. You can't just grind out 1 grueling set and exit the gym. And you can't skip through the weight room with a set of pretty pink dumbbells and expect to grow (ladies, listen up).

Will these stimulate some growth? Sure, but "some" isn't what we want here.

If you're going to hit the gym, *make it count.*

2. RECOVER AND REBUILD

After hitting our muscles in the gym, they - and our body as a whole - need time to regroup, recharge, and rebuild or OVER-build to lay down new muscle tissue.

We will also create clean space in our workout schedule for our body as a whole to perform at its best and set the stage for us to enjoy other areas of our life as well.

Solid nutrition, proper all around programming/scheduling, and sound recovery habits are big points in this step.

We grow outside of the gym. Remember this.

Deloading and taking complete time off is also a must to ensure that our mind and body recovers properly from the training being thrown at it. You can't go hard all the time, and if you try, you sure as hell won't be for much longer.

3. CONSISTENTLY PROVIDE MORE STIMULUS UNTIL DESIRED SIZE IS ACHIEVED

Making gains is about making progress.

To grow, in the gym or in life, you've got to keep facing new challenges and overcoming them. You can do this by adding more weight, reps, or sets. Weight *within the effective rep range* is the most efficient and most important, and that's the one we'll put most of our attention on here.

MAXIM OF AESTHETICS:
IF OVER TIME YOU AREN'T ADDING WEIGHT TO THE BAR, OVER TIME YOU AREN'T GOING VERY FAR.

This is what's known as progressive overload.

- ❧ It's not about the calorie burn.
- ❧ It's not about the pump.
- ❧ It's not about how sore you are.

Are you **objectively** *improving* over time following the workouts? THIS is the true measure of gym success when your goal is making gains.

The exercises and tactics you use can rotate in and out of your training, and the pump/grind are all parts of the lifting experience, but if you're not stacking weight on the bar in between your birthday candles based on some objective measure, something is horribly wrong.

Progressive OVERLOAD is King. Not progressive burnitude or progressive pumpitude.

When you've got the first two training principles down pat, progressive overload should come smoothly and naturally. When it doesn't, we'll handle it.

SUMMING UP OUR WEIGHT TRAINING OBJECTIVES

And there you have it. Train smart, rest up, and hit it harder the next go ' round. That's how gains are made, ladies and gentlemen.

Equipped with these fundamentals, we can now dig into the delicious details of how to make that happen most efficiently via:

- ❧ Intensity (How hard)
- ❧ Workout volume (How much)
- ❧ Workout frequency (How often)
- ❧ Exercise selection
- ❧ Exercise variations

IN THAT ORDER.

These will be the foundations for our workout programming and schedule that'll take you where you wanna go.

MUSCLE SPECIFICITY

For the rest of our discussion over training, keep in mind that this is *specific for the muscle* that is being trained.

It's easy to get lost in the shuffle and think of hypertrophy as just "one thing", but muscle growth is a *local process*, so understand these concepts as they pertain to *each individual muscle* on your physique rather than a blanket that covers it all.

In other words, don't just think about training legs. You don't have one huge "leg muscle". Think about quads, hamstrings, glutes, and calves and how these concepts will apply to them. Each muscle is like a unique state in a country.

If there are multiple muscles in those groups (calves are comprised of the soleus and gastrocnemius which have 2 different personalities, for example), think about each. These are the cities in those states. Think about overlap. You're going to have to put your mind to work here. Embrace it. That's what it's there for.

Lastly, the information I dish out here will be for *optimal* solutions for growth based on *general guidelines*, so use them to gain solid knowledge and then adjust them to your individual needs and goals.

I will give you tips on how to do that, but if you don't know how to adjust them based on sound practices, then don't. Stick to what I recommend before you think you're in expert mode and can fly solo. You'll either crash or never even get off the ground.

To enable you to form the right mental bridges and understand why I am recommending what I do in context of the bigger picture, take a look at the chart below with the conclusions we will arrive at.

FACTOR	RECOMMENDATION	NOTES
INTENSITY	6-15RM split up for 80% of the work	Within 1-3 reps of failure
REST TIMES	As much as necessary to perform next set(s) Usually 2-3 min.	Heavier and/or compounds longer, lighter and/or isolations shorter
VOLUME	8-12 weekly sets = ~4-6 sets/ ~30-60 reps per muscle per session	Starting point - start low Consider overlap
FREQUENCY	2-3x/7-10 days per muscle group !Factor in total volume!	Depends on lifter, status, and overall training volume for the muscle Consider overlap/full recovery

12

INTENSITY

OW HARD DO YOU HAVE TO GO to grow? Setting up the right intensity is the first step in putting your workouts in motion, and it'll make or break the rest. With that in mind, let's look at the factors influencing intensity to get moving in the right direction.

WEIGHTS AND REPS

You can't just waltz into the weight room, screw around with some pink dumbbells, and expect to make your best gains. If you could, the whole world would be jacked. Muscles are *built* to handle light work all day, every day.

You've got to *challenge the muscle* to push it to adapt and put on size optimally [1,2]. However, muscle growth can be seen across high, medium, **and** low rep ranges when volume is equated [3,4], and they've got all got their ins and outs, so we've got to narrow this down to determine what's best for *our* goals of slapping size on our statue for maximal hypertrophy by optimizing efficiency, volume, and frequency. Lift heavy or lift light...what's right?

Let's break down the rep ranges and get to the bottom of this. For sake of discussion, we will be assuming weights used that provide the maximum number of the repetitions listed.

← REP RANGE CONTINUUM →

1-5 Reps	6-10	12-15	15+
85%+ of 1RM			< 65% of 1RM
More	75-85% of 1RM	65-75% of 1RM	*More*
Strength			**Endurance**

given rep ranges assume sets taken to failure
1RM = 1 rep maximum

Going heavy (1-5) is an attractive range for lots of young guns. After all, you get to slam the weights and post videos on the internet of how strong you are. However, this is an inferior choice for hypertrophy.

Low rep ranges are all about maximizing *strength* [3,4,5,6,7].

Your body must quite literally figure out how to somehow lift that massive object by improving movement coordination and neural efficiency. It does *not* get better at this through growth per se, but rather learning *how to use* what's already there better. Size is just a side effect.

In fact, you can improve strength monumentally without growing *at all* simply through neurological adaptations and improved technique. Think of it like overriding the chip and improving the alignment on your car to hit max speeds.

Lifting heavy also has many downsides:

- Hard on the mind, joints, and body as a whole
- Higher risk of chronic injury and vacations to Snap City
- Requires longer warm-ups and workouts to have a productive training session with adequate volume for optimal growth.
- Higher intensity that impacts recovery

Contrast the total time and life force investment required to successfully prepare for and knock out 3 sets of 10 vs. 10 sets of 3 at peak loads. And that's for a small volume of 30 total reps.

Could you truly withstand much more than this? Could you do this often and sustainably? Think back to the triangle I presented. The answer is no.

Going light (15+) gets laughed at and ignored for its small size, but as it turns out, it also is effective at packing on size [4].

High rep ranges are effective for stimulating Type I fibers, help in working around injuries, and let you get in a good training stimulus without the load on the joints. This makes it a very viable option for specific applications in your training.

On the other hand, they miss out on enough tension to make productive strength gains and stimulating all of the muscle fibers from the get-go because the weight is simply too light [4,8]. This isn't as efficient for our goals.

Perceptually, high rep ranges also make for torturous sets and unnecessarily grueling workouts for no real extra added benefit – especially on larger muscle groups and compound movements. Go do a set of squats with your 20 rep max and tell me how you feel after you get brought back to life.

For these reasons, they are not the best route to take for the bulk of the work, all things considered. They are best for smaller muscle groups and isolation movements when used sparingly.

Moderate rep ranges (6-15) provide the best of both worlds. They will get you full motor unit recruitment either immediately or early on depending on how heavy you go, are light enough to keep form tight, and generate good amounts of intra-set fatigue from keeping enough tension on the muscle by doing enough repetitions in one set. They're also very efficient for generating productive volume, the biggest driver of hypertrophy. They are useful across the board of exercises and muscle groups.

	PROS	CONS
Heavy (1-5)	Raw strength	Less time efficient Hard on mind/body
Light (15+)	Recovery Type I fibers	Grueling sets Little strength gains
Moderate (6-15)	Effective and accessible Efficient for volume	Not optimal for max strength or endurance adaptations

These conclusions lead us to:

REP RANGE RECOMMENDATIONS

Contrary to anything else out there that claims otherwise, there is no 'perfect' number of reps per set for growth. Instead, we'll be looking at a *range* to draw from and utilize for our artwork [9].

> They say "jack of all trades, master of none", but when it comes to mixing up the specific reps you do, you are master of one: muscle growth.

With that in mind, the majority (~80%+) of your training should be spread across the range of **6-15 repetitions**. The remaining 20% *can be* done in the lower or higher ranges if and when appropriate for the muscle, movement, and trainee.

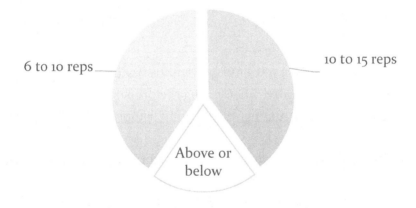

6 to 10 reps

10 to 15 reps

Above or below

These ranges can vary by muscle group and be split up within the workout (heavier first) and/or across workouts and training cycles in a periodized fashion and will depend on the exercise being done and the lifter. Main compounds lend themselves best to 10 and below, and isolations and accessory movements are typically best in the 10-15 rep range.

For example, you could do 6-10 repetitions for one exercise/day and 10-15 for the next. You could do 6-10 for squats and 10+ for lunges since high rep squats are called physical torture. The reps reside on a continuum, so including some lower repetitions and higher repetitions are better than one in isolation. This will also mix in some variety and freshness into the workout routine.

Females tend to do best starting at slightly higher rep ranges (8+). This is for psychological as well as structural reasons.

Ultimately, put most of your effort on the rep range that enables you to perform your best work to carry your volume requirements out sustainably. Within a certain range, there is no need to stress it, and you'll be mixing them up over time to maximize gains.

HOW HARD

So that's how *heavy* you should go, but how hard *with that weight* should you go? As stated when giving the proper rep range, the rep ranges given were assuming sets taken to complete muscle failure.

But going all the way to muscle failure is not necessary for growth, and you absolutely do not want to train to failure all the time if you know what's good for you [10,11,12,13,14]. Why not? Let's see.

THE FEMME FATALE OF FAILURE

Muscle failure is a tricky temptress. She reels you in with sweet songs and offers of amazing gains, but if you're not careful, she'll pull you under like the sirens of the sea and dig her fangs into you that sap your sarcoplasmic soul.

Muscle failure is when you cannot - under any circumstances - complete your current rep or another rep should you so attempt it with clean form and without the use of assistance.

Muscle failure can ensure you maximize your effort in each set, but if you take your sets to failure early or often, you'll be sucked dry of energy and see a huge drop-off in your performance both during the workout and over time that plants the sinister seeds for overtraining and purgatory plateaus. It's very stressful to your body.

This is a terrible idea because it will hurt your ability to perform enough quality work to achieve the volume goals required for optimal growth. You won't be able to lift as heavy afterwards, and your work capacity both in the workout and across the week will take a major blow. Consider going to failure on your first set here:

WEIGHT	REPS (to failure)	REPS (not to failure)
225	10	7
225	7	7
225	5	7
225	3	7
225	2	7
VOLUME LOAD	6075lbs	7875lbs

The effects are diminished with lower volume or Reverse Pyramid, but we must factor in the neural fatigue, workout killmenow factor, and recovery implications.

To top things off, flirting with failure under heavy loads can open up the possibility for injury as you try to grind out reps towards your upper ceiling, and that's not optimal for growth by anyone's standard.

Therefore, we will keep ourselves in check and make sure that we're not overexerting ourselves when we train at our own expense. You absolutely do not need to go all out to have a good workout. Get that out of your head right now.

How will we do this?

REPS IN THE TANK (RITTs)

Using weights at a certain % of your 1RM (1 rep max) can be a good starting point in choosing your weights, but this doesn't necessarily tell the whole story about how hard you're working in every set.

To give you a *better picture* of what's going on, you should set your weights and intensity based on how many repetitions you can perform all out in the set with clean form.

For example, if you know that you can do 10 reps all out to failure on a particular exercise, then you will know what your upper limit is for performing your sets and how to dance around it to set yourself up for optimal growth by only doing 7 or 8 instead.

This is the basis of the RPE (Rate of Perceived Effort) scale and Repetitions in Reserve (RIR), and it's a highly effective way to set your intensity levels in the weight room for optimal performance [15].

For mental simplicity and verbal repetition purposes, I will refer to these as Reps in the Tank (RITTs) moving forward. It's easier to say in practice than the tongue twister of "repetitions in reserve" or growling at people by saying "RIR", and there's no mental math steps involved like in RPE scales where you would have to subtract the RPE from 10 to get the practical number (an RPE of 8 means there's about 2 reps left in your system).

USING RITTS

In the rep range of 6-15, you predominately want to use weights that are heavy enough to put you at roughly 2-3 RITTs for your first set per exercise. By the end of the exercise, you will be at 1 RITT or brushing against muscle failure due to fatigue, depending on your overall total workload for the session. This can vary by person and exercise, but this is an excellent guideline.

Less reps in the tank will break you down over time and must be used wisely – if at all. More RITTs are for warm-ups or deloads.

For example, if you choose 225lbs for a lift and shoot for 3 sets of 8 reps but are hitting muscle failure after the 8th rep, that's 0 RITTs, and you've got to either lower the weight or aim for 6 reps instead (2 RITTs).

Over time, you will develop a 6th sense for how many RITTs you have on your sets. When this happens, you'll be able to auto-regulate your weights by either adding or subtracting weight on the bar to ensure you're staying in the sweet spot that will enable you to sustain your performance required for growth.

Remember that weight is just part of the growth equation, so ensuring you're doing quality work is more important than the number on the bar.

CHOOSING YOUR WEIGHTS

With the knowledge of rep ranges and RITTs, now you can determine which weights to use in your workouts.

Before beginning your workout routine, take the time to test where you are at in terms of your rep maxes for each exercise. If your program calls for 3 sets of 8 repetitions with 3 RITTs, then you will want to do an AMRAP (as many reps as possible) set that will put you at 11 reps all out in clean form. This will give you a good idea of where you should be starting out. The rest of the workout can be completed after this is done using the Reverse Pyramid approach presented in the chapter Making Gains to still get use from the day.

You will run through this with all of your exercises and record them. Over time, your AMRAPs will increase, and that means gains are being made. Achieving aesthetics is all about increasing your work capacity within the designated rep range.

Detailed instructions for finding your working weights can be found in the beginner section of the workout chapter.

What's your max, man?

Lastly, 1RMs (1 Rep Maxes) are an idiotic idea for hypertrophy, so don't do them. Hitting a 1RM is heavily reliant on technique and neural factors, so it is largely irrelevant if size is your goal and isn't worth the effort or risk. Use AMRAPs instead within your working rep range to gauge your progress and set your weights if necessary. If you want to impress people, do it with your physique. Don't be a tool; weights are the tool.

FLIRTING WITH FAILURE

Even though muscle failure is a sexy seductress, we can tame her wisely to harness her abilities for our cause.

In the chapter on how to make progress, you will see that we can go down to lower RITTs with our heavier compound movements by incorporating a Reverse Pyramid style of training and reducing the weight on each set or saving failure for when it won't affect us adversely by putting it at the end of our work sets.

Additionally, muscle failure can be hit on smaller muscle groups with isolation movements because they are safer, less coordinated, and don't sap the body as much as failure would a set of squats, for example.

We can also cheat failure by reaching the point of muscle failure and then incorporating rest pause techniques or drop sets to push past the point of defeat on a set. Let's look at these.

ஜ REST PAUSE

A rest pause is where you reach failure, end your set, rest for a period of a few seconds, and then resume the set by performing a couple more repetitions. This can be performed multiple times until the weight can no longer be done.

For example, you perform 10 reps of curls, rerack the weight and rest for 10 seconds, perform 3 more repetitions, rerack the weight and rest 10 more seconds, perform 2 extra repetitions, and so on.

ぺ DROP SET

A drop set is where you reach failure and then reduce the weight before proceeding to crank out more repetitions. This can then be repeated as you drop weight. It's effective at fully training the muscle [16] but can cause drop-offs in performance and should only be used judiciously.

These techniques are toying with the dark arts and must be used with great care and caution. They are to be executed only sparingly in your training programs and only when you are free from the grasp of the dangers Lady Failure can impose upon you. This primarily occurs at your last sets of an exercise and towards the tail end of the workout and training cycle where a looming workload no longer awaits you.

All in all, failure is just another tool in our tool belt, and it must be used for a purpose.

REST TIMES

As part of Intensity that ties us into volume, we now turn to how much time you should rest in between sets. This isn't doing any work per se, but it *does* impact the work that's done throughout the entire workout.

Shorter rest times might make you feel like you're working harder and getting more out of your workout, but they really only increase your muscular fatigue and *decrease* the weight and amount of work that you can do for *no* additional benefit [17,18,19]. Getting in enough quality volume is key, so this is a bad move to make.

Nevertheless, resting *too long* can drag a workout out, hurt momentum, and disperse all of the fatigue in the muscle that may be desirable both from a growth standpoint and workout enjoyment standpoint (the pump).

Therefore:

> Rest times should be as long as needed to knock out the next set *fully and in proper form* but not any longer.

This usually works out to:

- 6-10 reps: 2-3 minutes
- 10-15 reps+: 1-2 minutes

Don't live and die by these values. They are only there to guide you.

Keep a good eye on the clock during the workout to maintain consistency. This will ensure that your workout variables stay stable and can serve as a good gauge for progress. Record your rest times in your workout log to make sure it's taken into account.

If you must take 4-5 minutes after a set - especially on the most intense and important sets that you want to progress on at the beginning of a workout - then by all means do so.

Quality and progressive overload takes precedence over all.

GET THE MOST FROM YOUR TRAINING

Rest times do not mean idle times. Depending on the exercise, you can incorporate supersets and set fillers to squeeze more out of your gym time and drive up efficiency. It's your hour of power, so maximize your benefit.

SUPERSETS

Supersets are a sure-fire way to build efficiency into a program. They're also a great way to fine tune your posture, generate some cardio benefits, or even hammer out some helpful movement drills instead of floating around like a lost ghost in the gym between sets. They may have actual training benefits as well.

To superset, you simply perform one exercise, regroup for 0-120 seconds, and then perform the second.

The amount of time between your supersets will vary depending on the intensity of the exercise. Compound movements and bigger muscle groups require more, for obvious reasons.

❧ TRADITIONAL SUPERSETS

There are several ways to superset, but the most common is to alternate between antagonist muscle groups. This is incredibly effective and is an efficient way to split muscle groups, enhance performance, and generate some cardio benefit [20,21,22].

EXERCISE 1	EXERCISE 2
Chest	Back
Biceps	Triceps
Lateral Delts	Rear Delts*
Quad Isolation	Hamstring Isolation

not antagonist but still practical

For specialization of body parts, you can team up two completely distant body parts that don't interfere with each other, such as calves with an upper body exercise. There's extremely little overlap, and if the gym set-up works for it, give it a shot to amp up the intensity and efficiency. You may find this helps you set up your workout routine and schedule better.

EXERCISE 1	EXERCISE 2
Upper body	Calves
Glutes	Arms
Arms	Legs

For most workouts, do not incorporate supersets until the main heavy compound work of your workouts has been completed. The sets are more intense, and you want full recovery and focus here.

࿇ SET FILLERS

Set fillers are ways to perform corrective work in between your exercises. Posture and movement quality is very important for great moods, great workouts, and showcasing your physique as it should be [23]. However, this is an area everyone is lacking in these days.

Rather than sitting around on the bench and being an easy target for those more interested in working out their personal problems more than their muscles, you can knock out the following:

- ❧ LIGHT STRETCHING
- ❧ FOAM ROLLING
- ❧ MOBILITY DRILLS
- ❧ CORRECTIVE EXERCISES

For example, you can work on your lackluster hip mobility and leg stretching in between sets of Rows or arm exercises. You can roll out your tight pecs in between sets of squats.

These are individual-dependent, but when chosen correctly, exercise fillers are an awesome addition to any program that will squeeze more effectiveness out of your sacred hour of gym time to fine tune your physique to set you up for more long term success.

EXTRAS

Even without extra physical work in between your sets, put your mind to use by performing visualizations. Burn the image of your goals and motivation within your psyche and pull from it like a sweet well to fire you up and spark life into your training.

If nothing else, pace back and forth the gym like a ravenous tiger in a cage ready to rip apart the next set when that gate opens. Keep up your rhythm. Get that blood flowing. Prepare to kill it.

13

VOLUME

$\mathcal{H}$ OW MUCH WORK at the given intensity is optimal for growth? Volume is, simply put:

WEIGHT x REPS x SETS

And when you put that in play with *full* range of motion and consistent, *effective* exercises*, it is the **biggest driver of muscle growth** there is [1-6]. We've got the weight and reps down with our Intensity, but how many sets should you do to achieve optimal growth?

*you could perform more weight with partial ranges of motion or by using machines (i.e leg press vs. squats), but this does not mean it is better for muscle growth. Nice try. A better measure would be weight x reps x sets x (ROM multiplier) x (proximity to failure multiplier) x (muscle effectiveness factor). We'll keep it simple here.

VOLUME DOSAGE

As cool as that'd be, one set isn't going to cut it if you want to make the best gains. You've got to be able to push the muscle enough to grow the best by giving it enough work to challenge it and force it to adapt by increasing in size.

Yet in the rep range of 6-15 repetitions as recommended in the last chapter with properly set RITTs, you could do a wide range of sets in a workout without getting totally thrashed. How many should you do for optimal, sustainable progress?

5? 10? 100?

We need to tighten up our scope and find the optimal volume.

If you do too little volume, you won't grow well, and the research is crystal clear that adding more and more volume will lead to more and more growth [2,3,4,5].

...but if you do *too much*, it's overkill and you're wasting your time alongside setting yourself up for plateaus, overtraining, injury, and excessively grueling and lengthy workouts for *no extra gains* that will only hurt your recovery and the optimal frequency for growth. In fact, you will see LESS gains from pushing too far [6].

More volume *is* better, but only **up to a point.**

The key to volume lies in finding the sweet spot that marches you to growth in a way that fits snug with your goals and lifestyle.

V O L U M E
B E N E F I T

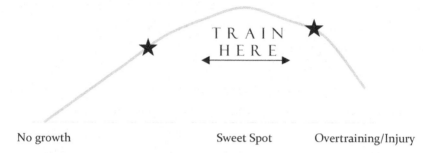

| No growth | Sweet Spot | Overtraining/Injury |

See Chapter on How to Progress. We will use a double progression by increasing weight and reps and then add sets as necessary once enough strength is reached.

As you can see, the growth benefit from extra volume rises steadily, begins to level off, peaks, tapers down, and then drops rapidly as the body can't keep up with the demands and recover. I have placed the range at the points where most of your training should occur.

The first point shows up just before where the benefit begins to level off and diminishing returns appear, and the second point is placed before a rapid drop-off appears. The aim is to be within the middle.

But how do you know where you should be?

Determining your ideal volume can take experience and comes over time, so to give you something to run with, check out the recommendations and continue on to adjusting your volume to find the amount that will suit you best to maximize your progress.

VOLUME RECOMMENDATIONS

As a good *starting point*, aim to perform **8-12 sets per week** per muscle group in the rep range of 6-15 repetitions within 1-3 reps of failure on your sets [3,6]. As you'll see in the next Chapter, the ideal workout frequency is at least 2x/week, so this will put you at ~4-6 sets per workout per muscle group.

A 2007 systematic review [6] analyzing data from several studies on muscle growth of the quads and biceps demonstrated that on average, 4-6 sets per workout per muscle between ~30-60 total repetitions 2-3x/week is the sweet spot for maximizing hypertrophy before seeing a decline in the rate of muscle growth. Later meta-analyses lend support to meeting this amount [3,4].

However, this was based primarily on moderate repetition ranges over periods of time, and in your training, you will be incorporating different ranges for different days and even within the same workout that can provide drastically different rep totals. Therefore:

- ⇘ When working in a moderate to high rep range with mixed sets, stick to **number of sets** for your volume level. The rep totals will vary wildly, but effort and muscle growth won't. (4x8 vs. 4x15, for example).
- ⇘ If incorporating heavier, low rep work, ensure that you stay within the rep total target. This can be as easy as doing your low rep work with a set or two of a higher rep range tacked on for a little extra volume if need be. (4x4 vs. 4x4+2x10)

As weekly volume requirements increase due to either training age or a periodized approach, these per session targets become less important, as you'll be spreading your volume out more strategically throughout the week. More information on this can be found in the chapters of frequency and periodization.

These recommendations are also a nice blend between per session effort, workout scheduling, and exercise variety that I regularly see success with in my own personal and practical experience and in many effective training approaches over the years.

VOLUME PER MUSCLE GROUP

	SETS	REPS
PER WORKOUT	4-6	30-60
PER WEEK (2-3x)	8-12	60-120

SAMPLE WORKOUT FOR A MUSCLE GROUP

	SETS	REPS
EXERCISE A	3	8
EXERCISE B	2	12
TOTAL:	5	48

This volume prescription varies depending on the muscle group [6], training status, nutrition, and your lifestyle factors. If you are sleeping well, eating well, and have a low-stress life, you will recover better and can tolerate more volume [7,8].

If you don't have those factors fine-tuned, you'll need to do less to avoid burnout. Because of this, custom tailoring it to you is a **must.** *Keep reading to see where to set this.*

START LOW AND BUILD

Volume is like a drug. One helluva drug. It follows a *dose-response* relationship, so generally speaking, beginners do better with less volume, and advanced lifters need more to get the same growth response due to their level of adaptation and the effect that any given training stimulus provides. There's a lot of personal variation at play here as well, and different individuals may need more or less than this. Therefore, with these volume recommendations:

Do as little volume as you need to progress and add in more as you become more advanced and stop responding to that stimulus. Start on the low end and work your way up over time.

Start low (4 sets/workout/muscle group 2 times per week). You can always add more in later, and starting low gives a good glimpse as to how receptive you are to that training dosage. It's more dangerous to do too much than too little.

Remember that volume is **Weight x Reps x Sets**, so if you're progressing by increasing the first two and riding the gain train full steam ahead with no bumps to speak of, don't mess with success.

MAXIM OF AESTHETICS: LESS IS MORE. PUSH FORWARD ONLY WHEN THERE IS GROUND TO GAIN.

As you gain experience and learn how you react to training, you can start to increase your total volume through more sets to see how you adapt and establish an 'upper limit' to how much you can tolerate and progress off of. I will go over this in more detail in the chapter on periodization.

REMEMBER THE COMPOUNDS

For smaller muscle groups, compound exercises can eat this number up such that *zero or very minimal training* must be explicitly done for them.

There is overlap with these exercises, so you may only need 1/3-1/2 of those volume requirements for smaller body parts, and that's why compounds are the all-stars. Bench will work triceps and shoulders to some extent, so they need less direct work, for example.

Even then, it's usually just to hit the muscles a bit more directly and effectively than they are utilized in the major movements (overhead triceps extensions to better target the long head of the triceps.)

ADJUSTING THE VOLUME

If you're ambitious and observant, you may be wondering:

If volume is the key, then why shouldn't I just do more? What if I'm not doing enough and not living up to my potential?

And you'd be entirely correct. More volume *is* better, so long as you can recover from it and don't slip into your doom on the other side of the volume curve. So let's look at how to go about fine tuning your volumage.

Once you set your volume and are following the protocol I gave in the section over intensity by keeping your failure in check, test it out and see how you respond over at least 3-4 weeks. Make sure you have your nutrition, life, and recovery on point like I recommend. These things are extremely important or else these questions for adjusting volume won't work the way they're meant to. Once you've got that down, ask yourself:

1. AM I MAKING GAINS?

The entire point behind training is progression towards a concrete goal. As such, your performance should be improving over time and is the most pertinent thing to monitor.

In the chapter Making Gains, you will see that through a double progression scheme, you'll be increasing your reps and weight on the bar over time. In the beginner and intermediate range, you should be improving on your main compound lifts by at least 5lbs every 1-2 weeks or so.

2. HOW DO I FEEL?

Next, you've got to look at the other side of the equation: Recovery. Recovery is more tricky to tackle because it's subjective by nature, so you are the most qualified person to know this. Pay very close attention to how you feel *on all* levels.

How is your mood? How do your joints feel? How do you feel throughout the day? Your body will let you know how hard you are pushing things. Learn to listen to it.

&ᴏ FEELING GOOD

If you're feeling fresh and good to go, then add in an extra set per workout (2 per week), and then go from there to repeat the process.

&ralig; FEELING BANGED UP

If you're feeling like the workouts are too much to handle and you're getting worn out, then you may be pushing it too much. Deload and subtract 1 set per workout (2 per week) and repeat the process again. You should always feel like you have more sets in the tank per workout and throughout the week.

By doing this over time, you will get a better feel over time for how you respond to certain volumes of training. This will allow you to set different thresholds for your workouts as you learn how your muscles respond to various volumes.

IMPLICATIONS

As you can see, these volume recommendations are far away from the popular 30 set marathon workouts posted up all over the place, but trust me, if you're *actually* working hard in the weight room, you're right where you need to be and will be making gains all over the place.

Because of this relatively low volume compared to most popular programs, you can easily team this up with multiple body parts in one day to be more efficient and allow for more days off and enjoyment of your life outside the gym. You will see training set-ups in more detail later on.

Lastly, these volume recommendations are for *optimal* progress, so if you don't want to grow a particular muscle group to its full potential, stay on the low end. This is key for maintaining proportion and optimizing overall outcomes.

14

FREQUENCY

HOW OFTEN ARE YOU HITTING IT IN THE GYM? Frequency deals with the number of times that you're hitting a muscle group per week, and it also has to do with how often you're in the gym overall.

Let's take a look at what goes into this.

GROWTH AND RECOVERY

After you train the targeted muscle group, the body is thrust into motion to recover, grow, and get stronger. It's soaking up nutrients, churning its molecular machinery, and doing what it does best - ADAPT.

But is this a stairway into infinity?

No. The muscle will fully recover within 24-72 hours [1,2,3,4] and be ready and stronger than ever to handle a new challenge assuming your nutrition and recovery are on point – which they will be if you're reading this book and putting it in practice.

Your muscles won't vanish into thin air by waiting around a week to train them again, but by waiting so long between workouts, you are missing out on your opportunity for extra growth. Research consistently demonstrates the superiority of more frequent sessions *even when total volume is the same* [5,6,7].

In other words, 10 sets on one day is not as good as 5 on two days. However, 3 may not be better than 2, so focus on getting your weekly volume in and only split it up over more days if you need to.

GROWTH FROM ONE WORKOUT VS. TWO PER WEEK

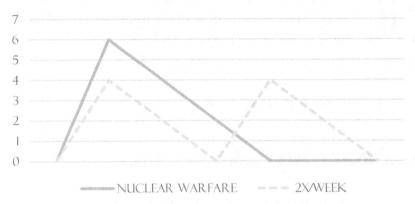

To illustrate a point only.

Blitzing, blasting, and bombarding muscles once a week is not as effective a strategy as splitting the volume up. You're doing more work with more effort for less payoff. Sound good to you?

Take home point: *Work each muscle group more than 1x/week*

SKILLS THAT KILL

Lifting weights takes *skills*. It's a synchronization of mental processes, muscle movements, coordination, and breathing, all of which contribute to that intense concentration and state of *flow* - that dream-like state where you're on top of the world and time comes to a standstill as you get lost in the moment. That's the euphoria that a great workout can achieve.

To develop a skill, frequent exposure delivers the goods. Think of it like digging a hole. If you dig a little bit infrequently, it'll fill right back up by the next time you dig. You've got to dig often enough. Then someday you'll hit gold.

By training more frequently, you will refine your form, technique, and comfort with the lift. The exercises will become like second nature, and this will make you stronger and better at them that will translate into more gains on your frame.

This is also why switching exercises all over the place to chase 'muscle confusion' is a horrendous idea. You're spread too thin and can never master any of them.

Build your physique off of a handful of solid exercises and leave the variety for your workout playlist.

VOLUME SPLIT

Total volume is another factor to take into account when calculating frequency. How should you split it up to make it most manageable and high quality based on your schedule?

Additionally, the volume recommendations in the previous chapter were *starting points*, but as you get more advanced, more volume dosage becomes necessary to get results.

Because of this, splitting the volume from 2 into 3 weekly sessions can be a solid idea to avoid cramming it all into 2 days and the fatiguing physical and mental aspect to training this can generate. You can only do so much in one day before you burn out or start just going through the motions.

DAY	SETS 2DAY/WK	SETS 3 DAY/WK
Monday	10	7
Tuesday	-	-
Wednesday	-	6
Thursday	-	-
Friday	10	7
Saturday	-	-
Sunday	-	-
TOTALS:	20 sets	20 sets

Furthermore, these sessions can be periodized with heavy/light or heavy/light/medium days to alter the intensities and allow for better performance and training variety.

For most, 2-3 sessions per muscle group per week is best, and splitting is not practical until you start going over 7-8 sets/session.

SYSTEM WIDE AFFAIR

The above points are speaking very highly of a higher frequency, but there's one final thing to make note of when it comes to training frequency:

Our *muscles* will recover in just a couple of days, but lifting weights is a *full-body* affair.

You've got to look out for your joints and nervous system to ensure you stay strong and healthy all around because the muscle itself isn't the only factor involved in pushing those weights.

The total recovery ability of the whole body is less than the total recovery ability of the sum of all the muscle groups.

You can hit every muscle group hard *on their own*, but you can't hit *everything* hard day in and day out across the board. Think back to the analogy of marbles I gave in an earlier chapter. You only have so much to go around.

RECOVERY CAPACITY

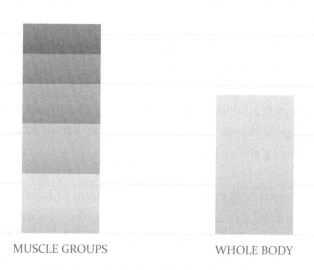

MUSCLE GROUPS   WHOLE BODY

Assuming optimal volume; for sake of example only

There is also tremendous overlap across the body, and body parts used in one exercise on one day will still be in use for completely different ones on the next. The core, shoulders, knees, elbows, and grip are heavily involved across the board. This can be reduced through proper exercise selection and scheduling, but the principle remains:

> Let some daylight shine through your workout schedule and include some off days in the workout week to allow for more recovery and lifestyle.

FREQUENCY RECOMMENDATION

Given all of those factors, for optimal growth you should be splitting your training volume for each muscle group into 2-3 sessions/week on average.

Larger muscles should be hit less frequently to factor in the higher workload to the system and smaller *can be* hit more frequently. For some with recovery/joint constraints, once every 5th day may be more favorable to allow for extra recovery.

Females can potentially do better off of 3x per body part per week for optimal gains due to physiological reasons related to their quicker recovery ability [6,8,9,10].

Beginners should perform each main movement at least 2x/week because they need the extra exposure time in the weight room to dial in their exercise patterns and set the foundations for their training as they get more advanced.

LOW TO HIGH

Just like with volume, start on the low end and work your way up. Even with equated volume, your body needs time to adjust to a higher frequency. If you jump up too fast, you'll start hearing from your joints in no time.

Therefore, my practical recommendation is to start at 2x/week per muscle group and only break your volume into thirds once your volume requirements get so large that doing it all in 2 sessions would be over-fatiguing and less quality (around 7-8 sets per session).

NO DAYS OFF?

No matter what you do, make sure that you take at least 2 days off per week in your lifting schedule to allow for full recovery across the body, preferably mixed into your week and not back to back.

This will keep your mental zest for the gym up as well. 3-5 total workouts per calendar week is best for most people to make consistent progress while enjoying the process.

Absence makes the heart grow fonder, and this will ensure you're always coming back stronger.

SUMMARY OF TRAINING PRINCIPLES

- Muscle growth is specific from other weight lifting goals and dependent upon several factors.
- Progressive overload across the factors of growth (leading ultimately to increases in working weight) is the key to improvement towards our goals
- Different rep ranges offer different degrees of benefits across a strength/endurance spectrum
- Failure is to be used wisely. Never as an ego boost
- Training must always consider factors outside of the gym to provide consistency and enjoyment in life.

OPTIMAL GROWTH GUIDELINES

FACTOR	RECOMMENDATION	NOTES
INTENSITY	6-15RM split up for 80% of the work	Within 1-3 reps of failure
REST TIMES	As much as necessary to perform next set(s) Usually 2-3 min.	Heavier and/or compounds longer, lighter and/or isolations shorter
VOLUME	8-12 weekly sets = ~4-6 sets/ ~30-60 reps per muscle per session	Starting point - start low Consider overlap
FREQUENCY	2-3x/7-10 days per muscle group !Factor in total volume!	Depends on lifter, status, and overall training volume for the muscle Consider overlap/full recovery

15

EXERCISE
SELECTION

E'VE JUST ESTABLISHED WHAT IS NECESSARY to grow: Intensity, volume, and the frequency thereof. The exercises you perform under progressive loading are *the tools* in your kit to carry out those principles and achieve your goal of muscle size to create an aesthetic physique. So when it comes to exercise selection, you've got to pick the right tools for the job based on where you want to sculpt your statue.

Certain exercises may look cool or be useful for increasing performance in specific sports, but the gym isn't a playground, so before dabbling in the voodoo you need to ask yourself if they truly even do something for **your** goals.

You have to be specific towards your goal of muscle growth.

HOW TO CHOOSE AN EXERCISE

For any given exercise you want to add to your arsenal, ask yourself:

1. CAN YOU DO IT SAFELY?

You can have the greatest exercise in the world, but if it isn't safe for you to perform at your fullest potential, then you need to find something else.

Lifting weights is a *long-term process*, and **no** gains are worth acute or chronic injury on your body. It's all about making progress *and sustaining* those results.

If a spotter is necessary and you don't have access to one, then you will need to find a work around. Either do them in a power rack with properly set safety bars or find an alternative exercise that still targets the muscle effectively.

2. DOES IT WORK FOR YOUR BODY?

We've all got our own unique architecture and battle scars, so some exercises just plain tend to work better for some than others. You can't fit a square peg into a round hole, and a cookie cutter approach is never a good idea for *anyone* when it comes to training and nutrition.

A wrong selection here can lead to injury issues and lackluster gains in the gym. If you have excellent form and can't seem to make an exercise work, go for another. Not everyone is built to back squat or overhead press.

3. IS IT MOST EFFECTIVE FOR THE MUSCLE YOU'RE TARGETING?

People often choose their exercises based on how heavy they can go, how alpha they look, or what they've simply been taught to believe is good. This is bad.

The whole point of the exercise for hypertrophy is to *effectively target the specific muscle(s)* that you want to grow. If they're not doing a good job at that, they're fired. The exercise needs to be able to...

1. Stimulate as many fibers of the targeted muscle(s) as possible
2. ...with as much weight as possible
3. ...through as large of a safe range of motion as possible

...within the rep ranges that have been designated. That'll lead to your best growth.

In line with this, stay away from exercises that prevent you from accomplishing those 3 things as effectively as possible.

In other words, you must make sure that the *muscle* gives out before anything else causes you to end your set early or reduce the effectiveness of the exercise. Here are common examples of exercise blockers and their solutions:

LIMITATION	SOLUTION
Grip strength	Straps, chalk, gloves
Core Strength	Seated or supported variation
Balance	Bilateral Variation

In most cases such as squats or rows, these will resolve themselves as you grow and adapt to the training, but if they don't, you must either find a way around it or choose different exercises that enable you to get a better training effect.

4. IS IT EFFICIENT?

Your exercises must not only be effective; they must be *efficient*. This means that they must:

- MAXIMIZE BENEFIT
- ELIMINATE OR REDUCE WASTE

As you'll see, compound movements kill many birds with one stone and increase workout efficiency monumentally. For the price in time and effort of one exercise, you've effectively targeted *multiple*.

On the other hand, you also want to eliminate waste from your exercises by kicking out intruding muscle groups that aren't doing anything towards the growth you want and interfere in other areas or overall recovery. Remember: the body only has so much capacity to go around.

For example, heavy conventional deadlifts are a great exercise that'll build your glutes and hamstrings, but because they incorporate all sorts of other muscle groups that generate fatigue and throttle the system, don't work them through a full ROM, and don't have a nice eccentric portion (lowering the weight), they're typically a *bad* choice for a hypertrophy program when you're really pushing the envelope for optimal growth across all areas.

Additionally, most dumbbell movements involve a lot of extracurricular activity in setting up and getting into position for your sets that can wear you out and limit your true potential on an exercise, so unless you're the Napoleon of the gym and have your peons fetch your weights for you, you have to factor this in.

Bent over rows incorporate a lot of core and lower back. And so on. You don't have to kick 'em out completely, be but cognizant of them and determine your tradeoffs. Find workarounds if necessary. Do them for lighter sets, get a chest-support, etc.

5. CAN YOU LOAD IT PROGRESSIVELY?

Progressive overload is the key to gaining muscle mass, so whichever exercise you choose needs to lend itself to progression or you aren't going anywhere.

You can find an exercise that'll give you a sick pump 6 ways 'til Sunday, but if you can't load it up in small, precise increments over time, it's a poor choice that's got to go. Remember the maxim:

MAXIM OF AESTHETICS: YOU MUST BE ABLE TO SATISFACTORILY JUSTIFY EVERYTHING IN YOUR WORKOUT, DIET PROGRAM, AND LIFE.

With that in mind, let's look at exercise types and how they're done to pick the tools that you'll be using to sculpt your physique.

COMPOUND LIFTS

Compound exercises are multi-joint movements that work several muscle groups at the same time. They'll be your main money makers over the course of your lifting career that'll slap the most size on your frame.

With compound lifts you will:

- Generate maximum strength and power to target the muscles being worked
- Optimize efficiency by simultaneously working multiple muscle groups effectively
- Define a firm standard with which you can progressively overload over time
- Assist in joint integrity by distributing the load across several structures

You can get a full body workout and build an impressive physique with compound lifts alone [1,2]. With a couple of specific isolation lifts to follow up and fill in the gaps, you're good.

EXAMPLES OF COMPOUND LIFTS

LEGS/GLUTES	CHEST/SHOULDERS/TRICEPS	BACK/REAR DELTS/BIS
Squat Variations Deadlift Variations* Lunges	Bench Press Dumbbell Press Machine Press Pushup variations	Rows Pullups Pulldowns

*we will do **Romanian** deadlifts, a single joint movement that still hits multiple muscles effectively*

SINGLE-JOINT/ISOLATION LIFTS

Isolation exercises are single joint exercises that isolate one muscle group explicitly at a time and are better suited higher rep ranges than traditional compound work (8-10+) because the load isn't as evenly distributed across the body.

They aren't as efficient for a complete workout (why do 3 isolations when you can do 1 compound), but they definitely have their uses, so let's look at them and determine how they'll be implemented.

FILL IN THE GAPS

Compound lifts will work most of the major muscles of the body, but you can still choose to concentrate a bit further on particular muscles that aren't hit evenly enough or adequately with the compound movement.

For example:

- If you do your rows with an overhand grip, then a set of underhand curls can help to round out your biceps training.
- Bench presses work the triceps, but the long head of the triceps is optimally worked in overhead positions.
- Bench press also works the shoulder, but the anterior portions gets the bulk of the work, and the lateral deltoids are not as effectively worked in this movement

*Caveat: If you include different grips in your workouts, then you may need **zero** additional direct work.*

SINGLE OUT

You may also choose to single out a certain muscle without involving others that get worked in a compound movement.

-   If you want to do more chest work but don't want to fry your triceps and delts, you can throw in some chest flyes to work the pecs without involving the other muscle groups.
-   Hip thrusts are the best glute exercise you could possibly do, and they do a great job at hammering the glutes without the extra stress placed on the rest of the legs and body.

SPECIALIZE

Once you've built a strong base and are getting more advanced, isolations are a good choice to specialize for any lagging body parts.

For example, if you are pleased with your back development but need more size on your biceps to become more proportional, you should hit your biceps on their own outside of any back work with isolation movements so that they can get full direct stimulation without any fatigue from back exercises interfering with your performance.

You'll learn more about this later in the book when we go over specialization.

SUPERSET THEM

Isolations are the exercises that lend best to supersets and dropsets, should they be incorporated.

They are not as draining on the body, and most isolation work is done towards the tail end of a workout with higher repetitions, so switching back and forth without compromising performance is no problem and can generate a pleasureful pump, non-harmful intensity, and a bit of cardio benefit that can enhance the workout experience with little drawback.

LESS IS MORE

Don't fall into the trap of adding tremendous amounts of isolation work on top of the compound lifts. The reason you do compounds in the first place is for their ability to hit multiple muscles effectively at the same time [1,2].

Isolation work is the icing on the cake, not the cake itself.

Besides female glute work and the calves who aren't trained much at all through other exercises, 1-3 sets at most is more than adequate for most muscle groups, if even needed at all.

Build up the basics. Outside of specialization, only 20-30% max of your exercises for a muscle group should be isolations.

FAVORITE ISOLATIONS:

- Tricep extensions (particularly overhead)
- Bicep Curls
- Calf raises: Bent-knee and straight leg
- Lateral Raises
- Rear Delt Flyes
- Hip thrusts

EXERCISE ADJUSTMENTS

Once you understand compounds and isolations, now you can look
at different adjustments to the way that they're performed.

The body moves in space across several different angles from
several different positions, so by making adjustments here, you will
target different areas of the muscles to different degrees. For
aesthetics, the goal is a *well-rounded physique*, so by providing
variety to the movements, you will ensure maximal development all
around [3,4]. Additionally, modifications to the movements can
help to work around problem areas and individual differences in
biomechanics to get the most from training.

ANGLES AND PLANES

Changing the angle and plane of motion that you subject the
muscle to under load will change the area of the muscle(s) being
worked. For example:

- Incline bench will work the clavicular head of the pecs more
  than flat bench.
- Pull-ups and pulldowns will put the lats in a vertical line of
  pull whereas rows will target them horizontally
- Front, angled, and side lunges will all target the legs, quads,
  and glutes differently
- The deltoids have 3 heads that are best stimulated in front,
  side, or rear variations of motion

For this reason, incorporating some variety into the exercises that
you choose to train the muscle groups will ensure that the entire
muscle is being worked effectively.

UNILATERAL AND BILATERAL

Before you get intimidated by the unusual words, unilateral means that each side is working *independently* to move the weight, and bilateral means that both sides are *working together* to move it. Each has their pros and cons:

> ❧ UNILATERAL

By going unilateral, you will be incorporating more stability into the movement, ironing out side imbalances, and offering variety and a change of pace to your training.

Additionally, for certain movements, going unilateral means less overall load on your frame and better effective range of motion. For example, lunges or split squats will reduce the loads on the spine, and dumbbell bench will allow you more freedom and depth.

> ❧ BILATERAL

Bilateral movements will enable you to generate more force because the load is distributed evenly, and the muscle group doesn't have to worry about balance or stability as much as when it's working in isolation. This makes it a good choice for your main lifts to progress.

STANCES AND GRIPS

The stances and grips that you use to perform the movement will affect the results of the exercise. This refers to the way that you place your hands and feet.

◈ MOVEMENT QUALITY

Adjusting your stance or grip can help you to perform the exercise better. For example, some people can get into a better squat to target their legs by adopting a wider stance, and others with shoulder problems can get more out of their bench work by using methods with a neutral grip or more from their lateral raises by gripping the dumbbells with their thumbs turned slightly upwards to externally rotate the shoulder better and allow for more space under the acromion.

◈ MOVEMENT EFFECTIVENESS

Secondly, different stances and grips will target the muscle in varying ways. For example, varying them will alter the arm muscles, lower body muscles, and even the emphasis on calf exercises by altering the positioning of the feet [5].

TAKE HOME POINTS

1. Incorporate movements that target the muscle in different angles and planes
2. Incorporate both unilateral and bilateral variations to exercises
3. Alter your stance and grips to allow you to perform the exercises safely and effectively and target the muscle fully and preferentially.

EXERCISE VARIATIONS

With the loading parameters defined, now we will we look at the various ways to use the equipment on hand in the gym to perform them optimally.

BARBELLS

With barbells, both sides of your body will work in unison (bilateral) since the bar will spread the weight distribution evenly. This will allow you to generate a lot of force and really load up the targeted muscles to do a lot of good, quality work to spur growth.

Barbell exercises are great for compound movements, and as I mentioned before, this will work several muscles at the same time, so you get more bang for your buck per exercise.

Because of these factors, compound exercises on barbells will be the traditional starting point and mainstay for every workout and program.

❧ RESTRICTIONS

For certain individuals, barbells can be a problem due to movement restrictions. Barbell bench and back squats can irritate the shoulder, for example. Other options will need to be considered if barbells prevent you from training safely and effectively.

DUMBBELLS

Dumbbells have the benefit of providing extra range of motion across a wider area of movement. Barbells can be limiting in this regard, and those with any movement restrictions or joint issues may find that dumbbells are a better option for performing the exercises.

Dumbbells also have the effect of forcing each muscle group to work by itself without the assistance of the other side to provide balance across the weight.

This will work the supporting musculature much more and ensure that the strong side isn't taking over as can be the case for barbell movements where the load is evenly distributed on the bar. Symmetry is a very important issue when it comes to developing the body aesthetically.

For bench press variations, dumbbells can be a good option for those who don't have access to a spotter while lifting, and for those with shoulder or back issues, dumbbell split squats can be performed to work the legs effectively without the loading on the shoulder joint.

NOTES:

When using dumbbells, it's important to note that the amount of weight you can do compared to the barbell will be lower because you are handling each side of the body independently and must work harder to set up/stabilize to perform the exercise.

And because dumbbells generally jump in increments of 5, the total load will move in increments of 10, so the progression scheme will be different than that of a barbell where you can slap on 2.5lb plates to steadily add progressive overload. In a double progression scheme that I discussed earlier, rather than adding 2 repetitions before adding weight, you will need to add 4.

For heavy sets, dumbbells can become a nuisance and wear you down. Having to go to the rack and pull off 100lb dumbbells and bring them back to the bench is not the same as loading a barbell up. Having to go through this entire process as you warm up is inefficient and a lot of extra work for heavy dumbbells. They are best suited for the lighter sets or having a training partner split the set-up with you.

MACHINES

Machines get a bad rap despite making life easy all over the place, but they, too, can have their place in a properly structured workout. Nothing is bad per se; only the use thereof. For sake of discussion, when I refer to machines, I am not including cable movements and movements such as pulldowns or pull throughs that use a machine, but rather fixed movement patterns.

Machines take away much of the pressure away from supporting musculature and can allow you to focus exclusively on the muscles you are aiming to work. Spotting is also typically not necessary on these, so you can flirt with failure more worry-free.

On top of that, because many machines are loaded up by simply inserting a pin into the rack, you can get to work quickly without having to fiddle with weight plates. This has important implications for supersets, drop sets, time-saving techniques, and so forth.

Because of these considerations, they are more useful for those with certain movement restrictions or for the lighter work when supporting muscles may be fatigued but we still want to target the main muscles effectively and safely.

One of the potential downsides of the machine is that it creates a fixed plane of motion, so always ensure that the machine and seat settings are set to where you can perform the movement optimally, making notes in your training log if necessary so that you can have the same conditions every time.

CABLES

Cables provide tension across the entire movement for the positive and negative part of the lift and allow free range of motion. They require coordination but are very effective at isolating the muscles.

You can attach several different attachments to cables and fix them at many different angles and planes of motion, so they are very versatile and useful at hitting the muscles in unique ways that other exercise variations can't do. Because cables are loaded with a pin in a rack, like machines, they can be great when doing supersets, drop sets, and the like.

Besides pulldowns, they're typically not the best for heavier movements, but cables can provide variety and an excellent training effect for triceps extensions, curls, lateral/rear delt raises, chest flys, glute pull throughs, glute kickbacks, and many other potent exercises in your arsenal.

EXERCISE ORDERING

When designing your workout programs, you have to take into account the order that you do your exercises in. To do that, follow these simple rules:

RULES OF EXERCISE ORDER

1. PRIORITIES FIRST

You are going to be your freshest at the beginning of a workout, so the muscle groups that you want to focus on need to be done at the beginning. If not, you will not be able to target them as effectively in a fatigued state. Growth is better if you prioritize [6,7].

2. LIMITERS FIRST

Any exercise that could limit exercise effectiveness or safety of any exercises that come after it need to be done beforehand.

This means that isolations come after compounds with the same muscle groups, you go heavy before you go light, and you do your free weight movements before machines.

SPLIT

If you are unable to do this in the same workout, then you will need to organize your workout split accordingly. You will see this in the workout section.

PRACTICAL RECOMMENDATIONS

Your main exercises should come from primarily compound bilateral barbell movements with other variations mixed in to round out the training and target the musculature effectively.

Compounds should be done before single-joints/isolations unless there is a specific specialization reason for advanced trainees and it doesn't interfere with performance or safety *(see workout routine chapter)* [6,7].

Machines and cables should only be utilized for secondary or isolation exercises unless there is an injury or physical constraint present that makes traditional free weight movements a less favorable idea.

By doing this, you'll be accomplishing all of the training goals efficiently and effectively and setting yourself up for the best short and long-term progress that you can.

VARIATION

I know you'd like to bundle up all of the exercises and work them into your workout, but you only have so much workout capacity, and spreading yourself so thin on all of them will make it difficult to master them to move the best poundages you can.

Therefore, pick a core of 2-3 exercise configurations per muscle group to incorporate into your training and use the techniques given in the chapter on Periodization to rotate them in and out of your training to take advantage of the full effect of variation.

LOWER BODY EXERCISES

MAJOR EXERCISE	ASSISTANCE/ISOLATION

QUADS

Squat variations	Lunge variations
Leg press	Leg extensions

HAMSTRINGS

Romanian deadlifts	Leg curls
	Cable pull-throughs

GLUTES

Hip thrusts	
Squat variations	Cable pull-throughs
Romanian deadlifts	Glute kickbacks
Lunges	Hip abductions

CALVES

Straight leg calf raises	
Seated bent-knee calf raises	Genetics

On this and the next page, you will see the exercises that I recommend for building a well-rounded physique to target all of the musculature based on the considerations that we've just discussed.

The major exercise is the exercise that will give you the most bang for your buck, and the assistance/isolation exercise is the exercise that will fill in the gaps to get you the well-rounded training effect.

If there are more than 1 major exercise listed, both can be done in the same workout, and the second can function as an assistance movement if desired. Explanations of the main exercises can be found in the next chapter.

UPPER BODY EXERCISES

MAJOR EXERCISE	ASSISTANCE/ISOLATION
CHEST	
Bench press variations	Incline movement Chest Fly
LATS	
Row variations Pulldowns Pullups	Straight arm pulldowns
BICEPS	
Curl variations	
TRICEPS	
Overhead Tricep Extensions Press-downs/Tricep Dips	
LATERAL DELTS	
Lateral Raises Overhead press*	
REAR DELTS	
Rear delt fly Face pulls	
TRAPS	
Shrugs (upper traps) Rows (mid/lower)	Isometric contractions for all handheld exercises (upper)
ABS	
Body fat levels	All standing exercises**

if biomechanically agreeable for the trainee
***You can train abs, but with the rest of these exercises, you won't notice much of a difference*

16

EXERCISE ALL-
STARS

HERE'S A PLETHORA OF EXERCISES to choose from out there. Some are great. Most are a waste of time. Here, we will run down the crème de la crème for building a world-class physique based on all the factors that go into aesthetics and selecting exercises that we've discussed thus far.

I'll tell you what they are and how to do them the right way, and these exercises are the ones that you'll see in the workout programs that follow.

Right here are the battle-tested basics. Get to know them well. They'll serve you loyally and get you mountains of gains for as long as you may lift.

SQUAT

Once upon a time, a young lifter asked the gym guru which exercise he needed to perform to maximize his lower body development. What do you think he responded? If you answered with anything other than squats, you need to go find yourself.

Squats are a fantastic lower body builder. They'll stack superb size on your quads and glutes and even contribute to building a stronger core and lower back.

HOW TO SQUAT

1. Out of a power rack, place yourself under the middle of the bar so that the bar rests snugly on the top of your traps. Grab the bar slightly further than shoulder width but not too wide. Most bars will have markers for this. This is high bar style and best for hypertrophy. Low bar squatting is more for powerlifting style squats. Squats can really dig into your upper back when things get heavy, so either wear a shirt that covers the area or for ladies, consider using a towel or pad to avoid the bar from roughing up your back as you build up your lower body.
2. Unrack the weight and walk back with the bar to provide enough space to perform the movement. No more than 4 steps, and no twinkle toes.
3. Brace your core and slowly lower the weight down as you squat into a nice, deep position. It is okay to go past knee level. Keep your entire back from your head to your glutes in a nice, neutral straight line.

4. Pause briefly at the bottom of the hole and then explode up by contracting your leg muscles until you are back in the top position

5. Take a breath, reset, and repeat until the indicated number of repetitions are done.

For all squatting besides split squats with dumbbells, either find a trusted spotter or perform them in a power rack with safety bars that are set in a position that will catch the weight in case there are any issues in completing the set. Know your limits.

Squats are best from 6-12 repetitions. Any more is very hard on the body and can become a big cardio drain that'll sabotage your workout.

FRONT/SPLIT SQUATS

Front squats and split squats are other excellent squatting options - especially for those with movement restrictions, shoulder problems, or lower back issues.

As you get more advanced, these can be done switched in and out over days or workout cycles to offer variety on different rep days.

ROMANIAN DEADLIFTS

I don't know if Dracula was jacked or had a Transylvanian training center, but Romanian deadlifts (RDLs) are hands down one of the absolute best exercises around that you can do for your glutes and hamstrings and work seamlessly into your program.

Regular deadlifts can be a grenade in a workout program because they involve so many large muscle groups and take a ton out of you when you start to push things heavier as you get more advanced.

This can throw a lot of other things out of whack across a workout week and adds in a lot of unnecessary fatigue that's better spent elsewhere. They are also only heavily focused on the concentric portion of the lift and miss out on the muscle building benefits of the eccentric portion.

Romanian deadlifts, on the other hand, offer much of the same benefits of regular deadlifts while working through both the concentric and eccentric portions and can allow you to use less weight and still get a solid training effect. They're excellent after your sets of squats that work the quads a bit more preferentially.

Holding the bar will also contribute to forearm strength and build the upper traps to resist the downward pull of the bar on the shoulder blades. And to top it all off, Romanian deadlifts are excellent for posture by training you to keep your chin tucked, weight on your heels, and building up the glutes that are too often weak and inhibited by tight hip flexors.

NOTE: Romanian deadlifts are not the same as Stiff-legged deadlifts (SLDLs). Do not do stiff legged deadlifts. The spine is rounded at the bottom position, and that's a great way to take a trip to Snap City when you're pushing an appreciable amount of weight. They're not worth the extra risk when Romanians get the job done like a pro.

HOW TO PERFORM THE ROMANIAN DEADLIFT:

1. Start from a locked-out deadlift position with the feet shoulder width apart.
2. Slowly lower the weight down with the bar grazing the front of your body. Your knees should be slightly bending as you descend, and the entire back should be in a nice, neutral position from top to bottom. No curved backs allowed. Keep your chin tucked and resist the urge to look up into the mirror with your head. Eyes only.
3. Once the weight is at about knee level or slightly below depending on your flexibility, pause and feel the stretch generated in your hamstrings. Do not let your back go to parallel. Keep it slightly angled upwards.
4. Contract the hamstrings and glutes by driving through the floor and power the weight back up to the starting position with a strong glute squeeze at the top of the lift. Do not go into lumbar hyperextension here.
5. Repeat until all of the indicated repetitions are completed.

Dumbbells can be used and even implemented for single-leg varieties, but barbells are the better option overall for loading and progressing the exercise for heavy work.

Many women prefer the dumbbell options to avoid scraping up their shins, and as long as the exercise is overloading and providing stimulus, there is nothing wrong with this, but long socks/leggings can just as easily be used to get around this and move maximum weight to build the glutes and hams.

Romanian deadlifts are better suited for 8 repetitions and up. Going heavy is harder to maintain good form and grip, and higher repetitions here allows for a better exercise groove and rhythm for maximum stimulation of the targeted muscles. Straps and chalk can be used to get more out of the exercise when grip starts to fail. Grip should never be the limiting factor for targeting the muscle appropriately.

HIP THRUSTS

If you want to maximize your glute development, look no further than the hip thrust. This a fantastic exercise for loading the glutes through a good range of motion. Many compound leg movements incorporate the glutes, but none are as effective as the hip thrust for maximal glute development. You're doing yourself a disservice if you don't work them in.

Glutes are a fundamental component of any aesthetic physique, especially for women. They anchor the body's midsection and are a powerful muscle group that is too often lazy and underdeveloped. Not anymore.

HOW TO PERFORM A HIP THRUST:

1. Sit on the floor with your upper back on the edge of a padded bench that isn't too high. Roll a barbell with bumper plates or 45s right above your waist. This is to ensure it can clear your legs and sit at the right height. Put a pad or towel here on the barbell to avoid it digging in and being uncomfortable.

2. Contract the glutes and bring the weight up to get into the starting position. Your shins should be perpendicular to the floor, and your back should be on the bench just below the shoulder blades. Your gaze should be at a point in front and slightly above you. Watch your neck posture.

3. Let your hips sink down with the weight to generate a great stretch on the glutes. Do not let your lower back round here, and be careful not to let your upper back slip and slide on the bench.

4. Forcefully contract the glutes to get back up into the top position like you're trying to shoot the bar all the way to Jupiter. Ensure a full lock out and squeeze at the top. Do not hyperextend the back.

5. Slowly lower the weight and repeat for the indicated number of repetitions.

You can place resistance bands at the knee and thighs to increase activation of the glutes. Hip thrusts are best from 8 repetitions upwards.

CALF RAISES

No physique is complete without a fine pair of diamond calves. They're far too often neglected, but they're a key area to balance the body visually in space, and if you don't build them up, you won't have that pristine physique you're looking for.

For guys, they'll make the body pop more in shorts and joggers, and for girls, it'll do the same in shorts, leggings, skirts, and dresses. They'll also give you a nicer set of legs in heels and avoid the stringy stiletto-induced look.

STRAIGHT AND BENT

Calf raises come in two varieties: Straight leg and bent-knee. Each one targets the calves, but they do so in different ways. Straight leg works the gastrocnemius and soleus, but bent-knee is more effective at isolating the soleus by putting the gastroc in a hampered position.

Do both to get the best pair of calves you can. You will see this expressed in the workouts I provide in the book.

You can perform the straight leg on a standing calf machine (preferred), a leg press, or holding dumbbells/barbells. Seated variations are done in a seated calf machine, but if there are none, a barbell or dumbbells supported over the knees can work. Consider a towel or pad underneath to avoid discomfort.

HOW TO DO CALF RAISES:

1. Start in a neutral position with your heels hanging slightly below level for a bit of a stretch on the calves
2. Push off from the balls of your feet by contracting the calves upwards until you are up on your tippy toes. Do not use your arms or shoulders to jerk the weight up. Let your calves get that work in.
3. Pause at the top and then slowly lower the weight back down to the starting position
4. Pause at the bottom and repeat for the indicated number of repetitions.

It is vital that you pause at the bottom of the calf exercises for a nice stretch. Bouncing the weight is highly ineffective on calves.

They're built to bounce and walk around all day efficiently, so you must make them work.

If you do them both in the same work out, start with the straight leg variation for sets of 6-10 repetitions and follow that up with a bent-knee variation for 10+ repetitions.

BENCH PRESS

The bench press is excellent at building total chest size and thickness alongside the shoulders and triceps, the biggest muscles of the arm that give you that full look.

HOW TO BENCH:

1. To bench, lay back on the bench so that your eyes are a couple of inches short from the middle of the bar.
2. Squeeze your shoulder blades back and down like you are trying to crush a penny into smithereens with your scapulae, and ensure that you brace your glutes and core and keep your feet firmly on the ground. This will ensure that you have a proper base of strength to push off from.
3. To perform your repetitions, grab the bar at roughly shoulder width. Don't go too wide. This will disrupt the proper form of the lift and piss off your shoulder.
4. Unrack the weight and position the bar above your chest. It's best to have a spotter hand off the bar to you so that you don't lose your tight base.
5. Lower the bar all the way down to your chest in a controlled fashion with your elbows tucked and not flared. Elbows flared will grind down your shoulders and lead to issues and

isn't best for maximum strength or muscle stimulation. Seek for a 45 degree angle instead.

6. After a light pause when the bar touches your chest, explode up by contracting your chest muscles and extending your arms to finish the lift. During this motion, don't let your shoulder blades unhinge. Keep them tucked and tight.

7. After each rep, pause, breathe, and remember to maintain your firm base before diving down for another rep. Repeat until the entire set is done.

I highly recommend that for your bench presses you have a trusted spotter. This can be a very dangerous lift, and if you get pinned with no one around, you're screwed. They will help you unrack/rerack the weight and help you out if you get in a pinch for whatever reason. If you don't have a spotter, you absolutely MUST NOT go near failure. A dumbbell variation would be a better option.

Because of the way the bar is gripped during bench presses, it can be a contraindicated exercise for those with shoulder problems. Dumbbells allow for a more neutral grip on the exercise and allow you to target the same muscles with more shoulder breathing room.

The same principles apply regarding form no matter which bench variation you do: barbell, machine, or dumbbell. Keep the shoulder blades tucked and tight and focus on squeezing the pecs.

Bench presses are very variable and can be done for 6 reps and up.

ROWS

Rows are a prime back builder that will get your lats wide that contribute to that stunning V-Taper necessary for an aesthetic physique, and they're excellent for building a thick, dense back.

The back has a ton of muscle mass with the potential to grow, and rows will also target your biceps and rear delts during the ride. Because of the heavy mid-back and posterior shoulder involvement, it's also a great exercise for postural health to get you standing tall and mighty.

HOW TO ROW

1. Hold the weight at a weight at a dead hang and your shoulder blades slightly protracted
2. Begin the lift from the middle back and contract the lats to pull the weight up towards the midline of your back. All of the movement should come from the back and arms. Do not let your lower back assist in the movement. This will shorten the lats and hyperextending the back is a poor idea.
3. Squeeze at the top and ensure that your shoulder blades are back and down. Do not let your elbow break far past the body leading to your shoulder slipping forward, and make sure that you do not let your neck jut outwards in an attempt to think you have pulled the weight back further. No cheating.
4. Slowly lower the weight back to the starting position and repeat for the indicated number of repetitions.

There are several ways to row. You can perform them with a barbell, dumbbells (uni/bilateral), or even machines and cables.

I recommend doing your rows in a supported fashion to take the lower back and legs out of the equation and focus on the task at hand. This can be done by using a chest-supported setup, using your opposite arm to brace you when doing unilateral dumbbell rows, or ensuring a tight, neutral core when doing standing cable rows. This one in particular is a personal favorite for posture, a little core work, and as a secondary back exercise.

Rows can start at 6 repetitions and higher, provided tight form.

PULLUPS/PULLDOWNS

Rows hit your back horizontally, but pulldowns work it vertically. Pulldowns will generate a great stretch on the lats, and the constant cable tension will really work the muscle like no other and allow for very stimulating eccentric portions of the lift. Pull ups can just as easily be done, and a chain weight belt can be added to continually add more resistance to the exercise.

HOW TO PERFORM PULLDOWNS:

1. Start with the bar overhead and your arms extended so that you feel a nice, deep stretch
2. Pull down by triggering the lats and finishing off with the biceps until the bar is all the way down. Do not use your back sway to jerk it down, and do not jut your chin out to convince yourself that you brought the bar down all the way.
3. Pause and then slowly let the weight lift back up into the starting position until all the tension in the cable is relieved
4. Complete for the indicated amount of reps

Those who don't have enough back strength to get an effective workout doing pull-ups are better off doing pulldowns instead. This will target the back more effectively and produce better form because there is no need to stabilize in free space like is necessary for pull-ups.

For either of these exercises, you can switch up your grip to provide a different training effect. Take this into consideration when choosing your curl variation for arms.

Pull-ups and pulldowns can be done for sets of 6 and up, although a bit higher may be necessary to avoid elbow wear and tear. 8-12 reps is a good practical range.

BICEP CURLS

Rows and pulldowns are excellent at targeting the biceps, but you can still benefit from an extra set or two of bicep curls done with a different grip to get a more well-rounded effect.

For example, if do your rows with an overhand grip, you'd do your curls with an underhand grip. If you do your pulldowns with an underhand grip, you could do your curls with an overhand or neutral grip.

You can use dumbbells to perform the movement to alter your grip a bit more and get a different contraction by adding in a twist.

HOW TO PERFORM CURLS:

1. Start with the weight in your hands either shoulder width or closer and your arms fully extended at your sides
2. Contract the biceps and bring the weight up until your arms are fully bent in the top position. Do not use your anterior delts to move the weight, and don't lean back like you're in the club to help move the weight. You want the emphasis to be on the biceps alone.
3. Squeeze at the top and then slowly lower the weight back down to the starting position
4. Repeat for the indicated number of repetitions.

Machines can help to ensure that you aren't cheating on the curl by using your deltoids or lower back sway to complete the lift, and these are useful for Supersets or drop sets towards the tail end of a workout. Cables facing away from the cable system are also very effective.

Bicep curls are best done starting at 8-10 repetitions and up, especially after back work.

TRICEP EXTENSIONS

The triceps are a three-headed monster that you will slay like Hercules. The tris make up most of the muscle mass of your upper arm. Chest press variations will torch these very well, but they benefit a lot from some additional training on the side to fully target them properly. The long head is left under-stimulated by chest work.

My preferred way is done standing and using a cable set-up with attachments that brings your arm overhead. You should feel a stretch in your lats and tricep. This places emphasis on the long head and will really fill out the arms well. This style is what I call the Apollo Press, and brownie points if you can figure out why.

HOW TO DO A TRICEP EXTENSION:

1. Start at the top position with your arm bent as if you were in the contracted position of a bicep curl. Your grip should be shoulder width or closer, depending on the attachment.
2. Contract the triceps forcefully to full extension, being careful not to lat the lats or any chest activity assist in the lift
3. Squeeze for a brief pause, and then slowly release the tension under control by allowing the weight to move back up to the top position so that you feel the stretch on the tricep.
4. Repeat for the number of indicated repetitions

If you do not have access to a cable system, you can do this by going overhead with the use of a spotter and a dumbbell or an EZ bar. 8 reps and up are advised here.

LATERAL RAISES

Bench press will work the front of the shoulders very well, but the lateral head of the deltoids needs a little more love. The side delts are critical for aesthetics in enhancing the V-taper and adding to the width of the physique that produces appealing proportions in men and women. Nicely capped delts are a sight to behold. The best exercise for this are lateral raises. Overhead presses can work as well, however some individuals are not good fits for them due to postural issues and/or movement restrictions.

Lateral raises are best done with a set of dumbbells or a low cable pulley set-up. Do not do them on a machine. This is an exercise where the shoulder needs its free range.

HOW TO LATERAL RAISE:

1. Start with the weight down at your sides with a neutral grip or slightly turned outwards to avoid impingement. Make sure you keep your arms straight with only as little bend in the elbow as necessary to complete the exercise
2. Contract the deltoids, being careful not to let the upper traps and backwards sway move the weight, and bring the weight up to roughly shoulder level or slightly below. Your shoulder blades should move as you bring up the weight, so don't keep you shoulder blades tucked. You want smooth scapular motion here. The path should be to the side but slightly in front of you at an angle can be easier on the shoulders by putting you in a different plane of motion.
3. Slowly lower the weight back down and repeat for the indicated number of reps

The dumbbell variation can be done with both sides simultaneously, but another great way to do lateral raises is by gripping the edge of a power rack or cable pulley station with your non-exercise hand and leaning to the side. This is especially powerful if you do this with the cable variation and will really keep maximum tension on the muscle for the entirety of the set.

Lateral raises are best done with 10+ repetitions. Less can be hard on the joint and cause form to break down.

REAR DELT FLY

If there is one muscle group that gets neglected most on the upper body, it would have to be the rear delts, and that's a shame.

A fine pair of rear delts will really round out the shoulders magnificently, and a set of plump rear delts is also a great thing for shoulder health that often goes out of whack from too much chest work and sedentary living. Back exercises will involve the rear delts, but they can benefit from a little extracurricular activity to really hammer them home.

To do rear delt flyes, you can use a set of dumbbells and bend over/lay supported on an low incline bench, or you may find that a standing cable set-up or rear delt fly machine works a bit better at isolating the rear delts properly.

HOW TO PERFORM A REAR DELT FLY

1. Start with the dumbbells/handles out in front of you at about chest-level for a good stretch. Use a neutral or overhand grip here, and allow for a little bit of a bend in your elbow.
2. Contract the rear delts and bring the weight out to your sides so that your chest is expanded
3. Squeeze briefly and then slowly lower the weight back down to the starting position
4. Repeat for the desired number of repetitions

Rear delts are best done in a relatively higher rep range from 10 repetitions upwards.

Alternatively, face-pulls can be done for rear delt work as well, and this will incorporate a heavy dose of work for the external rotators of the rotator cuff that's beneficial for shoulder health and balancing out the joint.

EXTRAS

These are just a handful of exercises, but through these exercises alone, you will build a spectacular physique that accomplishes all of the aesthetic goals. They cover the entire body effectively and are effective, efficient, and fit the bill for everything a stellar exercise must cover. They will also serve a solid foundation for other accessory movements to follow.

That being said, that isn't to say that other exercises are off limits entirely.

I've given you the tools to be able to judge an exercise's usefulness to you, so stick to the basics and if you're looking to accomplish a specific goal, you have what you need to determine the best way to go.

17

FORM

Excellence is an art won by training and habituation. We do not act rightly because we have virtue or excellence, but rather we have those because we have acted rightly. We are what we repeatedly do. Excellence, then, is not an act but a habit.
Aristotle

*L*IFTING WEIGHTS ISN'T JUST about getting the weights up. It's *how* you get the weights up that matters. Weights are the tool that you use to sculpt your physique, not the means in and of itself.

MAXIM OF AESTHETICS: STRIVE FOR EXCELLENCE WITH EVERY REP, JUST AS YOU WOULD STRIVE FOR EXCELLENCE WITH EVERY DAY YOU LIVE AND EVERYTHING THAT YOU DO.

Your life is just the sum of every day and moment you live. A towering castle is just the sum of the individual bricks and stones. Likewise, your training is simply the sum total of each rep and movement you make in the gym. Make it count, and make it great. Full range of motion. Full of focus.

WHAT IS GOOD FORM?

Good form demands performing the exercise with a *full, controlled* range of motion and maximum muscle stimulation of the targeted muscles while avoiding both acute and long-term injury [1].

- *All* the way down. Nice and steady. Don't let gravity do the work for you.
- *All* the way up. Explosive, yet controlled. Focus 100% on the targeted muscle(s) without any assistance from any muscle groups you aren't looking to train.

Don't concern yourself with specific tempos [2]. Move the way that I've outlined above, and tempo will take care of itself. This will ensure that you drain that exercise of every last succulent drop.

If you have to reduce the weight to ensure excellent form, then so be it. You don't lift or live for external validation. Know your goal, and get your ego out of the equation.

MAXIM OF AESTHETICS: THE NUMBERS ON THE BAR ARE NOT AS IMPORTANT AS THE EFFECTS THAT LIFTING THEM CORRECTLY ARE.

Learn the movements properly, execute them properly each and every time you're under the bar, and THEN you will have earned the right to add more weight.

HIT THE TEST TRACK

In the previous chapter, I gave you a breakdown of some all-star exercises and how to carry them out, but the best way to nail good form is to get your eyes on what the movement is supposed to look like & putting it into practice with proper guidance to get the right feel for it.

- Look up videos online and study how the exercises are performed.
- Watch experienced lifters in your gym perform them (correctly).
- Ask questions.
- Analyze.
- Seek coaching.
- Study the details.

After you've got an idea of how the movement is supposed to look, trying them out for yourself under zero to low loading is the only real way to get a feel for how they're done.

Do so under the watchful eye of a good trainer or experienced lifter and have them teach you the correct way and walk through the movement step by step to make sure that you are lifting correctly.

This is key for the compound movements like the squat, deadlift, bench, and rows that will get loaded and pushed for progression.

The heavier and more technical the movement, the more crucial form becomes.

Working on your form is a constant journey, and an important one at that. The more experienced you become, the better your form will get and should be.

Practice doesn't make perfect. PERFECT PRACTICE makes perfect.

MIND-MUSCLE CONNECTION

Maximum muscle stimulation is the objective, but many have trouble with stimulating the targeted muscle properly. This is where mind/muscle connection comes into play.

Throughout the exercise, shift your focus to the contraction of the targeted muscles. You must feel it activate and do the work of the movement as you perform the exercise. Simply moving the weight isn't enough.

This connection is important and will get you better results from your training. If you can't feel the lats when you row, then the lats aren't getting the targeted result. Your biceps will thank you, but great wings you will never have.

USE CUES

Certain cues are helpful for creating a better mind/muscle connection. For example, if your biceps are doing all of the work on rows, shift your attention to your lats. Visualize your back squeezing and pulling as if you were trying to pinch a penny between your shoulder blades. The arms are just along for the ride.

There is a learning curve to all of this, and it varies depending on the movement. You didn't hop out the womb and start sprinting, did you? I didn't think so. You wobble and sway as you stand and learn to walk. Eventually, it becomes second nature, and you have things down pat.

There are several tricks for different exercises that can help you form a mind/muscle connection and better stimulate the targeted muscles. You'll begin to figure these out for yourself as you progress and get more experienced, and soon you'll begin to wonder how you ever had any trouble with it at all.

FORM CHECKS

Keeping tight form is a must at all times, and to help us do so, we can use mirrors, training partners/coaches, and video primarily.

MIRRORS

Why do gyms have mirrors? To bathe in our narcissistic glow? To detect the hidden vampires in the weights section? To stare at some squat assets across the gym mid-set? None of the above.

The REAL reason that gyms have mirrors is so that we keep an eye on our form during our lifting. Utilize this tool, and ensure that you are performing the movements correctly. Depending on where you stand in the gym, you can take advantage of the front and side mirrors simultaneously to ensure that you are on track in all angles.

The lift may feel right, but the mirror doesn't lie. Pay attention to things like:

- the angle of your lower back
- whether you are slouched, swaying, or leaning
- the position of your head and neck

...and so forth. You may just be targeting your arms, but *your whole body* plays a role. You don't want to get into bad habits that'll take away from your performance or set the stage for bad posture or injury in the future.

The mirror can help you keep that on track. Use it as a tool to verify that your form is how it should be, but don't depend on it excessively at the expense of your workout quality.

The ultimate goal is to get a good feel for the movement and trust in your form. Being glued to it will take some of the effectiveness away from the exercise by matter of focus.

TRAINER/PARTNER

Having an experienced trainer or lifting partner is also of superb use here. Besides the other benefits these can have, they can see things that perhaps you can't see or aren't aware of in your lifting technique and help you to correct it. Using a mirror isn't practical for all lifts.

<u>VIDEO</u>

Finally, you can record yourself on video to make sure your form is on point. Going to this length typically isn't necessary or practical in many instances, however given the opportunity, this can be a great tool to use to analyze your lifting technique and record your best lifts and milestones.

You can set up your smart phone in the corner with a timer to record your sets and then review later. Pull it up, compare it to clips of how it should be done, and get some feedback from a knowledgeable source to fine tune your technique. You want to get things as spot on as you can and ingrain it until it becomes second nature.

GOOD FORM IS A LIFESTYLE

People tend to shift all our attention to good form during the exercise, but don't forget to transfer this to your warm-ups, set-ups for the exercise, and day to day life.

What good does it do to have picture perfect form on deadlifts but round your back like a frightened feline when you go to pick up the dumbbells to set up for some presses? Or picking up a pencil that slid off the table?

When you go to open a door, think good form. When you go to pick up a heavy box, think good form. Remember: lifting weights is a skill. Good form is a habit.

Most injuries are brewing in the depths far before they ever end up occurring in the gym or playing field, and they get their start in the minor things that get overlooked or deemed as unimportant, but the truth is that these things add up over time, and the moment of injury is simply the straw that broke the camel's back.

Listen to your body; it'll talk to you. Correct things when it's talking before it starts screaming. Make every movement count, and see everything as an opportunity to move the right way.

18

MAKING GAINS

NO MATTER HOW GREAT your workouts are, you MUST have a plan in place to push forward and progress. *Progressive overload is the key* to growth, so doing the same work day in and day out week after week isn't going to cut it. You're wasting valuable time and effort if you think anything else will get you some place.

In this chapter, we'll talk about progression schemes geared towards progressing in the gym and making gains to add quality size to your aesthetic physique.

PROGRESSION SCHEME

A progression scheme will set the map for how you're supposed to move forward each workout to keep getting bigger and stronger. For our purposes, we'll be sticking with a *double progression* scheme. In a double progression scheme, you simply take your working weight for a particular exercise and then:

1. Increase reps within a range
2. Increase the weight when you hit the upper limit of that range
3. Repeat

This will steadily march your volume up over time and get you the growth you're after. See below for a visual representation of how that happens. Reps increase, drop after adding weight, then rise again. Lather, rinse, repeat.

VOLUME ON DOUBLE PROGRESSION

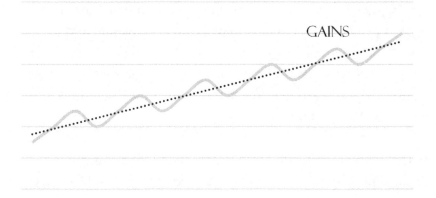

GAINS

To see examples of this, let's look at the two most commonly employed ways of approaching double progression: Straight Sets and the Reverse Pyramid.

For both of these, ensure you record your weight each and every workout during your workout after each set. It is a must.

STRAIGHT SETS

In a straight set system, you'll be picking a weight with ~2-3 RITTs on your first set (reps in the tank) and sticking to it for every set. This will allow you to perform all of the work you need to hit your volume requirements without drop-offs in performance. By the last set, the RITTs will reduce to roughly 0 or 1 due to fatigue.

Failure must be avoided on these sets, with the exception being the last set when hitting failure won't damage any sets that follow. For example:

You pick 185 lbs for 3 sets of 8 repetitions to start off with using a weight that you could do 11-12 times cleanly for one set. Once you are able to complete 3 sets of 10 repetitions, you increase the weight by 5lbs.

STRAIGHT SETS EXAMPLE

	WEIGHT	REPS
WORKOUT 1	185 LBS	8,8,8
WORKOUT 2	185 LBS	9,9,9
WORKOUT 3	185 LBS	10,10,10
WORKOUT 4	*190 LBS*	*8,8,8*

Using straight sets is an excellent way to maintain freshness across workouts and allow for more volume to be done within each individual workout. This is the default mode for beginners to avoid pushing too hard too fast, but it works well across the board.

REVERSE PYRAMID

Reverse Pyramid [1,2] style training starts with the heaviest weight (1-2 RITT) and then factors in the expected drop in performance by reducing the weight on each subsequent set and instead adding in repetitions.

REVERSE PYRAMID EXAMPLE

	WEIGHT	REPS	NOTES
SET 1	200lbs	6	1-2 RITT
SET 2	180lbs	8	-10% in weight; 1-2 RITT
SET 3	160lbs	10	-10% in weight, 0-1 RITT

The goal is to make improvements on the first set of each workout after proper warm ups. This is when you are at your freshest. Ascending pyramids suck and are for warm-ups only. By the time you climb to the top, you're already wasted.

A 10% reduction per set is typically enough to keep performance high. This will depend on the exercise and the lifter. You can use large ranges (6-10) or more narrow ranges (6-8). Progression with the Reverse Pyramid is just like straight sets:

	WEIGHT	REPS
WORKOUT 1	200, 180,160	6,8,10
WORKOUT 2	200, 180, 160	7,9,11
WORKOUT 3	200, 180, 160	8, 10, 12
WORKOUT 4	*205, 185, 160*	*6, 8, 10*

Note that if you're handling dumbbells or heavy weights, the set-up between sets can get old fast and take away from workout momentum and energy.

SET PROGRESSION

For smaller muscles and isolation movements, you will reach your limits faster and find that a double progression scheme leads you to stall. No worries. When this happens, consider adding an extra set instead to keep overload going until you are able to go up in weight.

PROGRESSION RATES

The examples shown are *just examples*, and you might not make such fast jumps week in and week out. Outside of nailing your recovery and nutrition, that's to be expected.

In general, you'll be making the fastest gains on the biggest muscle groups and the compound movements. Beginners will progress faster than advanced trainees.

Finally, dumbbell or machine variations will call for you to use a wider range before adding weight. Dumbbells go up in increments of 5 lbs for each side rather than 2.5, and machines can make jumps of 15 pounds between levels.

To get around this, you would need to shoot for adding 4 repetitions before adding weight, and this may be less effective at increasing strength at the optimal rate, so take this into account when planning your exercises and workouts.

Alternatively, some gyms have small rubber weighs that fit into the weight stack to allow for smaller progression jumps on machine stacks. Take advantage.

SUMMARY

Each of these ways to approach double progression have their pros and cons, and the one that is chosen is dependent on the training status of the individual, the movement, the goal, and their psychological dispositions.

These are very methodical, step-by-step ways to approach progress. And that's what make them so damn effective. There are no rapid, huge gains overnight. But with one small step at a time, you will look back and marvel at how many gains you have made.

5-10lbs average in weight spikes per month with 8 gaining phase months per year will yield 40-80 pounds of strength gain in your target rep range within a year.

Do you wager you'd be looking much bigger being able to push 80lbs more on your main lifts? Just imagine your leg transformation after pushing 135 for 8 reps vs. 215 for 8 reps.

This rate of progression will wane over time, but the fact remains:

Step by step, you will go far.

MAXIM OF AESTHETICS: FOCUS ON PROGRESSION, NOT PERFECTION.

19

PERIODIZATION

You must not fight too often with one enemy, or you will teach him all your art of war.
Napoleon Bonaparte

*P*ERIODIZATION IS SWITCHING UP your training variables in a determined way over time. This is a sure-fire way to pursue progress, avoid stagnation, and offer variety to a program.

No one said you must keep the same style of training forever, and by strategically manipulating the various training variables, you will be able to reap the benefits from a wider range of stimuli [1,2,3,4]. In this chapter, we will focus on manipulating reps, volume, frequency, and exercise selection to keep you marching towards success sustainably.

REPS

As you saw in the chapter on Intensity, the rep ranges exist on a continuum of strength and endurance that each offer their own benefits, so changing up your rep schemes is a trusty tactic for your training to maximize your results.

WITHIN THE WORKOUT

Although not typically thought of when it comes to periodization, mixing up your rep ranges within the workout already provides many of the benefits of more deliberate periodization approaches.

EXERCISE A	6-10 reps
EXERCISE B	10-15 reps

For earlier stages of your lifting career, this gets the job done like a charm, but when the weights start getting heavy, it can be wise to give more focus to ranges in particular in each individual workout through workout day/week.

ACROSS A WORKOUT WEEK

When you periodize within the week, the rep ranges will vary depending on the workout day. For example, on Workout 1 you'll be hitting rep ranges on the lower end of the spectrum, and on Workout 2 you'll be hitting the ranges in the higher end, or vice versa.

WORKOUT A	6-10 reps
WORKOUT B	10-15 reps

If you have more than 2, you will bounce back and forth or include a middle day.

WORKOUT A	4-6
WORKOUT B	8-12
WORKOUT C	15-20

This style of training is most useful for more advanced trainees who have larger volumes and the practicality of incorporating their main compound work and higher rep work in the same workout would prove to be a disaster for recovery and training quality.

ACROSS A CYCLE(S)

Lastly, you can adjust reps across weeks of your current training cycle. One week, you may do lower reps, the next higher, and the next medium. Each can enable you to focus on different ranges. I am not a fan of this approach for making optimal progress outside of small spurts of lighter lifting when there are joint flare-ups or vacations. Changing rep scheme emphasis across numerous cycles is more promising. 6-10 reps for one 2 month block, 10-15 for another, and so forth.

SUMMARY

For all of these methods of manipulating reps, ensure that you factor in total volume unless specifically periodizing volume, as you'll see next. Unless you're a late intermediate or more advanced, stick to within the workout and across the week. This will enable you to have a steady gauge for your progress on your main exercises. Periodization can get very technical, and I don't want you trying things out before you're ready to that will only distract you.

VOLUME

Volume is another factor that can be manipulated for progress. In the chapter on volume, I gave you a starting point for hitting your volume. That figure is based on *averages over periods of time*, and volume follows a *dose-response* relationship, so there is value in manipulating training volumes during and over training cycles to maximize growth in relation to your potential. This will ensure that you optimize progress while keeping recovery and the risk of overtraining in check.

Additionally, when you get more advanced, it may simply be unsustainable to train at such a high volume for sustained periods, so strategically reaching your peaks by accepting small gains early in the training cycle, ramping things up to squeeze the max gains you can for brief periods, and then deloading is a better way to go.

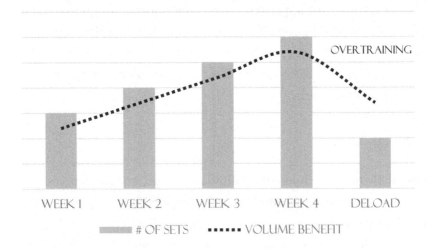

Progression through double progression is still key, but here volume is being increased deterministically by the # of weekly sets. The number of weeks may vary.

VOLUME RAMPS

WEEK NUMBER	NUMBER OF SETS
WEEK 1	10
WEEK 2	12
WEEK 3	14
WEEK 4	16
WEEK 5 : DELOAD	6

In general, you do not want to go drastically over your normal effective workload when periodizing volume. ~50% over normal is a good starting point, but start mild. Short periods of high volume overreaching can be effective when making progress, however they *must always* be followed by a deload or 'taper' so that you can adapt and super-compensate to respond to the training demand.

In your progress log, make note of how you feel along with your workout progressions each week as you do this. It is critical that you be extremely observant as you start ramping up volume so that you can look back at how you respond to different volumes of training. This will allow you to see just how receptive you are to the volume dosage and better determine your individual volume curve.

IMPORTANT NOTICE

Doing this is better off limited to later intermediates or advanced lifters. Unless receiving specialized instruction, when you're a beginner or early intermediate, stick to the basics that I outlined and focus on progression through weight and reps on the bar while monitoring your volume tolerance and adjusting accordingly.

FREQUENCY

Outside of optimizing growth cycles, manipulating frequency by itself is likely not going to do you much good on its own, but periodizing frequency *can be* a helpful tactic for bringing about those changes in volume and making for more manageable, high quality workout sessions.

In the previous example on volume, weeks 1 and 2 may only require 2 weekly sessions per muscle to hit your volume requirements, but as you get into week 3 or 4, it may be more helpful to split that up over 3 days. Advanced trainees may even need to push for 4 to allow for the quality work to be done.

FREQUENCY

WEEK NUMBER	NUMBER OF SETS	SESSIONS	SETS/SESSION
WEEK 1	10	2	5
WEEK 2	12	2	6
WEEK 3	14	3	4-5
WEEK 4	16	4	4
WEEK 5 : DELOAD	6	2	3

Beyond 7-8 sets for a muscle group per workout is when you will begin to note a drop off in performance and workout quality, assuming adequate intensity and challenging movements.

When altering frequency, consider periodizing your reps as well.

SWITCHING EXERCISES

Finally, you can periodize through exercise selection by swapping exercises from one workout or cycle to the next. Beginners are better off choosing solid compound movements best for them and progressing on those in frequent training sessions for the reasons mentioned earlier related to motor learning until they graduate to a more intermediate level of training.

EXAMPLES OF EXERCISE SWAPPING:

EXERCISE 1	EXERCISE 2
Back Squat	Front Squat
Bench Press	DB Bench Press
EZ Bar Curl	Supinated DB Curl
Lunges	Split Squat
Rows	Pulldown

Different ways of performing a movement may give preferential emphasis to different muscle groups that can allow for progression on the original lift and uniform size growth [3,4]. Front squats will shift the loading of the movement and target different portions of the quad, wide-grip rows will work the back horizontally whereas pulldowns will do so vertically - thus triggering more mid back. You get the idea.

In addition, trying new exercises can allow for a bit more spice and variety to the training program, and that keeps things fun and interesting, which is why muscle confusion has always been such an attractive idea to so many people - just not at the expense of focusing on what really matters and maintaining an objective standard of training progress to avoid screwing around in the gym.

HOW TO SWITCH UP THE EXERCISES

Switching up the main exercises can be done across a workout week (7-10 days) for the different workouts or across different training cycles (6-8 weeks). There is a motor component of the exercises you perform, so this shouldn't be taken as an excuse to get excessively liberal.

Pick 2 exercises and alternate with a PLAN. Switching things all over the place will erase your standard of progress and lead to inconsistency and waste. For example:

Barbell Bench on Workout 1 and Dumbbell Bench on Workout 2. This may or may not be accompanied by different rep scheme emphasis as explained in the previous section on periodization (Heavy on Workout 1, Lighter on Workout 2). So Barbell Bench for 6-8 on Day 1 and Dumbbell Bench for 12 on Day 2.

ACROSS TRAINING CYCLES

Additionally, you don't want to completely revamp your training routine across larger training cycles. Keep at least one of your main exercises constant from one cycle to the next. After the second cycle, you can switch it out for something else while keeping the new exercise you added in as the constant.

This ensures that you still maintain some of the stimulus and standard for progress alive and don't radically change your program. If you're renovating a building, you always leave some of the main structure there as you make changes.

Training Cycle	Exercises
1	Back squat Side lunges
2	Back squat *Reverse lunges*
3	*Front squat* Reverse lunges
4	Front squat *Side lunges*

AUTOREGULATED PERIODIZATION

As you gain experience in your lifting career, you will learn your body on a very intimate level. You'll make note of your energy levels, any aches and pains, and be alert to when your exercises simply aren't feeling like they should. When this happens, you can autoregulate your training and reactively periodize.

- If you're set to lift heavy that day but had a draining day, do the same workout in a higher rep range.
- If you just can't get into your groove on an exercise, go do another so that you can have a productive training session.

These are all effective examples of ways that you can weave flexibility into your program based on the real-world conditions [5]. If you start to notice a trend over time, it's a sign of something in your program that needs to change, so don't make every day a coin toss. You have a program for a reason. Monitor and adjust as needed.

20

THE WORKOUTS

ITH THE UNDERSTANDING OF AESTHETICS, the fundamental principles of training, and the exercises to perform them with laid out on the table, it is now up to you to determine what the best way is to combine them to achieve your goals.

You could have all the theory in the world, but if you aren't able to string it together in a cohesive, workable program, it will do you absolutely no good. Let's get it right.

With every optimal workout program, here are the things you need to do:

    I.   ACCOMPLISH TRAINING GOALS EFFICIENTLY
    II.   FACTOR IN TOTAL RECOVERY AND OVERLAP
    III.   CONSIDER THE OVERALL LIFESTYLE PICTURE
    IV.   LIGHT THE FIRE IN YOU

THE WINNING WORKOUT ROUTINE

I.   ACCOMPLISH TRAINING GOALS EFFICIENTLY

First and foremost, your training needs to be geared up through proper intensity, volume, frequency, and exercise selection in a way that will create a well-balanced physique with your ideal proportion, symmetry, flow, and meaning. This must be done taking your level of development into account. *See next section.*

II.   FACTOR IN TOTAL RECOVERY AND OVERLAP

Life is a limited resource, and you only have so much to give to your training. Your mind and body need a break to fire on all cylinders, and the body is interconnected, so one day's training must not impede on the next.

III.   CONSIDER THE OVERALL LIFESTYLE PICTURE

Working out is a way of life, but it is also just *a part* of life. You will give me one hour of power and then get out of my sight to spread your wings and live life to the fullest.

Your routine must be flexible and fit in with your schedule to ensure you get in and make the most of it each and every time.

IV.   LIGHT THE FIRE IN YOU

Lastly, you've got to *adore* heading into the weight room to train. For that one hour, you leave the world behind and enter into your metamorphosis. Nothing and no one can stop you. Because of this, throw a little fun and spice into the mix to keep things invigorating.

<u>H O W   A D V A N C E D   A R E   Y O U ?</u>

Your program needs to be calibrated to your level of development. A beginner should not train like they're advanced and vice versa.

See below for a rough overview of different training statuses from beginner to advanced. If you can achieve those standards as estimated by a 1RM calculator, then you can then think about graduating to the next level. Elite levels (~5+ years of solid, consistent training) are not discussed.

T R A I N I N G   S T A T U S   C H A R T

RANK	TIME LIFTING *CORRECTLY*	STRENGTH*
BEGINNER	6 months - 1 year	Bench: 1 (M), 0.5 (F) Squat: 1.25 (M), 1 (F) Deadlift: 1.5 (M), 1 (F)
INTERMEDIATE	1- 3 years	Bench: 1.25 (M), 0.75 (F) Squat: 1.5 (M), 1.25 (F) Deadlift: 2 (M), 1.5 (F)
ADVANCED	3 years+	Bench: 1.5 (M), 1 (F) Squat: 2 (M), 1.5 (F) Deadlift: 2.5 (M), 2 (F)

Factor is to be multiplied by lean body weight
Achieve ⅔
M=male, F=female

This chart is based on *rough estimations* to provide a reasonable frame of view in determining where you stand as it pertains to lifting level. The ideal would be basing training status based on the lifter's proximity to their genetic potential, but these are good proxies. People vary wildly in terms of where they start out, how fast they progress, and until what point.

Additionally, resist the temptation to be constrained by the time frames and numbers listed. As long as you are progressing and achieving your goals with the current program, there is no need to "graduate" to the next level. You get more complex as needed, not on a whim or because you're bored.

When understanding the following workout split examples, keep these things in mind:

- The examples given are only examples and should be custom tailored to the person. Generic templates and exercise prescriptions suck and should only be used to give you a good idea to start. Don't waste your money on them.
- All workouts are to be done following a proper warm-up as outlined in the book. *See chapter entitled Before Battle.*
- These are far from exhaustive and have been chosen to best suit the 3Ps of physiology, psychology, and practicality
- These are the starting base and open to periodized approaches for optimal progress (see Chapter)

And lastly, there will be no fancy bells and whistles with these programs. You will get the tried and true goods that are effective and based on sound training principles. If you want to be impressed and dazzled, go take a pre-workout and watch Japanese cartoons.

MAXIM OF AESTHETICS: EITHER YOUR PROGRAM OR YOUR RESULTS CAN BE FLASHY, BUT RARELY WILL YOU GET BOTH. AND EVEN IF YOU DO, THERE WAS PROBABLY A BETTER WAY.

Now let's proceed.

BEGINNER PROGRAM

So you're new to lifting and aren't quite sure how to get your journey rolling. Most programs out there are designed to look fancy and impressive. That might get you clicks, likes, and sales, but they're all sparkle and no substance.

Your goal as a beginner in pursuit of aesthetics is to form a solid, firm foundation to set you up for success. This means:

BEGINNER PROGRAM GOALS

- ❧ Ironing out any postural/mobility problems before you're pushing heavy weight
- ❧ Perfecting your form in the main movements that will serve you throughout your lifting career
- ❧ Forming the neural adaptations to lifting
- ❧ Developing a powerful mind/muscle connection
- ❧ Driving your strength up to progress into a more intermediate program
- ❧ Accustoming your joints and frame to lifting
- ❧ Building good habits in and out of the weight room
- ❧ Cultivating that love for the iron

There is no sense in pushing for optimal hypertrophy in a higher volume, complex routine if your body isn't even geared to handle that type of training yet.

You have to get strong enough all around and develop the proper foundations first. You don't build a skyscraper on a bunch of quicksand.

BEGINNER

DAY 1: LOWER A

EXERCISE	SETS	REPS	RITT	NOTES
Squats	3	6	2-3	
RDL	3	8	2-3	
Lunge	2	10	1-2	Or leg ext
SL Calves	5	6	2-3	Straight leg

DAY 2: UPPER A

EXERCISE	SETS	REPS	RITT	NOTES
Bench	3	6	2-3	
Row	3	6	2-3	Supported
Incline Press	2	10	1-2	DB optional
Pulldown	2	10	1-2	
SS Shoulders	3,2	10	1-2	Lat./Rear Delt
SS Arms	2,1	10	1-2	Tri Overhead/Bi

DAY 3: LOWER B

EXERCISE	SETS	REPS	RITT	NOTES
Squats	3	6	2-3	
RDL	3	8	2-3	
Leg Curl	2	10	1-2	
BK Calves	4	12	2-3	Bent-Knee

DAY 4: UPPER B

EXERCISE	SETS	REPS	RITT	NOTES
Bench	3	6	2-3	
Row	3	6	2-3	Supported
Chest Fly	2	12	1-2	DB or cables
Pulldown	2	12	1-2	
SS Shoulders	3,2	15	1-2	Lat./Rear Delt
SS Arms	2,1	12, 15	1-2	Tri OH/Bi

Supersets (SS): Rest 60-90 sec between each exercise.

RITT: Reps in the Tank for your first set.

HOW TO SCHEDULE

You will be doing this workout routine on a schedule of 3-4x per
week. You may perform an Upper and Lower day back to back, but
do not work out more than 2 days in a row. See the various
schedule options below.

M	T	W	Th	F	S	Su
1	2	-	3	4	-	-
1	-	2	-	3	4	-
1	2	-	-	3	4	-
1	-	2	-	3	-	-

On the last option, you would begin the next week with workout 4
and continue accordingly. This 3 day/week set-up is for those who
have schedule conflicts or soreness:

M	T	W	Th	F	S	Su
1	-	2	-	3	-	-
4	-	1	-	2	-	-
3	-	4	-	1	-	-
2	-	3	-	4	-	-

The schedule begins on Monday, but you can have workout #1 on
any day of the week you choose and go from there.

You do not have to do this on the same set schedule every week. As
long as you stick to the rules, you are good to go.

COMMENTARY

This program is designed to drive strength through the roof while also putting on size where we want it to go. It is flexible, simple, and accessible to lay down the bricks of the proper, well-rounded aesthetic physique. As a beginner, *it's all about the basics.*

ೞ STRONG BASE

As you can see, the main movement patterns along the entire body are being hit in the same way 2x/week. The reason for this is to enhance motor learning and form a strong base of relevant strength that will allow for more success in the future when volume is increased.

ೞ TEMPERED VOLUME

As a beginner, you do not need much volume to make gains. Your muscles are new to being trained in such a way, and keeping volume low will give your body a chance to adjust across the board. Too much volume will also lead to excessive muscle damage and soreness that we want to avoid. Here, you're doing ~10 sets per muscle per week.

ೞ A LITTLE VARIETY

Lastly, there's a little variety in the mix to ensure that the muscles are being worked effectively and entirely. You will gain a little exposure to some different movements and get to tour the gym a bit that keeps things fresh and interesting.

SELECTING YOUR WEIGHTS

To choose the weights that you will be using, find the weight on each exercise that puts you at the number of RITTs listed.

For example, on exercises that say "2-3 RITT", select a weight for the exercise that you can perform 2 to 3 more times with crisp, clean form before hitting muscle failure. This will make sure that you are leaving yourself enough energy to complete the workout, perform the exercises correctly, and avoid burn-out.

EXERCISE	SETS	REPS	RITT	NOTES
Squats	3	6	2-3	

Here, you will be finding a weight that you can do 8-9 times. You can perform an AMRAP set to do this (As Many Reps As Possible):

1. After proper warm-ups, begin each exercise with light weights for 1-3 reps and then begin to add weight to the bar until you start to feel that you are facing resistance that you estimate you can only do 8 or 9 times before failure.
2. Complete a set aiming to get as many reps as you can in clean form. For exercises such as bench press variations or squats, find a spotter or set the safety bars in a power rack when you are ready to do your AMRAP set.

If you over or undershoot your actual results, you have two options: Either adjust by 5lbs up/down or rest 3-5 minutes and try again with a different amount of weight.

Record the values you get in a notebook or application on your phone. These will serve as the starting weights of your lifting career.

HOW TO PROGRESS

WORKOUT	WEIGHT	REPS
1	100	6,6,6
2	100	7,7,7
3	100	8,8,8
4	*105*	*6,6,6*

As you can see, you are using a double progression scheme. Each workout, you try to increase the repetitions, and once you get to the upper limit across the board, you increase the weight by 5 pounds and start again.

Depending on your starting point, you will be making *rapid* improvements on your main exercises. If you can improve more than 1 rep per set while keeping your reps in the tank under control as listed, don't hold back. This is simply the progression *scheme*.

Record your results!

Record your workout progress *each and every* workout. Do this after *every set that you do* so that you don't forget. This will cement your efforts in time and show you exactly where you're at for progression. You'll look back at these someday and be amazed of how far you've come.

HOW LONG TO FOLLOW

Following this program will add size and strength linearly until you end up getting strong enough to where moving to a more advanced routine would be better to continue growing and progressing favorably. This will typically happen at the 6 month - 1 year mark.

OTHER NOTES FOR BEGINNERS

Your first trips to the gym can be intimidating, but don't be afraid to ask for help from a trainer or other lifters in the gym to spot you on your movements, help you figure out how to set up the equipment, or check out your form. This is the time to form great foundations in lifting, and they'd be happy to. If not, hit me up and I'll make some calls to my Russian friends.

Optimize your nutrition and recovery based on the guidelines in the nutritional part of the book. Getting enough calories, protein, and rest is *vital* to your success at this stage in your lifting career. You will be growing around the clock, so make your growth and repair a **priority.**

Some soreness is to be expected. On your off days, stay in line with my daily activity recommendations in the book and get up and get moving for at least 30 minutes a day at a low, leisurely intensity.

Work hard. Be patient. Focus on progression. And enjoy the tsunami of gains that's coming full blast your way.

FEMALE CONSIDERATIONS

Women can do well starting at 8 repetitions on the main lifts if it suits them better, provided RITTs are kept in check.

Don't fear the upper body work. As far as I know and fortunately for me, women do not have telekinetic powers and still have upper body muscles to move and use. It is **essential** for your well-proportioned physique, and you will be better for it. Trust in me.

INTERMEDIATES

After a certain level running the beginner routine, the gains slow down and you begin to plateau. This is where you want to increase the volume dosage for each of the body parts with more focus and specificity to get the growth gears churning again.

Here is also where the programs for men and women start to separate more to veer off in their different directions. The base is built, and now you'll be looking to chase your ideal proportions more.

INTERMEDIATE MEN

Men are going to take the base built by the beginner routine and add more volume to continue growing across the entire body proportionally. This will be split into lower and higher rep days to allow for proper intensity and emphasis.

INTERMEDIATE WOMEN

When women get into the intermediate stage, more of their training budget is going to go towards the legs and glutes to hone that hourglass figure for the aesthetic female physique.

The entire upper body is still going to be hit 2x per week, but the emphasis will be more on a gentle V-taper with preferential treatment towards building a strong back and nicely capped shoulders.

INTERMEDIATE MEN

LEGS A

EXERCISE	SETS	REPS	NOTES
Squat	3	6	
RDL	3	8	
Single Leg	3	8	Lunge/Split Squat
Leg Curl	3	8	
Str. Leg Calf	5	6	

UPPER A

EXERCISE	SETS	REPS	NOTES
Bench	3	6	
Horiz. Row	3	6	
Incline DB	3	8	
Pulldown	3	8	
SS Shoulders	2,1	10	Lat/Rear delt fly
SS Arm	2,1	10	OH Tri/Bicep

LEGS B

EXERCISE	SETS	REPS	NOTES
RDL	3	10	
LP	3	10	
Hip Thrust	3	10	Or Pull Through
Leg Curl	3	12	
Bent Knee Calf	4	12	

UPPER B

EXERCISE	SETS	REPS	NOTES
Bench	3	10	Can be DB
Pulldown	3	10	Alt. Grip from A
Chest Fly	3	12	Cable, Incline
Horiz. Row	3	12	Unilateral
SS Shoulders	3,2	15	Lat/Rear delt fly
Superset Arm	2,1	15	OH Tri/Bicep

SCHEDULING

M	T	W	Th	F	S	Su
LA	UA	-	LB	UB	-	-
LA	-	UA	-	LB	UB	-
-	LA	UA	-	-	LB	UB
LA	-	UA	LB	-	UB	-

The spacing here is very similar to the beginner routine. You'll be lifting 4x per week and ensuring clean spaces for rest and recovery.

COMMENTARY

As you can see, you're expanding upon the beginner routine by adding in a little more volume and variety.

By this point, you'll be getting strong, so you're going to be doing periodizing your rep ranges and body part emphasis a bit more by having a heavy and light day.

In later phases, here is also where it can be advantageous to periodize further with regards to volume and reps as you reach into the upper intermediate stages.

INTERMEDIATE WOMEN

DAY 1

EXERCISE	SETS	REPS	NOTES
Squat	3	8	
Single Leg	3	10	Split Squat, (Side) Lunge
Leg Curl	3	10	Or Pull-through
Glute Iso.	2	12	Kickback/Hip Abductions
SL Calf	5	8	Straight leg

DAY 2

EXERCISE	SETS	REPS	NOTES
Chest Press	4	8	Bench variation
Horiz. Row	3	8	Bilateral
1 arm row	2	10	Cable or DB
Lateral Raise	3	10	Can superset next
Tricep Ext.	3	12	Can superset
Rear Delts	2	12	Fly/Facepull

DAY 3

EXERCISE	SETS	REPS	NOTES
RDL	3	8	
Hip Thrust	3	10	Banded Optional
Leg Press	3	12	Or Lunge Variant
Leg Curl	3	15	
Bent Knee Calf	4	15	

DAY 4

EXERCISE	SETS	REPS	NOTES
Pulldowns	4	10	
Chest	3	12	Bench, Incline, Fly
Overhead Press	3	12	Or lateral raise
Rear Delts	2	15	Fly or facepull
Bicep Curl	2	15	Alt. DB

HOW TO SCHEDULE

M	T	W	Th	F	S	Su
1	2	-	3	-	4	-
1	-	2	3	-	4	-
-	1	2	-	3	-	4

You'll be hitting the gym 4x/week with a modified upper/lower split. Always ensure 2 days between workout 1 and 3.

COMMENTARY

- The glute volume on this routine is quite high, but it has been managed appropriately through frequency and exercise selection so that you can handle it maximally. This will add size to the glutes magnificently, and the addition of more hip abduction will assist in widening the hips and creating those killer curves. On Day 1, the Glute isolations can be supersetted on a cable machine if desired based on work tolerance
- Quads, Hams, and Calves are getting a nice even split at medium dosage.
- Upper body is now leaning heavily on back and shoulders for the subtle V-taper, and chest work takes more of a backseat role to free up bandwidth in your barbell budget for more quality work on your assets and better proportions.

WORKOUTS FOR MAINTENANCE

Maintenance phases are a key part of your physical journey. They provide you with the opportunity to establish a new baseline for your physique to prime it for the next phase, regenerate and repair fully, and mentally regain clarity and passion for pursuing more training goals.

We've looked at working out for growth, but things switch up a bit when your goal is to maintain your current size.

CORE PRINCIPLES

During periods where the goal is to maintain muscle mass, the principles are as follows:

    I.   PERFORM THE SAME EXERCISES
    II.   MAINTAIN INTENSITY
    III. REDUCE VOLUME AND FREQUENCY

Now let's look at each in further detail.

I.   PERFORM THE SAME EXERCISES

This should come as no surprise. If you got your lavish lower body from a steady diet of squats and RDLs, to keep your gains, guess what you'll be doing.

Do not go around trying new exercises for fun here unless you already have a proven track record with the movements from training with them in your gaining cycles. If you want to add variety, do it on your accessory and isolation movements.

II.   MAINTAIN INTENSITY

Keep lifting weights heavy enough to challenge you (~1-2 RITTs on first set to factor in the lower volume you'll see below). This will ensure you're still stimulating the muscle enough to continue sending the signal for retention of muscle mass, even if you dabble in different rep ranges to give the body a break from heavy loads.

III.   REDUCE VOLUME AND FREQUENCY

When you are in a gaining phase, *you are overloading on purpose* to make gains, so when your goal is simply to maintain, you need nowhere near as much volume. And because frequency most often spikes to accommodate that extra volume and maximize growth rates, that'll go down as well. Therefore:

1.   Volume can be cut by up to 2/3 [1]
2.   Frequency can be reduced to 1x per calendar week

...provided you are using the same exercises and intensity I've outlined. For example, if you were training at a total of 15 hard sets per muscle group spread over 2x/week, you can perform 5 hard sets every 7 days and maintain your gains. If you get an unclean number, always round up. If you do multiple exercises, keep the volume reductions *per exercise* to maintain the same training effect with them.

And yes. You read all of that right. Maintenance should be a breeze. Your workouts may only last 30 minutes during a maintenance phase. That's perfectly acceptable, so don't push it for feeling guilty about not living in the gym. Maintaining your gains is like guerrilla warfare. Get in, be effective, get out. Win the war.

WORKOUTS FOR CUTTING

After a long and successful gaining phase with plenty of productive training, you're now looking to get lean and bring out the crisp, carved details of your physique and the enhanced proportion and separation that come along for the ride.

The goals during this period are:

1. DROP BODY FAT TO ENHANCE THE PHYSIQUE
2. MAINTAIN YOUR MUSCLE MASS

The first goal is going to be done by *your diet* with very minor contributions from cardio. <u>Not training</u>. Reread that 300 times until it sinks in nice and deep.

The second goal is where our attention here lies.

TRAINING PRINCIPLES OF CUTTING

To design your training routine for cutting, there are 3 very simple principles you have to carry out:

1. PROVIDE A STRUCTURED OVERLOAD
2. REDUCE THAT OVERLOAD AS NEEDED
3. AVOID EXCESS EFFORT

Here, we will be building upon the concepts of the two previous sections of training for gaining and maintaining, as you'll soon see.

Let's take these items one by one.

I. PROVIDE A STRUCTURED OVERLOAD

During a cutting phase, you are going to be in a caloric deficit. As you'll see later in the Nutritional Section of the book, this means that your body will be burning stored energy for fuel to keep up with the energy demands of the body.

However, this is not just limited to burning body fat. The body can also break down *muscle tissue* to do this. You will greatly reduce the extent of this happening by adopting a <u>modest</u> caloric deficit (0.5-1% of body weight lost/week) and increasing your protein intake (1.2-1.5g/lb. bodyweight), but those two things do nothing to speak for your actual training. Nutrition is just an *enabler*.

Therefore, you want to continue sending a strong signal to your body to keep holding onto the quality size you've built over your gaining phase by continuing to train how you built it in the first place, even if your diet doesn't lay you up to grow from it.

But that's not the end of the story. A caloric deficit is also a *recovery deficit*.

You simply don't have the nutritional firepower to go full blast anymore, so the amount of quality training that you can perform will *decrease* on a cut. Because of this, adjust your training by dropping ~25-33% of your training volume right out of the gate. Frequency should be set at 2x every 7-10 days or so per muscle.

For example, if you were doing 10 weekly sets for a muscle group, you would only be doing 7-8. This will maintain your gains and mitigate the need for frequent deloads, a topic we'll touch on at the end of the section.

2. REDUCE THAT OVERLOAD AS NEEDED

Although you will still be training hard on your cut, you will need to *reduce* that over time the further along you get in your diet.

As you get leaner, the body becomes more resistant to change and more rebellious against your aesthetic goals. Being in a caloric deficit at a low body fat percentage and moving heavy weights at high volumes is not in the cards for the best physical conditions.

Hormones start to drop, energy levels get low, and performance capacity can take a hit. These do not speak good things for retaining muscle mass, do they?

If you were to continue training the same way, you would soon discover yourself in an overtrained state and unable to maintain the same performance in the gym to retain the most muscle mass you can. The reps, sets, and weight on the bar will start to go down, and your muscles are right behind it.

To get around this, you will need to drop some of that volume as time goes along to allow for proper recovery. How much?

As you saw in the previous section of the chapter for maintenance phases, you can safely reduce the volume you do by up to 2/3 and still maintain your gains, provided you maintain the same intensity on the same exercises you used to build your physique. For cuts, in practicality I like to see this at ~50% while leaving 2/3 in reserve based on performance and psychological feedback.

Monitor how you feel both during and in between workouts judged against performance, and reduce volume accordingly if necessary.

3. AVOID EXCESS EFFORT

What's the first thing that comes to mind when people hear the word "cutting"? Unless you live on another planet, Princess Cardio is sitting smug on the top of that list. Let's knock her down.

As I've made quite clear, on a cut your goal is to train hard to maintain muscle in the face of an energy deficit. It should be no surprise to you that adding in a bunch of extracurricular activity is something you should avoid. This will only take away from your training budget.

Bring out cardio only if you need to, and make sure that it is low intensity and done away from your training on off days or separated from your workout time. High intensity interval training (HIIT) such as sprints is very popular and might seem like a logical idea to cut up and maintain muscle, but the truth is that this is very taxing on the body, generates very weak caloric burn, and will only interfere with training and recovery.

A NOTE ON DELOADS

Lastly, by reducing the training volume while cutting, your need for deloads will decrease as well. However, if you are looking at a diet lasting longer than 10-12 weeks, incorporate a 1-2 week deload with maintenance calories to recharge and stabilize.

This may sound counterintuitive to cutting, but you will be much better off for it physically *and* mentally. Start your cuts earlier and optimize your process. A little forethought goes a long way.

Deload before your cut kicks off, and prepare to train to sustain.

SPECIALIZATION: ADVANCED

When you are beyond the ranks of the beginners and intermediates, trying to improve everything at once will be a suicide mission diving headfirst into a sea of Spartan soldiers.

Instead, you will *maintain* your gains and pick *specific* areas to target with full focus. This will shift your resources from a more even arrangement to a concentrated, laser-like emphasis. Observe:

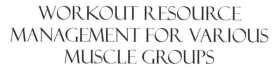

WORKOUT RESOURCE MANAGEMENT FOR VARIOUS MUSCLE GROUPS

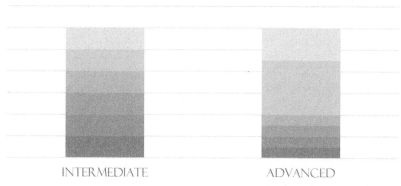

INTERMEDIATE   ADVANCED

For the overeager: You have *no business* trying to specialize until you have already milked your gains and are in a late intermediate to advanced stage of lifting. How can you say you need to bring up your arms when you can't even bench a decent amount of weight for reps?

Trick question. You can't.

PRINCIPLES OF SPECIALIZATION

I.   Do not specialize more than 1-2 muscle groups at a time

II. Maintain non-specialized muscle groups with reduced frequency and volume in a way that won't overlap or interfere with specialized muscle groups

III. Give targeted emphasis to specialized muscle groups with proper volume and frequency by performing them when you are fresh and uninhibited. Be careful not to overdo it on compound movements that involve lots of other musculature

Where you give to one area, you must take from another. We'll factor this in by following the principles as outlined in the previous section on maintenance.

DETERMINING THE PROTOCOL

The first thing you need to do is assess the situation you're dealing with.

❧ LAGGING

Why are you trying to specialize this muscle group?
Is it truly lagging or are you just pushing for enhanced proportion?

In many cases, the muscle group isn't lagging at all. You may only have tunnel vision in the mirror out of a special interest in that area. Every guy wants bigger biceps, and every girl wants better glutes. You must stand back and see the bigger picture.

☙ TRAINING HISTORY

Next, you need to look at the training history of the muscle group in question. Have you been giving it the attention it deserves?

- ☙ How much volume are you giving it?
- ☙ How frequently?
- ☙ Where are you placing it in your workout day and week?

These are based on my earlier recommendations of volume for 8-12 weekly sets spread out over at least 2 days. Based on those questions, you'll fall into 1 of 3 groups:

1. DEADBEAT

If you have been neglecting the area, then you are going to start small by prioritizing it first in your workouts, giving it proper training dosage, and seeing how it responds.

2. GOOD SOLDIER

If you have been giving it the right attention but either want to push it bigger or still can't get the growth gears churning, then you will be looking at increasing volume and frequency to carry that out. A periodized approach of heavy/medium/light and volume ramps is particularly useful here.

3. OVERKILL

If you have been doing too much, then you will simply need to scale things back. Too much volume is just as bad as too little.

SPECIALIZATION EXAMPLES

Now to look at some examples. These are not the only way to do it, but they will show you the rationale behind it. Exercise selection, periodization, and the other principles we've discussed still hold.

	M	T	W	T	F	S	S
2x	Chest	Lower		Chest		Back	
3x	Chest	Lower		Chest		Upper	

Here you can see how chest is scheduled to either target it 2 or 3x per week. On the 3x per week setup, chest is hit first and the rest of the upper body is hit afterwards for maintenance afterwards.

Be careful not to burn out triceps on this protocol. Aim to include good amounts of chest isolation exercises such as flyes to make up the volume.

The chest days can easily be replaced by back following a similar set up as outlined.

	M	T	W	T	F	S	S
2x	Glutes		Upper		Lower		
3x	Glutes		Lower		Glutes	Upper	

On the glute days, there would be a good dosage of glute exercises that do not involve the other large leg muscles. These days would include lots of hip thrusts, kickbacks/extensions.

The lower body day will be maintenance volume for squats, RDLs, and your other main movements. Although these hit the glutes, you don't want to push these for recovery purposes. Afterwards, higher repetition glute work would be done that do not involve the legs.

	M	T	W	T	F	S	S
2x	Arms		Lower		Upper		
3x	Arms		Lower	Arms		Upper	

This goes for any of the muscles of the shoulders or arms.
Remember to factor in the volume for them on Upper days.

	M	T	W	T	F	S	S
2x	Q/H		Upper		Lower		
3x	Q/H		Lower		Q/H	Upper	

Specializing the legs can always be tricky due to overlap, but stick
to the principles of exercise selection and aim to utilize more
squatting movements for quads and Romanian deadlifts for
hamstrings with more single-joint movements to hit your volume.
To further allow for work capacity, shift to machinery that will
allow you to decouple other body parts from the movement that
increase the intensity (i.e leg press rather than more squats).

CALVES

Remember that the calves are crucial as a cornerstone of the
aesthetic physique for both men and women. They are often
underdeveloped and ignored, but we won't let that happen.

The calves can be specialized earlier on and placed virtually in any
workout without the need for a dedicated specialization cycle. For
programming simplicity, I've placed them on lower body days in
the sample routines I've given earlier in the chapter, but you could
experiment by putting them before, supersetted within, or even on
a separate day from Upper or Lower body training, provided it
doesn't interfere with performance in other areas. Start at 2x per
week and bump it up to 3x/week if necessary.

❧ TWO PRONGED APPROACH

To do this, you will want to choose both a straight leg and a seated bent-knee calf variation, as these exercises target the calves in different ways. Begin with the straight leg movement for 3-5 sets of 6-10 and follow this up with the seated bent-knee variation for 3 sets 10+ repetitions.

	M	T	W	T	F	S	S
2x	L	U+C		L	U	C	
3x	L+C	U		L+C	U	C	

NUTRITIONAL CONSIDERATIONS

As you'll see in the Nutrition section of the book, the rate of muscle gain is slower for more advanced lifters.

Therefore, you will put a larger surplus on specialization training days and the day after to ensure you maximize your training and growth potential on these days.

You're only specifically targeting a specific area 2-3 days per week, so deploy all of your nutritional resources to ensure that no stone is left uncovered when you're bringing these body parts up.

Don't fear this. You will shred the minor fat gain with no problems at all with after with a better body to show for it. But of course, if you *really are* advanced and reading this, you knew that already.

21

BEFORE BATTLE

Victorious warriors win first and then go to war, whereas defeated warriors go to war first and then seek to win.
Sun Tzu

WHAT SEPARATES A KICKASS WORKOUT or night out from a forgettable one? It's all in the pregame and the march up to it.

Here, we will discuss:

- ᔓ Pre-workout nutrition and supplementation
- ᔓ Specific warm-ups and
- ᔓ Mental techniques to prime you for the workout ahead

...in that order.

PRE-WORKOUT NUTRITION

The right pre-workout nutrition is a *must* before making a date with the weights. 1-3 hours max beforehand, consume a small to moderate sized meal consisting of protein, carbohydrates, and some fiber and fat to round it out.

The smaller the meal, the closer to your training it should be. ~0.4-0.5g/kg body weight or roughly 20% of your daily protein intake (~1g/lb body weight for gaining) is how much to shoot for during this meal [1].

WEIGHT	PROTEIN PRE-WORKOUT
120lbs	25g
150lbs	30g
180lbs	35g

At least

A protein bar, a protein shake and a banana, a sandwich and an apple, or even a regular meal that falls nicely in line with your training time are all workable options of what to include here.

A pre-workout stimulant or caffeine can help to provide an extra boost, and this should be taken 15-20 minutes before the start of the workout itself – not the start of warmups. Assess your tolerance.

Doing this will make sure you're giving your body everything it needs to fuel your session and ignite that growth response.

For more detail on pre-workout nutrition, take a glance at the section over Meal Timing in the Nutrition Section of the book.

MUSIC

As soon as you step foot in that weight room, you enter a whole new world.

This is your bubble and your sanctuary, so as you plug into your new reality, plug your earbuds into your ears and enter a new mental state fueled by sound. The outside world is now a thing of the past. This is what you've been waiting for all day. Live it up.

Get your beats thumping and pumping during warm-ups to prime your inner state for handling the weights. So much effort is given to feeding our muscles, but not enough is given towards giving our minds the proper fuel it needs. Music is a must [2].

MUSIC SELECTION

For your warm-ups, pick out tracks that boost your mood but don't deliver the full dosage of pure power just yet. Keep them at an enjoyable but modest volume.

This will create contrast between your warm-ups and the major work of the workout itself. You don't want to be hyped and riled up when you're in your warm-up phase or else that juicy musical impact it has will lose its potency where it really matters.

When it's time to let the real workout rip, switch from the pre-workout tracks to the prestige tracks on your playlist, and bump up the volume.

The contrast it creates will make things bang like a brutal bullet.

BODY TEMPERATURE

Before doing a thing in the gym, you need to ensure that the body and muscles are warm and ready for the workout ahead. There are several options here:

- Hop in a hot shower. This will get your body temperature up and help make you loose and limber. It also works because of the effect of coming into the workout feeling and smelling fresh & rejuvenated. When you feel like a slob, you act like one. It doesn't have to be a long shower. 5 minutes can do the trick just fine.
- Hopping in the sauna for a bit also works for the same reasons, and most commercial gyms have one.
- A heating pad can add more targeted heat that can also work in bringing heat to the muscles you are preparing to train. Working out cold and tight is a recipe for disaster.
- Get on the treadmill for a couple minutes and walk at a brisk pace. Notice here I said treadmill - not stationary bike. The gym is no place to sit around.

The goal here is to get up, get moving, and shuttle blood to the muscles and joints.

These tricks are especially useful in the mornings, colder winter months, and after long periods of being sedentary or relatively inactive to warm & wake the body up a bit to prepare for the pre-workout preparations and warmups.

If you already have an active lifestyle and are not going from sedentary to gym level intensity, this is an optional step.

FOAM ROLLING

There are very few people who are structurally sound enough to dive straight into the weights. That's where these next steps assist.

A brief, 2-3 minute circuit of foam rolling, gliding over muscles with a lacrosse or tennis ball placed against a wall, or even using a massage cane pre-workout are excellent methods for preparing your muscle tissues for the workout ahead and enhancing mobility and range of motion.

Pre-workout foam rolls don't need to be excessive or all-encompassing. 5-10 good rolls over the main muscle groups will do the trick, and you'll note an improvement in how you feel and move both immediately and progressively over time as you continue the practice. *You will learn more about foam rolling later in the book.*

STRETCHING

Once you've done the foam rolling, you will feel more refreshed and limber. This is where you need to move your muscle across its new range of motion to build good motor patterns. The first step in this is very light, short stretching.

Stretching your hip flexors, calves, pecs, and lats in particular will allow you to perform better over the functional range of your core exercises.

Do them gently, and hold them for no more than 5-10 seconds. Your goal is not to lengthen the muscle. It is to move it through its range of motion to allow you to have a productive training bout.

MOVEMENT/ACTIVATION DRILLS

Some movement drills before a workout will get the body activated and moving through its planes of motion the correct way. The things that should be firing are, and the things that shouldn't are behaving. Run through the following:

MOBILITY CIRCUIT

T-Spine Extensions	2-3 reps each section
Glute bridges (banded)	8-10 repetitions
Walking Lunges w/ Rotation	5 reps each side
Wall Slides	8-10 repetitions
Chin Tucks	8-10 repetitions

Detailed explanations can be found in the section on mobility in a later Chapter of the book.

These should be done at least once a day, and the pre-workout warm up can be a good place to include them. Done circuit style, you'll be done in 2 minutes. Do them.

Some may find that they do better by including them throughout the day as well - in morning before kicking off their day and at night after the day has thrown them out of whack, for example. This will aid in aligning poor posture, help you feel and move better throughout the day, and straighten you out before bed and a deep night's sleep.

WORKING WEIGHT RAMP UPS

After all of the above has been performed, now we can get into the real weights. The body is loose, limber, firing where it's supposed to be, and ready to start handling the workout movements properly while adding weight to get ready for the hard sets.

A lot of lifters get themselves into trouble here. Weight warm ups such as the following are not uncommon:

<u>Squats with a working weight of 225lbs</u>

135 X 12

155 X 10

185 x 8

205 x 6

215 X 2

Working sets

If your goal is to get a workout in and sap your potential before your real workout even begins, then that's a great way to do it.

The main goal of weight warm-ups is to prepare the body and central nervous system for the REAL workout ahead. You want just enough to calibrate your movements for the exercise through good form and proper muscle activation and prepare the nervous system for the heavier weight looming in the distance.

Consider this weight warm-up for contrast:

<u>Squats with a working weight of 225lbs</u>

Bar x 10 (optional)
135 x 6
185 x 4
205 x 2
225 x 1 (optional)
Working sets

This is *much* more effective.

If any additional warm-up work needs to be done, then it needs to be handled in the steps leading up to the weight warm-ups.

Lift the weight properly with pristine form and fire off like it was your working set. The last warm-up set can be of the working weight simply to feel the weight in your hands and acclimate to the weight before doing the real thing. As an old saying goes:

MAXIM OF AESTHETICS: WHEN IT'S LIGHT, TREAT IT LIKE IT'S HEAVY. WHEN IT'S HEAVY TREAT IT LIKE IT'S LIGHT.

When combining multiple compound movements and large muscle groups in the same workout, you'd perform the above for both.

Warm-ups for the secondary or isolation exercises typically isn't necessary unless it's a different movement type (think pull-downs after barbell rows), but if you feel the need, go for it to get in your groove and calibrate your body better.

SMALLER MOVEMENTS

Finally, some individuals may find that grabbing a pair of 5lb dumbbells and knocking out some curls, lateral raises, or kickbacks can help prepare their joints a bit better for the work ahead.

This is individual and can usually be accomplished with the regular exercises themselves, but it is worth mentioning for its utility with those who do need it. It'll send more blood to these areas and help in preparing the joints for peak performance.

GET YOUR MIND RIGHT

The final important component of our warmups are our visualizations and mental focus. You can't simply go from your regular day into an intense workout. Just as you prep your body, you must prep your mind before heading into battle [3,4].

REFRESH YOUR MOTIVATION

Everyone needs to have a motivation folder on their phone in or in their wallet. It should be on hand at all times and include pictures of your goals, desires, and quotes that motivate you. Prior to and even during your workouts, look at these things and connect with their message.

Focus intensely, and picture yourself really achieving these things. Make them a part of your reality right now in the current moment. Imagine yourself already there and living it. See it. Feel it. Taste it. Experience it. You are synchronizing your present moment with your future.

<u>DIG DEEP</u>

Discover the things that move you intensely. Your anger, your hate, your frustrations, and your deepest desires can create tidal waves of intense emotions that can compel you to act with fervent force and relentlessness. We must control these wisely or they will destroy us, create suffering, and stifle us. During our workout, we can release the beast within us and harness its strength to tap into forces we never knew possible.

These are powerful techniques, and we can utilize them before and even during our sets to ignite the fire deep within us that can move mountains and take us to new heights.

SHUT OUT DISTRACTIONS

The phone has turned from a medium of communication to a medium of gratification. The only function your phone should be serving during a workout is to fuel your music, provide your dose of motivation, double as a stopwatch, and look up/record your workouts.

Put it on silent/do not disturb, and go into your notification settings to turn off any unnecessary lock screen notifications that may distract your attention when going to change your song or check the time.

Which ones are unnecessary? All of them.

Outside of an emergency, the world can wait. This is your time to disconnect from the world and pour yourself into your workout.

ALL DAY, EVERY DAY

All of these recommendations have dealt with the more immediate time periods pre-workout, but the cold hard truth is that a fantastic workout is slow-cooking all day and night. Just like a hearty Winter stew from the crockpot, it takes time for all the flavors to seep out and mix together.

Your daily life, relationships, passions, habits, and so on will strongly influence your workout quality. Work on them.

This is often overlooked, but someone's overall life has a huge impact on their physical performance, and you will do your best when you are firing on all cylinders everywhere you go.

SUMMARY: PRE-WORKOUT

To help you in carrying out your warm up properly and in order, let's condense that down to a workable pre-workout checklist:

1. NAIL YOUR PRE-WORKOUT NUTRITION
2. DIAL UP THE MUSIC
3. WARM UP THE BODY
4. FOAM ROLL
5. LIGHT STRETCHING
6. MOBILITY DRILLS AND MUSCLE ACTIVATIONS
7. WORKING WEIGHT RAMP UPS
8. GET YOUR MIND RIGHT
9. SHUT OUT ALL DISTRACTIONS
10. CONQUER

This shouldn't take any more than 10-15 minutes to perform. Anything more than that is just playing around and would be better spent being addressed in other areas of your life and daily routine.

Work through steps 3-6 on your off days with special attention. This is also applicable during deloads and time off (see next chapter). Steps 5-6 can be done lightly as needed throughout the day to keep you grooving in tip top shape.

The workout itself will only take an hour tops, so there's *no* excuses why you can't fit in a solid warm-up protocol before your workouts and get a solid hour of greatness out of it.

Make it happen and *make it a habit.*

22

DELOADS AND
TIME OFF

*I*N AN IDEAL UNIVERSE, you'd be able to go full blast
170% of the time without any repercussions. You'd be bullet-
proof. Invincible. You'd pound that gym like a war drum and
see steady progress forever and ever.

Yet this isn't the case. You are pushing hard in the gym to *overload*
the muscles and stimulate growth, so you're bound to get banged
up, beat down, and stagnate as the workouts take their toll on the
body.

What's the solution?

You'll be including deloads and time off. Avoid them at your own
peril.

MAXIM OF AESTHETICS: REST IS JUST AS IMPORTANT AS ROUTINE

DELOAD PRINCIPLES

A deload is a period of time in which the training is deliberately light and easy to allow for rest and full recovery to take place.

This allows the mind and body to "catch up" and fully adapt to the stress that's been placed on it through overloading training. You can't go hard forever, and every program needs to factor in the need to get fresh and harden up the gains that have been made.

Incorporating deloads regularly will enable you to:

- Sidestep plateaus
- Allow for full, proper recovery and adaptation
- Safeguard against overtraining and overuse injuries
- Assist in joint health
- Provide psychological relief and contrast

HOW OFTEN

On average, if you're training hard via my recommendations, every 6-8 weeks *at most* a deload must be implemented.

The more frequent and intense the training, the more frequent and necessary the deload. The longer the periods between deloads, the longer they need to be. A 3:1 training:deload ratio is a good starting point.

Don't fear losing your gains by deloading [1,2,3]. Although it sounds counterintuitive, by resting up, you'll be driving *up* your capacity to make more gains.

Outside of these planned deloads, if you find yourself stalling or grinding down, deload and bring yourself back up to speed.

HOW TO DELOAD

During a deload, reduce the working weights by 20% for 1-2 weeks and perform the rest of the workout as usual. When done over 2 week stretches, the first week will be 20%, and the second week will be 10%. If you have added in extra sets for more volume or are implementing drop sets or burn outs, then these need to be scaled back. During a deload, go nowhere near fatigue or failure (5+ RITTs easily). That defeats the purpose.

For example, if your working weight for an exercise is 200 lbs, on the first week of a deload you would do the same work with 160lbs. On the second week, you would bump that to 180 lbs. Then on the third week, you will be in a new cycle starting off at your working weight from the last week of your previous cycle.

As you do this, bring your full attention back to the movements and focus on fine tuning your form. The weights are lighter, so use this as an opportunity to really refine and polish your technique and focus on the muscles that are doing the work. Develop that mind-muscle connection and be aware of your entire body during the movement to cut out any unnecessary motion or bad habits. These catch up on you over time, and deloads are an excellent time to pull the weeds.

SWAPPING OUT EXERCISES

If you are going to switch out exercises in your program, it is during the deload that they should be done.

This will allow you to re-program your body and mind for the new lifts before you hit them hard for the next training cycle. You need to calibrate and coordinate your movement patterns to reap the maximum benefit from your lifts.

GET FRESH

Deloads are not lazy periods. During your deload, continue all of the other things you should be doing to take care of yourself structurally.

Continue foam rolling, working on your corrective drills, working out any kinks or tender areas, and get re-aligned and in tip top shape to handle the next training cycle. Take daily walks, get up and move, and destress your life by clearing up anything on your agenda that may have been put on the backburner due to training hard. Spend time with friends and family, and use this as an opportunity to shift priorities.

This will rejuvenate you and when you feel better, are structurally sound, and have your life firing on all cylinders, you'll be able to harvest more from your workouts in the next phase of your training.

DELOADS DURING DIETING

With a lower training volume training routine for cutting that I've proposed, deloads aren't going to be as frequently necessary. However, that is not to say you should wipe them off the table altogether. If you are looking at prolonged periods of dieting of 8 weeks or more, deloads are an excellent tool to enlist.

For 1-2 weeks, bring your calories back to maintenance levels and deload following the principles given in this chapter. At least 1 workout for each muscle group during this period should be at regular intensity to take advantage of the higher calories.

This will allow you to maintain your performance levels better and intersperse your periods of a caloric deficit with periods of regular caloric intake that put you in a prime position to weave more enjoyment into the process.

DELOADS DURING MAINTENANCE

During prolonged maintenance phases, your volume and frequency in the gym will be lower, so a deload is required only once every 3 months or thereabouts.

You aren't pushing yourself as hard in the gym, so the stress to your system isn't high enough to warrant frequent deloads. You're deloading in between your workouts all the time.

Complete time off counts for these periods, and more information on this can be found later in the Chapter.

REACTIVE DELOADING

As you progress in your training career, you will form a tight bond with your body and learn to decipher the signals it gives you via your performance and how you feel in and out of the gym.

If you begin to note signs of overtraining, injury and irritation flaring up, or general lack of desire to train, implement a reactive deload outside of your regularly scheduled programming.

There is little lost by dipping out early to recharge, but there is a tremendous amount to lose if you stay stubborn and push forward.

TIME OFF

Outside of formal deloads, take complete time off from the gym at least twice per year for a week. Time *completely off.*

You won't be touching the weights, but you can and should still be active doing things that you enjoy year-round. The focus is to take a break mentally and physically from the weights. Don't be afraid; you won't shrink and wither away from staying away from the weights for a while.

Continue doing your foam rolling. Continue some simple mobility drills. Continue your stretches. Enjoy more hot baths, eat well, and sleep a little more than usual. Schedule yourself a good massage. Discover a new interest or hobby. Go out to eat or the movies with friends. Live life and get fresh. That's what this is all for anyways.

23

CARDIO

Heaven cannot brook two suns, nor earth two masters.
Alexander the Great

Walk into the gym at any time of the day, and you're sure to see people lined up on the cardio equipment chugging away. Seeing this day in and day out, and you're sure to start to question whether you should be one of them. Maybe you even feel guilty as you see them all working hard while you stroll right by to crush your workout. Should you? What's up with cardio?

REMEMBER YOUR MISSION

The very first thing you need to do when thinking about cardio is to refer back to the analogy I gave in the earlier chapter of the Objective of Training regarding putting your marbles in the right buckets. You only have so many to go around, and where you place them will determine your results. Your training must be specific to your goal and how you organize your training must support your goal. Secondly, think of what we have gone over regarding training intensity, volume, frequency, and exercise selection. Where was cardio in all of this? Oh wait. It wasn't there.

Therefore, when you look at cardio, you must first understand that it is *doing nothing* for your goal of muscle hypertrophy, and by including it, you are necessarily taking away from your time, energy, and potential in other areas – including your life. Understanding this is the crucial first step. But is that enough? No. Because not only does cardio not contribute to muscle growth, it also *opposes it*. Let's look at why.

WISHFUL THINKING

It would be pretty badass to be in two places at once. I mean, think of all the cool things you do and what you could get away with. Maybe someday in the future we'll have the technology to make that happen, but as for right now, you can only be in one place and move in one direction at a time. The same things apply in training and nutrition.

You see, the adaptations to cardio and weight training operate via distinct mechanisms that oppose each other. Numerous studies have demonstrated that lots of cardio and weight training will reduce your gains and lead to inferior results in both [1,2]. You can't have it all. If you want to be great at something, you need to specialize.

FAT LOSS FLAWS

But what about fat loss? It doesn't take a genius to realize that most people trickling onto the treadmills are doing so to burn calories and torch fat. Surely you can't kill princess cardio altogether! Watch me. Cardio for fat loss is also a shaky proposition.

The amount of calories burned from cardio are actually very low - depressingly so when you look at the time and effort involved. For a 150lb individual, 30 minutes of running at a good pace will only burn 300 calories, and 30 minutes of brisk walking will burn half that at most, with only 150 calories being burnt.

Now consider that you can demolish 300 calories in 3 minutes by what you put on your dinner plate. Is that a good trade off to you? To really drive this home, that same 150lb person will burn over **1600** calories just by their natural processes of staying alive.

Moral of the story? Get your diet straight before you even think about cardio.

HEALTH

Last but certainly not least, you must be wondering about cardio for health reasons. All that muscle is good, but it means nothing if you're not healthy. I agree 100%.

But weight! Something that no one seems to realize is that *weight lifting generates cardiovascular benefit too* [3,4]. Intuitively, you already knew this from experience but the word 'cardio' threw you off. 30 seconds a set for an hour is a form of cardio in its own right.

Add supersets, and you will understand this even more. Staying healthy is more of a function of *being active* than doing cardio.

In fact, I would argue that a properly structured resistance training regimen is superior to cardio alone because it not only generates cardiovascular benefit but also contributes to muscle, bone, and joint health.

AESTHETIC USE OF CARDIO

If there's anything left, let's look at what we've got so far. Cardio:

- Does not contribute to optimal hypertrophy
- Eats into recovery space and time
- Actually opposes hypertrophic adaptations
- Is an inefficient fat loss tool
- Is not necessary for overall health

Well damn. Is there any use for cardio at all or should we just go ahead and exile it from the kingdom altogether?

No. You're an architect of aesthetics and you realize that *everything can have its place.* And despite being ugly, cardio is not entirely useless. Cardio can:

- Help alleviate stiffness and soreness
- Boost moods and well-being
- Assist in a structured dieting phase

Therefore, small amounts can be just fine in the bigger picture. But small amounts of *what kind*? That is the question.

TYPES OF CARDIO

There are 3 forms of cardio that are commonly performed out there: High Intensity Interval Training (HIIT), Moderate Intensity Steady State (MISS), and Low Intensity Steady State (LISS).

HIIT IT AND QUIT IT?

HIIT is a style of cardio characterized by near all-out effort followed by complete rest or very light effort. Sprints for 15-30 seconds followed by a 60-90 second rest interval for a 15-20 minute duration are a commonly used approach. It is often touted as the best method by being time efficient and getting rid of the interference effect of cardio and lifting, but HIIT is hard on the body and can impede recovery – especially while dieting. Not good if lifting at peak performance is your goal.

SWING AND A MISS

MISS is more in the endurance realm of things and involves sustained intensities of 30+ minutes. Long runs, lengthy cycling, and many team sports are examples of this. Here, the interference effect is most pronounced, and large amounts of this will absolutely impair optimal hypertrophy adaptations.

LISS IS MORE

LISS is light, low-level exercise like walking, bike rides, leisurely swimming, and day to day activities. It is easy on the mind and body and can be done every day for 45 minutes-1hr+ with minimal interference that will damage gains or recovery. Based on this, you can see which would be best for your goals.

THE VERDICT

For the reasons outlined here, formal cardio is vastly overrated and even counterproductive to maximizing hypertrophy if often used.

If you're going to incorporate any at all, simply incorporate some easy LISS on your off days for a little daily exercise. 20-30 minutes on these days is just fine, and you can break it up however you like. You should not feel drained or expending much effort with this, and if you are, you need to pull back.

MISS can be done for leisure 2-3x/week if it suits your lifestyle, but make it something you enjoy, keep it easy on the body, and keep it separate from training by several hours or on your off days [2].

CUTTING CONSIDERATIONS

For a little extra calorie burn to contribute to your caloric deficit or in sidestepping cutting plateaus, cardio can come in handy, but diet should always be looked at before adding in dedicated cardio sessions, and the least amount should be done to generate the rate of fat loss that you need.

2-3x/week for a little extra calorie burn is more than enough [5], and the specific time you do it when it comes to fat loss is largely unimportant outside of individual preference [6], so long as it is away from your weight training sessions. Off days or several hours away from training are your best bet.

For both of these applications, make sure to calculate your estimated caloric burn via an online calculator per activity and factor it into your caloric intake that you'll learn about next:

PART IV: NUTRITION

24

FOUNDATIONS OF NUTRITION

Let thy food be thy medicine and thy medicine be thy food.
Hippocrates

ITTING THE GYM IS A WASTE OF TIME IF you don't match your workout kills with your kitchen skills. Nutrition is unequivocally the most vital component of the body composition puzzle and profoundly affects our overall health, mood, mental function, workout performance, and physique construction goals.

NO TRAINING ROUTINE WILL OUTPERFORM A BAD DIET.

Here, we will optimize your nutrition to maximize your results.

GOALS OF NUTRITION

Ultimately, the optimal diet accomplishes *all* of the following goals:

I.   Provide the body with the energy & nutrients for optimal mental/physical functioning and health
II. Satisfying and enjoyable
III. Simple, flexible, sustainable
IV. Support our physique & performance goals

Not one. Not two. *ALL*. Food is more than just fuel. It's a key part of life. You will use it to optimize your results, but no matter what, you **must** make sure that you keep things in perspective to get *and maintain* your results. If you ever have any questions about what to do with your nutrition, make sure it resonates **with all 4.**

FACTORS OF NUTRITION

In order to achieve the above goals, there are a few factors at your disposal that you can manipulate and optimize. These key factors of nutrition, listed in order of importance to your physique goals, are:

I.   CALORIC INTAKE
II. MACRONUTRIENT COMPOSITION
III. MEAL SPLIT (SIZE/TIMING/FREQUENCY)
IV. FOOD/MEAL CHOICE
V.   MICRONUTRIENT/FLUID INTAKE
VI. SUPPLEMENTATION

This is the order that we will attack the beast of nutrition and go about setting up the optimal plan.

I. CALORIC INTAKE

Calories are #1 when it comes to nutrition. If any diet works, it's because it bows down to King Calorie and manages them properly. Calories will determine your entire dietary budget.

II. MACRONUTRIENT COMPOSITION

The macronutrients, protein, carbs, fats, and alcohol, are what you will *spend* those calories on. The amount you spend on each will vary and help you optimize your physique goals.

III. MEAL SPLIT (SIZE/TIMING/FREQUENCY)

The way you split those calories and macros up and spread them across the day is what is known as your meal split.

IV. FOOD/MEAL CHOICE

Within that meal split, you'll be eating different kinds of foods and combining them into meals to accomplish your goals effectively.

V. MICRONUTRIENT/FLUID INTAKE

Not to be forgotten, every solid diet needs to factor in vitamins, minerals, and the amount of fluids you're drinking. This is what allows your body to carry out all of the things it needs for optimal health and functioning.

VI. SUPPLEMENTATION

Lastly, supplements are there for any deficiencies or minor boosts.

STEP BY STEP NUTRITIONAL ATTACK STRATEGY

What is your goal?

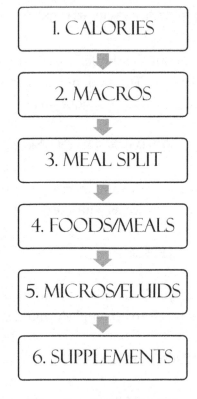

1. CALORIES

2. MACROS

3. MEAL SPLIT

4. FOODS/MEALS

5. MICROS/FLUIDS

6. SUPPLEMENTS

R E S U L T S

This is the recipe, but to ensure that the essence of this is really hammered home, take a glance at the pie chart on the next page to see just how these factors stack up against each other when it comes to forging the ideal physique.

IMPORTANCE FOR PHYSIQUE CONSTRUCTION

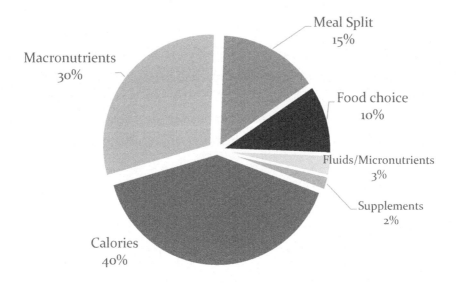

Meal Split
15%

Macronutrients
30%

Food choice
10%

Fluids/Micronutrients
3%

Supplements
2%

Calories
40%

Although this is the hierarchy of importance, ALL of these nutritional factors are important and form a piece of the physical puzzle. None are to be neglected if you desire the best results.

CHECK YOURSELF

Whenever a factor of diet is brought up pertaining to physique goals, it needs to be looked at with regards to its position in the hierarchy.

If a slice of that chart is smaller than another section, it CAN NOT and WILL NOT make up for or undo the effect of the larger section.

In other words, don't stress or waste even a morsel of your time with philosophical questions or compulsive little manipulations about meal timing, food choice, or supplements before you've addressed calorie or macronutrient intake. You have to pass through the individual steps. You cannot fly.

Read it 10 times. 100 times. 1000 times if you have to. Record yourself reading out the order out loud and listen to it as you sleep like old school Learn X Language of Your Choice While You Sleep tapes as if you were going to be kidnapped by deranged clowns and tortured unless you could recite the order of importance to them.

That's how crucial this is to understand when it comes to nutrition.

REVIST THE 10 LAWS OF THE ARCHITECT OF AESTHETICS

Lastly before embarking on your nutritional quest, recall the 10 Laws of the Architect of Aesthetics:

I.	HONOR YOUR GOAL
II.	THE BODY OPERATES ON A SPECTRUM
III.	THE BODY ACTS IN PHASES
IV.	THERE ARE NO HARD RULES. ONLY TECHNIQUES AND TOOLS
V.	CONSIDER ALL OF THE VARIABLES ON HAND
VI.	THE BODY IS MASTERFULLY BUILT TO SURVIVE AND ADAPT
VII.	SIMPLICITY IS THE SOLUTION
VIII.	MAKE GOLD OF WHAT IS GIVEN
IX.	STAY HUMBLE
X.	NEVER FORGET THE HUMAN BEING

The field of nutrition is a bloody battlefield filled with legends, treachery, witchcraft, deceit, and more warring tribes than ancient Israel. Staying true to these 10 Laws will keep your mind right and allow see past the smoke and mirrors.

You will understand the components of nutrition for what they are and use this knowledge for your benefit and for your glory.

If not, it will be your downfall.

25

CALORIES

C ALORIC INTAKE IS THE MOST IMPORTANT
FACTOR of nutrition for sculpting the body. It's your
dietary budget and will influence what you eat, how much,
when, and how you'll look because of it.

Nothing else matters if you don't have your calories under control.
You won't make gains, you won't get shredded, and you're wasting
your time worrying about anything else diet related. Get it right or
pay the price. Calories are King.

WHAT ARE CALORIES?

Everywhere you go, you hear all this talk about calories.

Any of these sound familiar?

"This has a lot of calories"
"I burned a lot of calories at the gym"
"I'm trying to cut my calories."

...and all that jive. But what are they?

Look at it like this. Your body is a high-powered machine, and just like any magnificent machine, it needs energy to run. So you feed it that energy, and then it burns that energy up to do its thing and live life. Lather, rinse, repeat.

Well, calories are just a measure of that energy.

The foods you eat contain calories, and your body burns calories day and night, rain or shine. The balance between the calories you consume and the calories you burn is what you will use to bring about changes in your physique.

To understand why that's the case, let's look at something known as the energy balance equation.

THE ENERGY BALANCE EQUATION

We live in a Universe full of a bunch of laws, one of which is known as the First Law of Thermodynamics: *Energy cannot be created or destroyed. It can only change form.* In its simplest form:

ENERGY IN = ENERGY OUT

Because our body runs on energy, we're also bound by this law, and for our sake it looks like this:

CALORIES IN = CALORIES OUT + CHANGE IN BODY STORES

It holds true no matter which spooky little witch doctor argues otherwise. We're interested about the *Change in Body Stores* part, and we'll use the *Calories In* and *Calories Out* parts to do it.

You can rearrange the equation in all sorts of ways, but rather than whip you with all the math to see how this works, let's do something more practical instead:

OF MUSCLES AND MONEY

Visualize money.

To pay for the stuff you want and need (**calories out**), you offer value to the world to make money (**calories in**). If you don't have enough money to cover your costs, you've got to go to the bank and take some out of your account (**body storage**). If you make more money than you spend, then you can deposit it in your account (**store as fat**) or use it to invest (**store as muscle**).

This is more or less how calories work in the body. **Calories are dietary currency,** and 3500 calories add up to about 1lb of fat. On the other hand, 1lb of muscle costs about 3500 calories of energy and material to make.

Now let's take that analogy and apply it to getting aesthetic:

❧ CALORIE DEFICIT

When you burn more calories than you take in, your body will snatch those calories from its storage in the body to cover its needs.

- 301 -

This is how you burn fat and bring out the carved in detail and definition of your physique.

❧ CALORIE SURPLUS

When you take in more calories than you burn, those extra calories will get stored away. They can be stored as fat and muscle, but relax. By working out and setting up our diet right, we'll maximize our ability to put those extra calories towards solid muscle growth.

NET CHANGE OVER TIME

The energy balance is like a teeter totter and moves up and down all the time depending on how many calories you're eating and how many you're burning, so you are "depositing" and "withdrawing" all the time.

What really matters is the NET BALANCE over the course of an extended period of time. This will determine the long lasting changes of your body composition and is the reason why precision meal timing and meticulous cycling is a losing battle outside of subtle, general recommendations that I will show you.

In other words, you can be in a 1000 calorie surplus one week and gain weight, but if you are in a 1000 deficit the next, the net is 0 because the two weeks cancel each other out. Remember: the body works over periods of time, so focus on the long term changes when your goal is muscle gain or fat loss.

But how do we know what balance even is?

Excellent question. The calories in side is fairly simple. You simply choose how much food to consume. But determining how many calories are going out is a different story that's influenced by many things, so let's tackle it head on.

How many calories do we really burn and what impacts this?

FACTORS INFLUENCING CALORIE BURN

The *Calories Out* side of the Energy Balance Equation - also called caloric burn, caloric expenditure, or TDEE (total daily energy expenditure), is determined by a few driving factors to varying degrees:

BASAL METABOLIC RATE (BMR)

A wise man once said that the two truths to life are that you will pay taxes and that you will die. This is incomplete, for as it turns out, you also must eat because your body has energy requirements related to the mere fact of being alive.

Your Basal Metabolic Rate (BMR) is the amount of calories that your body burns by carrying out its regular functions necessary for life - independent of anything else you do such as eating, daily activity, and regular exercise.

This is the biggest generator of calorie burn there is unless you have ungodly levels of exercise throughout the day. BMR can account for 75% of your daily caloric expenditure if you are sedentary.

Gender, weight, and age (amongst other things) factor into how much is burned for your BMR. All things held equal, men burn more than women, heavier individuals burn more by default than lighter ones, and younger people burn more than older people.

It stays roughly constant, although prolonged dieting can also have the effect of lowering this slightly as the body becomes more efficient and down-regulates its energy expenditure.

TEF (THERMIC EFFECT OF FEEDING)

The thermic effect of feeding is the amount of energy that it takes for your body to process the food you intake. So not only does your body charge you for life, but it also institutes taxes. How sweet.

TEF accounts for around 10% of the ingested calories (200 calories for a 2000 calorie diet), but this varies slightly depending on the content of the diet. Higher protein diets have higher caloric burn in this department, but before you wet yourself and start dialing up magic proportions to eek out more calorie burn, the difference is not drastic, so use the rough estimate instead.

TEA (THERMIC EFFECT OF ACTIVITY)

The thermic effect of activity is the amount of energy you burn through your daily physical function - lifting weights, cardio, and day to day activities, for example. The more intense and longer the duration, the more calories are burned.

However, as you saw in the cardio Chapter, always keep in mind that the caloric burn from exercise is much lower than wishful thinking would have you believe.

For most people, their daily exercise is the biggest part of this unless you live a fast-paced lifestyle or are on your feet all day moving around for work. NOTE: Many consider regular daily activity outside of exercise to be NEAT, but for simplicity and visualization purposes, I'll be referring to it here as TEA. It's easier to calculate into the caloric burn estimates that you'll learn about.

Overall TEA can go down if you compensate for intense workouts by becoming a vegetable the rest of the day. This is worth noting. Especially for dieters getting very lean whose body wants to slow them down to burn less calories. This leads to our next point:

NEAT (NON EXERCISE ACTIVITY THERMOGENESIS)

NEAT refers to the all of the other little things that are hard to predict or factor in due to their inevitable variability amongst individuals. Sporadic moving around during the day, fidgeting, tapping your feet to the banger you heard on the radio, and other like things fall into this category. This is also called subconscious physical activity (SPA) but I prefer NEAT because it can swing like a monkey on espresso and is pretty damn "!NEAT!" to see happen.

When you think of someone with a "fast" or "slow" metabolism, it typically refers to the person's differences in this area. (And/or simply over/underestimating how many calories they're actually eating over time, but that's a tale for another day.)

When some people eat more, they simply subconsciously auto-regulate their activity and move around more to compensate and burn it off. Others don't. Genetics strike again [1].

HOW MANY CALORIES DO YOU NEED?

Before you can figure out how to build muscle or get lean, you need to figure out how many calories are needed to maintain your current body composition. There are several ways to figure out your maintenance, but here's my preferred option:

1. FIGURE OUT YOUR DAILY STANDARD CALORIE BURN
2. ADD EXTRA ACTIVITY/EXERCISE AS NEEDED

This is as good as it gets. By doing it this way, you have more flexibility, more precision, and more control between training days, off days, and so on.

Your energy requirements are *dynamic*, so to optimize progress, you want to ensure that the nutrition that is built off of that is as well.

WHAT YOU'LL NEED:

- Online calculators (TDEE and Calories burned per activity)
- Simple math

The calculators can easily be found by a simple web search. Some smartphone applications have this as well, so it's quick and easy.

STEP 1: FIGURE OUT YOUR DAILY STANDARD CALORIE BURN

For the first half of the equation, fire up the TDEE calculator and simply select the "Sedentary" (also seen as "No activity") option from the online calculator. Then plug in the necessary information such as your height, weight, age, gender, and so forth.

For example: after plugging in your information, the TDEE calculator determines your sedentary caloric expenditure to be 2000 calories. So:

OFF DAY: 2000 CALORIES

This is the baseline caloric intake if you were to chill all day and will serve as our platform to build off of. From here, depending on your daily routine, you can bump this value up to factor in for the extra activity you perform and use this as your standard for your off day by following the process in the next step.

STEP 2: ADD EXTRA ACTIVITY/EXERCISE AS NEEDED

Once you've got your standard intake figured out, you would add in the extra exercise or activity you perform above and beyond the usual.

If it's a training day and you had an intense gym session that burned 400 calories, you would add 400 calories to the figure produced by the calculator.

You can find out caloric estimates for activity and exercise burn based on your weight on other websites, but err on the side of conservatism because these can be overly optimistic. In general, weight lifting will only burn 300-400 calories max on average depending on your individual factors, volume, and the intensity of the session.

So now you've got:

TRAINING DAY: 2000 + 400 = 2400 CALORIES

If the day included being out running errands and making moves, you would add in the estimated activity burn for that. Let's assume you spent an hour and a half walking around the city and use 200 calories for sake of example.

BUSY DAY: 2000+200=2200 CALORIES

As noted, if you have a busy day every day, then this should be your standard "off day" intake.

If you did both, you would add in both the extra bouts of activity:

TRAINING DAY AND BUSY: 2000+400+200=2600 CALORIES

Easy. Check out the table below to see how everything stacks up:

	STANDARD CALORIES	CALORIES FROM EXTRA ACTIVITY	TOTAL CALORIC EXPENDITURE
REST DAY	2000	0	2000
TRAINING DAY	2000	400	2400
BUSY DAY	2000	200	2200
TRAINING AND BUSY	2000	400 + 200 = 600	2600

If you were to consume the same amount of calories as indicated by your expenditure, you would maintain your current weight.

These would be your calorie requirements on these days.

To maintain, you would consume the same amount of calories to match. To gain muscle, you would hit the weights and create a calorie surplus by consuming more calories than this. To burn fat, you would create a deficit by consuming less calories and/or increasing your requirements through more activity.

BODY WEIGHT AND ACTIVITY LEVEL CALCULATIONS

All of these calculations depend heavily on body weight and activity level, so get them as accurate as you can.

Body weight fluctuates day and night and throughout the week, so use an average of your weights unaffected by outside factors to get your starting point - every morning after a trip to the restroom and before any meals. This will also help you track the accuracy of your predictions.

Activity burn varies drastically depending on the activity, duration, and intensity. Online activity calculations can at times spit out radical, overly optimistic figures and need to be taken with a grain of salt, but for the most common activities (walking/running/lifting), they offer good estimates to work with. For those with an active daily life, pedometers are useful for tracking movement patterns- a clip on, smart watch, etc.

In the end, personal experience/results will dictate how we set this amount and for that reason, simply use these as starting points and adjust as needed, a common theme for everything training and nutrition.

SETTING THE SURPLUS/DEFICIT

Once you understand the energy balance equation and have your base calorie expenditure determined, you can start to look at how you would create a calorie surplus or deficit to provide the effect you're going after (put on muscle, burn fat, maintain cruising altitude).

Sure that sounds simple enough, but the question is, "how much of a surplus or deficit?"

- Too little, and progress will take forever for no good reason. This can be demoralizing and an easy way to erase progress by simple measurement or estimation errors.
- Too much, and you can get undesirable effects such as putting on too much fat in the case of muscle gain or losing muscle and becoming an irritable psycho in the case of fat loss.

Before we go any further, let's take a moment to clear up some common mistakes that are made when trying to determine the rate of change in body composition.

POUNDS

The most common recommendations given to people are to shoot for fixed, generic standards of 1lb of weight loss/weight gain per week in either direction.

"Gain muscle at a pound a week. Lose fat at a pound a week."

Sound familiar?

This is not how you do it.

First of all, 1 pound of muscle gain is different to a small female and a large man, and much different from a raw beginner to a more advanced lifter. There are different things going on within the body for different people that warrant a closer look at optimal rates to better *custom-fit* the nutritional approach *to the individual.*

Secondly, scale weight goes up and down like a bipolar basketball. You can lose or gain weight from 953 different reasons unrelated to the actual progress you want - *especially for women.* Taking averages over time can smooth this out, but the principle remains:

4lbs change on the scale is not necessarily 4lbs of fat or muscle.

And lastly, scale weight is not wholly indicative of physical appearance - and THAT'S our goal. Not impressing the scale. Scale weight is just ONE of the tools we have to measure progress. Pictures will tell the cold hard truth.

TIME FRAMES

Setting hard time frames is the next biggest mistake people make when determining their desired rate of change.

People always want to gain or lose 15 lbs or look a certain way within 10 weeks because of some trip, some fixed date in their head, or things of that nature, for example.

This creates a rigid guideline that creates too much mental investment, saps the process, and causes people to do ludicrous things that sabotage their progress when achieving that goal may even be physically impossible or very difficult mentally to do for that person in that time frame.

While no doubt it's good to establish a target to help in calculating a rate and setting goals, it's better to set a *range* based on a solid measure rather than a hard, fixed goal you plucked out of Wonderland. Start early, take things as they come, and do your thing.

9 pounds of progress may not be 10, but it's still 9.

This allows for some leeway due to error, more flexibility, stalls, and whatever else comes up without any undue mental stress. Kick back and relax. The progress will come.

% OF CHANGE

For these reasons, we'll be using the *rate of body weight change in relation to total body weight* (or lean body mass/ideal body mass in over or underweight individuals) when figuring out how to set your deficit or surplus. Doing so gives a much better standard for progress in our goals than hard time frames and random numbers.

We can use numbers as a guideline, but let's not forget they are only there to guide our main goal and must be used in conjunction with other measures (pictures, gym progress, etc.)

Keep these things in mind as we continue onwards.

MUSCLE GAIN

To stack on muscle optimally, you need a caloric surplus [2,3].

Can you gain muscle in at maintenance or in deficit? Absolutely. Is it optimal or sustainable? No way in hell.

AN ENERGY SURPLUS IS THE BIGGEST NUTRITIONAL FACTOR WE HAVE WHEN GROWTH IS THE GOAL.

If you do not eat enough, you will not grow. You do not filter feed from the air or use photosynthesis.

Raw beginners, lifters with higher body fat levels, and lifters coming back from injury or break can pull off some magic within the energy balance equation and build muscle without a surplus by using their stored energy to fuel growth, but that gain train doesn't last forever and gets harder and harder the leaner and more advanced you get.

Trying to grow without a calorie surplus is fighting an uphill battle with one hand behind your back. You might push forward for some time, but eventually you'll just end up stuck and falling down. Don't be afraid of getting fat. You will gain a *little* fat, but

1.   The added muscle will make you look better regardless
2.   It's necessary and will optimize your muscle gaining efforts.

We'll optimize that ratio and diet it off easily later.

Are you really going to push through those intense workouts and not even go anywhere from not eating enough? That's depressing.

PREPARE FOR LIFTOFF

If you're starting your aesthetic journey at a higher body fat percentage and are afraid of gaining more weight, diet down first by following the recommendations in the next section on Fat Loss while following a solid, structured training approach. Lean out to a level where you feel comfortable with your appearance, take a week or two to deload and eat at maintenance intake, and then push for growth by training hard and increasing your calories per my recommendations to capitalize.

Everyone else: Ensure you've been eating at maintenance for a couple of weeks and are well rested and fresh to hit the weights in pursuit of size gains. This is especially true if you've been cutting for a while. Doing so will ensure that your metabolism is firing on all cylinders and prepared for reaping the full benefits of the gaining phase ahead.

HOW MUCH OF A SURPLUS DO YOU NEED?

The conventional advice thrown around recklessly is "Eat big to get big".

This is terrible advice no matter who's giving it.

Do you want to just get big? Or do you want to be muscular and lean? No need to put on extra fat unnecessarily that'll just have to get dieted off later unless you have a fetish for caloric restriction.

As with most things in fitness, there is a law of diminishing returns when it comes to rate of muscle gain. No matter how nice it may be to think that a little fairy magically turns all the extra calories you eat into muscle, after you reach a certain caloric surplus, you're going to be slapping on fat like there's no tomorrow because hey - to your body, maybe there isn't.

WEIGHT GAIN

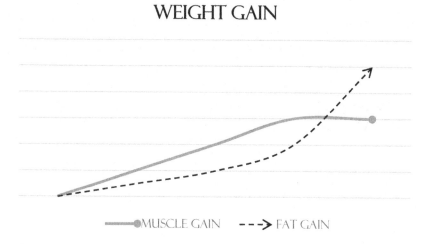

MUSCLE GAIN ---> FAT GAIN

As you increase your surplus, muscle gain tops out, and then it's nothing but fat gains.

Therefore, you want to consume enough calories to create a favorable anabolic environment and provide the necessary building blocks to MAXIMIZE muscle growth and MINIMIZE fat gain.

RATES FOR MUSCLE GAIN

With that in mind:

A good *starting point* for lean muscle gain is **0.25-0.5%** of total body weight gained per week for men. For women, roughly half of this (**0.125-0.25% weekly**) is a good measure, for although women have mighty muscular potential, women aren't physically equipped with the same machinery to put on muscle as quickly as men are.

The side you lean towards for the rate of muscle gain (0.25-0.5%) is most impacted by training status as judged by your performance ability in the gym and proximity to your genetic limits. The reason for this is due to the growth potential of the various training levels.

| 0.25%/WEEK | 0.375%/WEEK | 0.5%/WEEK |
| ADVANCED | INTERMEDIATE | BEGINNER |

When you're new to training, the body will soak up nutrients like a dehydrated sponge in the Sahara to adapt to the stress imposed by lifting, but the more your body has already adapted to training and progressed in strength and size, the less room there is to grow in relation to its growth potential. Therefore, the gains will be less plentiful and the caloric surplus should reflect that.

For this reason, beginners should lean towards the higher end of the spectrum to achieve maximal gains, and the more intermediate-advanced you get, the lower on the spectrum you will want to migrate to in order to keep the ratio of muscle: fat gain favorable.

Elite level lifters would theoretically need *even lower rates* of muscle gain, but this is tricky territory and won't be discussed here for practical purposes.

See below for how this would be reflected for lifters of various sizes and training levels.

% OF BODY WEIGHT GAINED PER WEEK BASED ON TRAINING STATUS

	0.25%	0.375%	0.5%
180lbs	0.45lbs/week	0.675lb/week	0.9lbs/week
150lbs	0.375lbs/week	0.563lbs/week	0.75lbs/week
120lbs	0.3lbs/week	0.45lbs/week	0.6lbs/week

*Women divide the above figures in half
Multiply by 3500 to get total weekly surplus

These values may seem low to many people conditioned to believe that rapid rates of muscle gain are achievable via natural means. However, recognize that over a year's span, the amount of muscle gained at these rates will make an undeniable impact on aesthetics.

This would produce about 20lbs of size added for men in their first year of training and roughly half that for women. This rate will decrease each year over time as you get more advanced and closer to your genetic limits.

See the chart for a graphical representation of how this goes down.

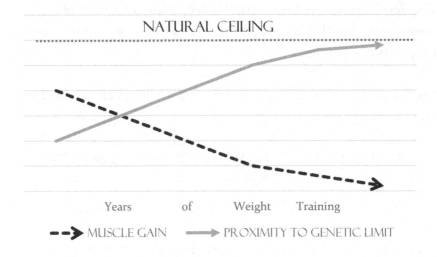

NATURAL CEILING

Years   of   Weight   Training

--→ MUSCLE GAIN   ━━→ PROXIMITY TO GENETIC LIMIT

THE GYM IS THE TRUE MEASURE

With the right training and dietary composition, adopting this rate of weight gain is a sound starting point to produce the results you want, but it *has got* to be analyzed against weight room progress and the various ways to measure body composition over time.

If you're not seeing gains in the gym, scale, and pictures while following a solid program like I've given in the book, you must add extra amounts of calories to adjust accordingly. 100 extra calories per day is a good place to start.

When in doubt for muscle gaining, it's better to stray on the side of caution and prefer to slightly overshoot the values to take advantage of your training. Short dieting stints done right will maintain the muscle while quickly stripping the fat gain - which will be minimized with such modest values in the first place.

Don't cut yourself short when it comes to adding mass.

HOW LONG?

I generally recommend alternating between longer gaining phases and shorter fat loss phases to keep people looking great year round while making gym progress and oscillating between different acceptable body fat percentages (8-12% for men, 16-20% for women). This is highly variable between people but any lower or higher, and you're not physiologically in the best situation for optimal rates of muscle gain and the muscle: fat gain ratio.

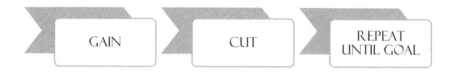

GAIN   CUT   REPEAT UNTIL GOAL

This will allow you to achieve maximal progress while keeping everything in harmony. If your ultimate goal is to have a lean physique, then you should live close to that every day and never get too far from it. That'll ensure you enjoy the whole process more and don't throw away your identity for no good reason. Determine your goal and start living in that neighborhood as soon as possible. This doesn't just stop at fitness.

Once you hit the upper limit of your body fat range, deload for at least a week, bring calories back down to maintenance, and then move into a cutting phase. This will stabilize your body and prepare you for the shred ahead.

Now let's look at fat loss.

FAT LOSS

Once you've built up some solid mass by lifting hard and feeding your body for prime muscle gain, it's time to trim up and get shredded, so you'll be diving into a fat loss phase. This will bring out the detail and definition in your muscles that will take an impressive physique into an astounding one. It will also bring out your natural facial structure, accentuate your proportions, and make your muscle shapes much more prominent to really round out your aesthetic appearance.

Let's see how it's done.

FAT LOSS FUNDAMENTALS

In order to lose fat effectively, you need to generate a caloric deficit. This can be achieved through:

- Dietary caloric restriction and/or
- Adding in additional activity such as cardio. (or nah)

DIET should *always* be looked at as the solution first BEFORE running to (get it) cardio because performing lots of cardio is nowhere near as efficient or practical and can interfere with weight training when done excessively.

You have better things to do with your life than watch daytime television on the treadmill like a hamster with hot flashes when you could make a simple swap in your diet, but it certainly can come in handy in certain contexts so let's not banish it to the Shadow Realm altogether now.

FACTORS INFLUENCING FAT LOSS

Cutting calories. Depressing, huh.

Well here's some refreshing news: The body can lose fat at a much faster rate than it can put on muscle. It may take 2 months to gain 4 pounds of muscle but half that to burn off the equivalent amount of fat. This is why you shouldn't fear the Fat Phantom when pushing for gains and eating in a moderate surplus.

However, you also have to balance this with maintaining performance and diet adherence/enjoyment. Cutting calories means eating less and moving more, so creating too large of a caloric deficit will lead you into trouble and make for a nightmarish experience at the expense of your hard work in the gym.

Why?

The higher your body fat percentage, the bigger a deficit you can get away with without hampering your workout performance, lifestyle, and sanity. The leaner you are, the smaller the deficit you can get away with.

The reason for this is because of the body's energy availability (food + energy stores) and the wide array of changes in the body that occur as a result of the level of that energy availability. Hormones and moods go haywire, and performance begins to nose dive.

The body's main objective is keeping you alive and well, not looking sexy, stacked, and shredded. So to the body, keeping a certain level of fat stores is a hot priority because if you get too low and food is scarce, you're SOL.

Bottom line is: More fat stores and more energy coming in, less problems. Less fat stores and less energy coming in, and your body is going to get pissed, so you must caress it like a delicate kitten to get the results you want. Therefore, the rule is this:

You want to lose fat as fast as you can while still enjoying the process and maintaining muscle/gym performance.

Very nice, how much? Let's look at the rates.

RATES FOR FAT LOSS

For fat loss, a good starting point is **0.5-1%** of body weight lost per week. The rate here should be set by body fat level [4,5].

As noted, your level of body fat will determine how fast you should aim to drop fat, so let's look at which side of the spectrum you should stay on.

I tend to break things down as such:

RATES OF BODY FAT LOSS BASED ON BODY FAT PERCENTAGE

Under 10% for men, 17% for women	0.5% of body weight per week
10-13% for men, 17-20% for women	0.75% of body weight per week
Above 13% for men, 20+% for women	1% of body weight per week

Use visual estimations. Calipers and handheld electric devices suck

You don't *have to* push for the maximal rate of fat loss you can get away with and can lose weight more slowly than this. Often times, *you may very well want to* for reasons of enjoyment and flexibility that I mentioned earlier. This simply represents the upper limit for sustained periods of dieting.

Also note that the rate of fat loss for women may also be slower in practice for various reasons that all the fine ladies reading this can nod their head to. Individual variation always plays a role here.

Now we can look at how that pans out for people of various weights:

RATES OF BODY FAT LOST PER WEEK

	0.5%	0.75%	1%
180lbs	0.9lb	1.35lbs	1.8lbs
150lbs	0.75lbs/week	1.13lbs/week	1.5lbs/week
120bs	0.6lbs/week	0.9lbs/week	1.2lbs/week

Multiply by 3500 to get total weekly deficit

These figures strike a good balance between a steady rate of fat loss, maintenance of performance/muscle, and diet adherence/satisfaction - all of which are crucial considerations for caloric restriction and the maintenance of the new body composition once you're down to your desired level of leanness.

When in doubt, opt for a slower rate.
Process beats all.

Individual factors are always most important, and slower rate allows for more flexibility. Dieting is nobody's favorite pastime. Slow and steady wins the race here. Big reason to stay lean enough in the first place.

As you lean out, remember to re-adjust your rate. If you start off at a higher body fat percentage and lose at 1% per week, you'll want to slow that down over time as you get leaner and leaner.

OTHER FAT LOSS CONSIDERATIONS

REFEEDS

The leaner you get when you are pursuing fat loss, the more it is in your best interest to start including what's known as 'refeeds'.

Simply put, refeeds are periods of higher calorie intake during a cutting phase where you are not in a deficit for that day. The purpose behind this is to provide a psychological break from the calorie deficit first and foremost by satisfying any little cravings and getting to enjoy a normalized diet with refilling muscle glycogen as a secondary benefit. I am not convinced there is a large benefit to metabolism or fat burning from refeeds, but they are still incredibly useful in the grand scheme of things, all things considered.

For refeeds, place calorie intake at maintenance or very mildly above (100-200 calories max). This should happen on training days and days of higher calories from social events or holidays that you will see next when we discuss Calorie Cycling. The extra calories from this day should come from a regular fat intake (if dropped from the values given in the Chapter on Macronutrients) and carbohydrates.

At 0.75-1% fat loss per week, you may need no refeeds. Once every 1-2 weeks is sufficient at the most, depending on how you are feeling. At 0.5% fat loss per week, a refeed should occur once per week, and if you are at very lean levels, there may be benefit in a refeed 2x/week. You will see how to incorporate refeeds in a calorie cycling setup later in the Chapter, and refeeds and diet breaks, our next topic, will be discussed again in the Chapter on Plateaus.

DIET BREAKS

Similar to refeeds, every 2-3 months a diet break should be taken [6]. This is a period of 1-2 weeks where you will eat at maintenance calorie intake with a 10% reduction factored in to adjust for any metabolic slowdown and normal dietary levels of carbohydrates and fat again.

This has many of the same benefits of refeeds, and after this period, you can either proceed with cutting again or slip into a maintenance phase or another gaining phase with a newly stabilized metabolism.

HOW LONG TO CUT

If you still have muscle mass to gain on the horizon, you should be cutting until you get to the lower level of your ideal determined body fat range. From here, you will eat at maintenance for a couple of weeks before jumping back into a gaining phase.

If you are cutting to get leaner than that, be very careful not to go too far. Very low body fat levels are not as aesthetically pleasing for the various reasons discussed in the chapter over aesthetics, and they bring with them several negative adaptations such as hormonal drops, adverse psychological effects, and unhealthy dietary habits. This is especially true for women.

If you have enough muscle mass, 7% for men and 14% for women is as low as you should ever reasonably go. If you need to get leaner than that, you're better off adding more muscle to improve your aesthetic appeal. You have been warned.

MORE CUTTING TIPS

Cutting will test your mental mantle and see what you're made of. Gaining is easy, but leaning out is where people fall flat. How often do you see folks with muscle? Often. How often do you see muscle *and* shreds? Exactly.

Stay patient, and stick to the sound principles I will lay out in the rest of the nutrition section of the book. Slow progress is better than no progress, so if you find yourself struggling, take a step back and weave more enjoyment and flexibility into the process, and do not forget how useful refeeds and diet breaks can be in getting to your goal.

Do not approach cutting with an attitude of restriction. You can still have a very satisfying diet even in a deficit. Stick to more filling foods and focus on enjoying your meals more.

To assist you with the mental aspect further, visit the Mindset section of the book, and learn to control your thoughts, feelings, and desires. You will be tempted by both your body and the world. Additionally, staying busy by managing your attention and staying firm to your goal will help you monumentally here. Cutting is an excellent time to ramp up your productivity and refine your mind.

SETTING THE TARGET CALORIES

So you've determined your rate of gain or loss.

To determine your weekly caloric deficit/surplus that you'll be adding to your maintenance calorie intake to accomplish your goal, simply take the figure produced and multiply by 3500, since as we saw earlier, 3500 calories is approximately how many calories are required to achieve one pound of fat loss or muscle gain.

For example, let's say you're a 160lb male beginner and want to stack on muscle. Your surplus could be figured out by the following:

(0.5% x 160lbs) x 3500
0.8lbs/week x 3500
= 2800 CALORIE SURPLUS PER WEEK

Once you've got that, it's best to divide this figure fairly evenly across the days of the week.

While the net is what's most important, there is also a limit to how much can be burned/gained in one day and running a huge surplus or deficit in one day to make up for it the next is not the wisest route to go down for psychological/lifestyle reasons, all things considered. So:

2800/7 = 400 CALORIE SURPLUS PER DAY *ON AVERAGE*

For a bit more fine tuning, you can opt for a 500 calorie training day and a 300 calorie surplus rest day, with calories more distributed around training - particularly after. You'll see that later in the chapter.

See. That wasn't so hard.

REMEMBER

As you go along in your process of gaining/losing weight, you must recalculate your maintenance level calories and the amount of calorie burn generated from activity.

Weight is a big factor in energy expenditure equations, so after losing/gaining, it is wise to rerun the numbers. Once every 2-4 weeks works well.

Let's look at some more examples now.

EXAMPLES OF CALCULATING CALORIE REQUIREMENTS

Achilles was one of the most badass warriors in history. Before becoming a hero of the Trojan War and seizing glory, he came to the architect of aesthetics to build his frame and put on strength. Let's see how we'd do that.

Achilles is 18 years old and sitting at 6'1, 170lbs and wants to put on muscle. He is a beginner and we've put him on a sound training program where he is lifting full body 3 times per week. He has an estimated caloric maintenance of 2600 calories on training days and 2300 calories on off days. How many calories should he consume daily to meet his goal?

$$((170 \times 0.5\%)(3500 \text{ calories}))/7$$
$$= (0.85 \text{lbs per week} \times 3500)/7$$
$$= 2975/7$$
$$= 425 \text{ EXTRA CALORIES PER DAY } _{ON\ AVERAGE}$$

Therefore, his calorie target will be:

TRAINING DAYS: 2600+ 425 = ~3025 CALORIES
OFF DAYS: 2300 + 425 = ~2725 CALORIES

Now let's say that Achilles hit 190lbs and wants to cut down and get diced. He is at 12% body fat, and his new maintenance intake is 2400 calories on off days and 2750 calories on training days.

How many calories should he consume?

$$(190 \times 0.75\%)(3500)/7$$
$$=(1.425)(3500)/7$$
$$=712.5 \text{ CALORIE DEFICIT PER DAY } \textit{ON AVERAGE}$$

For simplicity, we'll go ahead and round this to 700. Note here that this is the *maximum* rate of loss for Achilles. He may very well opt for a lower deficit but prolong his diet by a couple of weeks

This creates an interesting scenario because those 700 calories do not need to come from diet alone, and this is why dieters often incorporate cardio to avoid having to eat such few calories. In the following example, I'll offer an additional option that includes a LISS cardio session* estimated to burn 200 calories that adds to his energy expenditure per day so that his dietary reduction will only be 500 calories from his maintenance.

TRAINING DAYS: 2750 - 700 = 2050 calories per day
OFF DAYS: 2400 - 700 = 1700 calories per day
TRAINING DAYS WITH CARDIO: (2750+200)-700 = 2250 calories per day
OFF DAYS WITH CARDIO: (2400+200)-700 = 1900 calories per day

cardio is not a must and must be used sparingly.

As you can see, Achilles is only cutting his dietary calories by 500 in regards to his maintenance intake, but because he has done 200 calories worth of cardio, he is still creating the 700 calorie deficit.

And there you go. That's the way you set up a surplus or deficit to gain muscle or burn fat, and these are just the simple calculations. Now let's look at how you'd cycle calories.

CALORIE CYCLING

Our day to day lives are dynamic, and even with a relatively stable daily life, we still have to consider training days, off days, and the variances that this can produce for nutritional needs when it comes to optimizing our process. That's where cycling becomes incredibly powerful.

It is useful to:

- Keep fat gain in check during gaining phases
- Maintain muscle and enjoyment when dieting
- Stay lean and satisfied while maintaining
- Enjoy holidays, nights out, and social occasions
- Build in flexibility and offer variety to the diet
- Optimize desired outcomes via favorable nutrient partitioning and sensitivity

Picking one standard caloric intake for every day is the simplest, most standard option amongst the majority of aesthetics architects, but calorie cycling is an easy technique to carry out that delivers great benefits both physically and mentally.

On top of that, it gels marvelously with a moderate training frequency of 3-4 days/week as I've supported heavily in my routines thus far. This was no accident.

A comprehensive approach to physical development must be taken for an impactful 1-2 punch. Higher frequency (5+) training dilutes the effectiveness of cycling, but the base principles still remain.

SETTING UP THE CYCLING PATTERN

You've got your weekly rate established, so now it's up to you to decide how to split up your days. Here are some things to keep in mind when setting up your nutrition cycling plan:

TAKE THE GOAL AND LONG TERM INTO ACCOUNT

Based on your rate, we will be more focused on the *average* of a span of days rather than the individual days themselves. This means that:

- If your goal is to gain weight, the lower/higher values you select should allow for you to gain weight at the desired weekly rate.
- If your goal is to lose weight, the weekly outcome should have you losing weight at that weekly rate.
- If the goal is to maintain, your net balance should be 0.

HIGHER ON TRAINING DAYS AND SPECIAL OCCASIONS

Lifting weights is the biggest physical trigger there is for our aesthetic goals. You want to ensure that you have most of your calories around and after training for proper recovery and performance.

Therefore, training days and the day after should be higher calorie to take advantage of the effects of hitting the weights with the calories tapering off the further in distance you go from training. The way you schedule your calories in meals should follow suit.

Likewise, for maintenance and keeping your diet in check on special occasions or holidays, you should allot the space in your week so that you have a bigger calorie budget on this day. If you can schedule your training for that day, then it works out even better. However, don't make this a habit. Restricting your calories for the week to have very large spikes on the weekend is no way to live. Balance. Keep it mild or leave it for the big stuff.

AVOID LARGE SWINGS

When I say to go low-er and high-er in calories, this must be relatively mild.

Going 1000 calories over baseline and 1000 calories under baseline one day, going very high fat and low carbs then carb loading the next, and things of that nature are extreme variations in diet that should never be done outside of very specific protocols that are already pushing it and unnecessary.

Doing so has huge potential for generating eating disorders and cripples dietary flexibility and seamlessness, a very large component of any sustainable, well-rounded nutritional plan for making the acquisition of aesthetics a lifestyle that's enjoyable every day.

For special occasions coming up where you know there will be more calories, you should instead have a modest reduction in the days leading up to it or after.

All in all, calorie and macro cycling is an extremely effective, attractive method we have to get the results we want and maximally enjoy the process as well.

EXAMPLES OF CALORIE CYCLING

Below you will find examples of calorie cycling plans for various goals based on a lifter with a maintenance of 2400 calories on training days and 2000 on off days. They are intended to give you an idea of how the calorie distribution would work, and they are far from the only ways it can be done. The X here indicates a training day.

TRAINING 3 DAYS PER WEEK TO CUT

M	T	W	Th	F	S	Su	Total
1900	1500	1900	1500	1500	2400	1500	–
X	–	X	–	–	X	–	
-500	-500	-500	-500	-500	0	-500	-3000

Here you can see that there is a weekly deficit with a day of maintenance calories on Saturday for a training session. Ideally, this should be the hardest training session or favored muscle group. This is a "refeed" and is on a Saturday to account for any social occasions that may happen on this day.

To increase fat loss on the off days or allow for a bit higher intake on training days, a bit of cardio could be done. I recommend one complete off day per week, so 3 days of simple cardio for 200-300 calories burned would increase the weekly deficit without further cutting calories and can be a useful tactic when used sparingly and wisely.

Now let's look at 4x/week training with the goal of gaining.

TRAINING 4 DAYS PER WEEK TO GAIN

M	T	W	T	F	S	S	TOTAL
2900	2900	2300	2900	2300	3000	2300	
X	X	-	X	-	X	-	
+500	+500	+300	+500	+300	+600	+300	+3000

As you can see here, training days get the biggest dose of calories, and off days get less. Ideally, the major allotments of these calories are occurring around and after training especially and tapering off as time goes on. This is less important for beginners who are growing around the clock for days, but as you get advanced, it's worth taking a closer look. You'll see more about meal timing in a later chapter.

SET, ACT, OBSERVE, ADJUST

With all of the calculations and estimations out of the way, there's an important notice that must be made:

---

*Calorie requirements are a **moving target** - not an absolute, and any estimates or calculations will have to be adjusted based on the individual, alterations in daily activity, and the real-world results that are produced in the long run based on the starting values.*

Theoretically, everything may look freaking fantastic. But the TRUE TEST is what happens in real life. The numbers only give us a *target* to aim for. Energy expenditure is a dynamic beast.

IMPORTANT QUESTIONS

Once you set your caloric intake, check your progress every couple of weeks by asking yourself the following questions:

FOR GAINING:

- Are you gaining size as planned?
- Is gym progress going up?
- Is the scale weight going up over time?

FOR CUTTING:

- Are you losing fat?
- Are you maintaining strength?
- Is the scale weight dropping over time?

FOR MAINTAINING:

-   Is your appearance and performance remaining steady?
-   Is the scale remaining constant over time?

If yes, ensure that this is at the rate you want. Too much weight gain for muscle growth can indicate higher levels of fat gain, and too fast of fat loss can begin to hamper muscle retention.

If no, a change will have to be made. Add/subtract calories to your daily intake mildly to the tune of 100 calories. Look over your schedule and program carefully. There is no clear-cut answer for this, and experience is the best guide. Soon, you will learn your body better and refine your estimates and measurements make better progress, but until then, seeking counsel from a knowledgeable coach or seasoned lifter can help you pinpoint the potential problem areas.

As you saw in the section on Factors Influencing Calorie burn, there are several variables at play here that can affect the real-world results that take place. In addition, mismeasurements in calorie tracking from food intake can also lead to results that stray from what "should" happen in theory, so ensure that you are tracking your dietary intake carefully to rule that out.

A later chapter will go into how to measure and monitor your intake.

26

MACRONUTRIENTS

*F*OCUSING ON CALORIES and the energy balance alone will determine your *weight*, but we aren't concerned about weight alone. We're focused on health, performance, and what that weight looks like aesthetically, so we've got to go beyond mere calories and concentrate on what those calories are made of - the macronutrients.

To explain this, let's use another analogy about money.

TURN UP?

Based on the money you make, you can spend it on all sorts of things.

You can buy a giraffe. You can buy a first class trip to Dubai, complete with a 5 star hotel and a chauffeur to drive you around in a lavish limo. You can buy out all the bottles in the club and turn up like the apocalypse is coming. But if you don't leave money for your rent, groceries, and utilities, your life is going to go down the drain and you'll end up on a self-help infomercial at 3AM.

Now apply this concept to nutrition.

SPEND YOUR MACROS

The calorie intake you're shooting for based on the calculations in the previous chapter is your dietary budget. You can "spend it" by eating whatever you want, but if you don't allocate this budget properly based on your diet goals, you're not going to get the results you're shooting for.

This is where learning about the various macronutrients and how many you need comes into the picture so that you can be an educated buyer and avoid the late-night ridicule by sterile basement dwellers and cat ladies.

THE MACRONUTRIENT SQUAD

There are 3 main macronutrients and 1 additional one that plays ball a little bit differently. Each one of them does different things in the body. They are:

- PROTEIN (4 calories per gram)
- CARBOHYDRATES (4 calories per gram)
- FATS (9 calories per gram)
- ALCOHOL (7 calories per gram)

Different foods contain these macronutrients in various degrees. By selecting different foods to suit your tastes and needs, you will "spend your budget" and hit your calorie targets enjoyably while giving your body the things it needs to function properly and be "sculpted" in the way you're shooting for.

In other words, you'll get ride your giraffe to go buy your groceries AND to the club to turn up with the crew.

In what follows, we'll discuss each one of the macronutrients and their utilization in constructing our diets by providing some baseline recommendations- with the exception of Alcohol, as that will be treated on its own in a later Chapter.

This is an area that can get excessively scientificimical and technical, so instead of getting jumbled up in all that jargon, we'll hit the hot points and get more to the meat and potatoes (get it) with regards to practical recommendations for setting up your plan that you can do something with.

PROTEIN

When you think of nutrition for muscle, might, and aesthetics, protein is the first thing that comes to mind - and for good reason.

GAINS

Protein is the building block of muscle and getting enough is necessary for the growth and repair of muscle tissue following our training sessions [1,2]. In fact, it is *essential* for life and physical function, and the diet must provide adequate protein. For this reason, setting proper protein is a priority (say that 10 times real fast.)

SPARE ME, SIRE

For dieting phases, protein has muscle sparing properties. There is less energy available for the body to use in hypocaloric conditions, and we do not want to run the risk of the body breaking down muscle proteins for fuel. Higher dietary intake of protein can mitigate this to a certain extent [3].

SATISFACTION

In addition to its muscle building and muscle sparing properties, protein is also very filling. This is a crucial consideration for a satisfying diet and one of the reasons why a higher protein intake is such a good idea regardless of the actual growth benefit.

While the satiating effects of protein are most appreciated during a cutting phase (on top of maintaining gains), it's useful for periods of gaining and maintaining as well.

Overeating is not dependent on the caloric value of the diet alone, and unwarranted fat gain is something we want to avoid.

But all that protein...Is it safe...?

A lot of hype has been made about the safety of protein, but there is no reason to run in fear or consider it taboo. For healthy individuals, even extremely high intakes of protein intake have consistently shown to have zero adverse effects [4,5].

HOW MUCH

Protein needs fluctuate depending on other factors such as calorie intake, activity level/intensity, body fat level, and so on.

- The bigger your caloric deficit, the more you need.
- The more strenuous or extensive your activity, the more you need.
- The leaner you are, the more you need.

And vice versa.

To keep things simple, a useful way to think of protein needs is the more survival threatened you are, the more protein your body will require.

DIMINISHING RETURNS OF PROTEIN

Despite the above, the amount of protein ingested is also subject to a law of diminishing returns.

Protein needs will fluctuate based on these factors, but after a certain point, more is not better and no further amount will save you or get you more gains.

Your protein requirements simply "cap out" and another variable will have to be altered to make up for whatever goal you're hunting down - altering calories, another macronutrient, or in the case of muscle gain - simply being patient and letting time and hard work do the heavy lifting.

You'll see this reflected in the following recommendations:

PROTEIN RECOMMENDATIONS

The classical recommendation for protein intake is a stock-standard 1g/lb of bodyweight. There has been debate about the true requirements of protein intake amongst lifters, but when you look at the bigger picture, this is actually an excellent starting point.

PRACTICAL PROTEIN RECOMMENDATIONS

GAINING	MAINTAINING	CUTTING
0.8g-1.2g/lb bodyweight	0.8-1.2g/lb bodyweight	1.2-1.5g/lb bodyweight

For individuals with higher bodyfat levels, lean body mass (bodyweight - fat mass) should be used to calculate requirements.

To keep it simple mentally, shooting for the standard 1g/lb and placing your macros in a workable range (see end of chapter) is a simple, easy way to ensure you stay within these recommendations.

PROTEIN SOURCES

To get your dietary protein, there's a lot to choose from, but it's important that we look at them in a bit more detail:

	COMPLETE PROTEINS	INCOMPLETE PROTEINS
WHAT IT IS	Contains all the essential amino acids	Does not contain all the essential amino acids
PRACTICAL MEANING	Sufficient by itself	Must combine 2 or more
SOURCES	Meat, fish, eggs, dairy, protein powders, some plant sources	Most plant sources (fruits, vegetables, grains)

Calorie for calorie, dietary sources like meat, fish, eggs, and dairy are going to be a more efficient source of protein in your diet. Incomplete proteins still count, but they often don't provide enough protein per calorie and make meeting both your protein and overall calorie goals a difficult thing to balance.

Because of this, when choosing your protein sources, it's best to focus only on the complete sources, and you'll see this demonstrated in an easy fashion in the Macro Split diagram I present in a later chapter.

CARBOHYDRATES

Carbohydrates are perhaps the most plentiful macro in the standard diet and come in many different shapes and sizes that add a solid dose of variety and deliciousness to your plate. They primarily come from plant-based foods such as fruits, vegetables, and grains, although there is some in dairy as well, and because of these common sources, they provide lots of beneficial things to the body, such as fiber and micronutrients.

Carbs are a major energy source for the body - especially during high intensity activity such our workouts. Extra carbohydrates are stored as glycogen in the muscle and liver, and because of this, they contribute to that full, rounded look a muscle has.

FIBER

When we talk about carbohydrates, we also need to talk about something known as fiber. There is soluble and insoluble fiber, and it's important for digestive health in the body. Besides that, fibrous foods are also very satiating and help to make meals more satisfying while keeping you full longer.

Because of its importance and benefits, every main meal will include fiber to some degree. Too much is also to be avoided, as this can interfere with nutrient absorption. 30-60g per day is just fine. A good rule of thumb is to have at least 10-15g of fiber for every 1000 calories you eat. For reference, one 30 calorie serving of vegetables or berries has about 2g fiber. You'll hit this easily with a well-rounded diet including plenty of fruits and vegetables like I recommend.

WHAT ABOUT GLYCEMIC INDEX?

When you look at carbohydrates, the issue of glycemic index also surfaces. The glycemic index is essentially a rating of the quickness of digestion of various carbs, and from this, you've probably heard about the divide between simple and complex carbs.

Many people have lost their minds and micromanage the glycemic index rating of what they eat in hopes of heightened muscle gain or fat loss, but this is a losing proposition because insulin is regulated very well by the body, adding other items to a meal reduce the impact of the glycemic index, and it is only truly useful for those with certain conditions such as diabetes. Blood sugar is very well-regulated in the body.

In an active, healthy individual eating mixed meals with various macronutrients and fiber based on the recommendations in this book, this is a moot point and is one more variable to wipe off your mental plate. Unless you're a 2 a day athlete, that goes for post-workout, too.

Make your food decisions based on what you enjoy that satisfies you and covers your nutritional requirements. There is no need to run from sugar, bread, potatoes, or anything else. It's all a matter of perspective and how it works in the bigger picture.

CARBOHYDRATE RECOMMENDATIONS

Despite the large amount of carbohydrates in the typical diet, carbohydrates are actually not an essential nutrient unless you perform activity that requires them for fuel (like we do). However, weight training does not burn a tremendous amount of carbs compared to other sports like endurance training, so the total amount isn't freakishly high, and because of this, you can do just fine on a wide variety of carbohydrate intakes.

For practical purposes, 1g/lb body weight is a good starting point as a practical minimum, regardless of whether you're gaining, maintaining, or cutting.

Depending on how many calories you have to work with, after you factor in fat requirements you may end up with a carb intake of 2-4g/lb bodyweight.

For cutting down with lower calories, there may be less than this, but you should always aim to keep carbs as plentiful as you can while still getting the deficit you want.

FAT

Fat. The infamous F-word. When society at large thinks of fat, what do they think of?

- ➢ They think of jiggly jelly rolls flopping out from under your shirt.
- ➢ They think less sex-appeal.
- ➢ They think of ridicule and increased likelihood of disease and other health problems.

So when they think of fat regarding a diet, it's easy to see where they bridge a connection and think that they have to eliminate fat from their diets.

"If I eat fat, then I'll get fat, right? Isn't that where fat comes from? It only makes sense!"

Nah.

Dietary fat is not determinant of whether you will gain *body* fat or not. Energy balance is. Don't let the names get you confused.

Dietary fat actually serves very important uses in the body and makes for an enjoyable, well-rounded diet, so cutting it out and avoiding it altogether is a horrendous idea.

Don't fear the fat. Savor it.

FAT USES

Fats are important for optimal hormonal levels, vitamin absorption, and insulation of the body.

They also make the diet more juicy and savory. A diet with low fat is like eating chalk and cardboard because there's no mouth feel. More fat in your meals will make them more tasty and satisfying.

Lastly, dietary fat slows gastric emptying which means that not only will you enjoy the meal more, but you'll also stay fuller and more satisfied longer.

SOURCES OF FAT

Fat sources are everywhere to be found, and there are several different types. Avocado, fattier cuts of meat and fish, dairy, nuts and nut butters, seeds, high % dark chocolate, whole eggs, oils, oil based dressings all are viable options for incorporating some fat into your diet that'll get you what you need. In general, lean towards more plant-based fats for the majority of your fat intake.

Outside of these, there is a special kind of fat that you should look to get in your diet:

>   EPA/DHA

EPA/DHA are omega 3 fatty acids and can be naturally found in fatty fish like salmon, for example. These must come from the diet. However, unless you're a sushi fiend or eat these regularly, supplementation is required to make sure that you get the required amount and is much more economical as well.

To do this, aim for a combined ~2g of EPA/DHA daily. Depending on the fish oil supplement, the number of pills will vary. Check the label to make sure of the actual EPA/DHA content and not what is advertised as "fish oils", and make sure to count this into your total daily calorie intake. It typically works out to 60-100 calories per day depending on the supplement.

FAT INTAKE RECOMMENDATIONS

Fat intake can vary widely amongst individuals because outside of the essential fatty acids, they are not necessary either, but all things considered, here are some good starting points to make sure that the diet is optimized across all of the goals that we have defined:

- 0.45g/lb bodyweight
- 20-30% of the diet

The method you choose will depend on your calorie intake and you as an individual. For periods of higher calorie intake, I recommend sticking to the grams per pound of bodyweight measure while leaving the rest for carbs. In dieting situations, the percentage is often a better method of arriving at the total.

However, individual response and preference is key. Some may prefer higher fat intakes than this. Some may prefer lower. Women tend to do better on higher fat intakes (30-40% diet) approaching a more equal split between carbs and fats.

HOW TO SPEND YOUR MACROS

You've got your calorie budget and know the different macros you can spend them on. Now let's put the two together and develop your dietary spending plan.

When you're setting up your macros, it's best to look at our priorities to form a strong foundation and then build from there. The order in which we'll attack this is the following:

1. DETERMINE OVERALL CALORIE INTAKE
2. ENSURE ADEQUATE PROTEIN
3. SET CARBS AND FAT

From here, you can take your overall numbers and begin to look at meal splits to suit your goals and tastes. This can be modified to better suit your training and rest day needs. Let's take this step by step.

1. OVERALL CALORIE INTAKE

Our calorie target will set the stage for how much macro spending money we have. The table below are example calorie targets set by the calculations in the chapter on calories for a 170lb lifter on a training day.

GAINING	MAINTAINING	CUTTING
3000 calories	2600 calories	2000 calories

This is our dietary budget. Now to divide it up into the various macronutrients we'll spend it on.

2. ENSURE ADEQUATE PROTEIN

Protein is the name of the game when it comes to aesthetics. We want to ensure we get enough in the diet and make it a priority. In fact, the word itself comes from the Greek 'proteios', meaning 'first place' or 'primary'. Using the figures as outlined in the Chapter on Protein, we get roughly:

	GAINING	MAINTAINING	CUTTING
PROTEIN	170g	170g	200g
TOTAL CALORIES	700	700	800

After setting protein, we can figure out what we have left in the diet for carbs and dietary fat:

	GAINING	MAINTAINING	CUTTING
TOTAL CALORIES	3000	2600	2000
CALORIES FROM PROTEIN*	700	700	800
CALORIES FOR C/F LEFT	2300	1900	1200

*rounded up for sake of calculation

Boom. In many cases, *you could stop right here*. Once you hit calories and protein, the rest tends to fall in place due to personal preference alone, and managing the rest can start to become a pain in the ass.

Nevertheless, it's still a good idea to have a good starting point to see where you're at and add some structure if you want to optimize things. Let's carry on.

3. SET CARBS AND FAT

Remember that the amount of necessary carbohydrates and fats in the diet is something that is very low. Because of this, carbs and fat can swing wildly with little effect. The body will adjust.

In general for overall reasons pertaining to performance, mood, and meal habits, more space will be given to carbohydrates than fat. For women and certain individuals, they may prefer more of an equal split between carbs and fat.

For this example, we'll use a happy medium by using the recommended value for fat in the previous section (0.45g/lb body weight) and then allotting the rest for carbs. This is for maintaining and gaining, but for cutting, we will start here and then adjust a bit.

SUMMARY

With these calculations, we have a diet that looks as follows:

	GAINING	MAINTAINING	CUTTING
CALORIES	3000	2600	2000
PROTEIN	170g	170g	200g
CARBS	407g	307g	127g
FAT	77g	77g	77g

Clean and simple. In the case of Achilles, these numbers will serve as the rough targets to hit and he will track his intake through nutritional information on the various foods he consumes and food measurements to make sure he stays on track.

For off days, to factor in the reduced calorie expenditure, amounts will be deducted from carbohydrates primarily. In the cutting scenario, some may be taken from fats to allow a bit more carbs for dietary enjoyment.

These figures can be adjusted to suit his particular needs better, but they are good starting points to track intake.

Which brings us now to a very important topic: Dietary ranges.

USING DIETARY RANGES

As you go forward in your reading, you will discover how to choose your meal splits and what to consume at these meals. You will be using your calorie and macro goals to plan this.

However, you may find that planning perfect meals all the time to hit your numbers is more struggle than it's worth. I agree. For this reason, when planning your food choices and meal combinations:

> Use **ranges** and view your macro targets as a **guide** for your nutritional habits rather than an absolute number that must be hit.

Remember that the body does not work in black or white scenarios. You want to be *in the neighborhood*. You're not trying to win at the slot machines or snipe a terrorist from a spaceship. Minor differences are nothing to lose sleep over.

The range selected will depend on the macronutrient and its relative importance in the hierarchy. Let's take a look.

CALORIES

Because calories are the primary determinant of body composition and the rest of what we do nutritionally, overall calorie intake should be the most closely monitored number.

Get as close as you can to your calorie goal for the day. This will allow you to see if your calculations and estimations are on point. For maintenance phases or more broad goals, you can set a simple range of 100 calories in either direction, but stick to this as closely as you can.

PROTEIN

Protein should be the tightest range out of the macronutrients. Given my conservative protein recommendations, a 10-20g variation in either direction gets the job done.

Therefore, if Achilles needs 170g of protein daily, then ideally he will be in the daily range of 150-190g.

The low end of the range is closer to the upper level of conservative research, and the high end has no extra effect besides extra satiety in a properly setup program. Simple.

CARBS AND FAT

As mentioned, carbohydrates and fat are much more variable due to individual factors, so wider ranges can be used here.

Depending on the total calories you have to work with, carbs can swing by 20-40g as well and fats can go up and down by 10-20g (remember that fats are 9 calories per gram whereas carbs are 4 calories per gram).

So in this case, if Achilles' targets are 300g carbs and 77g fat, he would be looking to hit in the realm of roughly:

260-340g carbohydrates
60-90g fat

Plenty of breathing room.

As noted earlier, to make things easier you can forgo counting carbohydrates and fat at all and let the chips fall where they may. Calories and protein are the most essential, and if you nail these 2, the rest will fit by default, so these are just guidelines if you're looking to hit your numbers.

Personal preference alone will often lead to a favorable ratio between carbs and fat anyways. You can always tighten things up if need be.

SUMMARY

By looking at the diet this way, you are not bound by the numbers and have leeway due to variances in measurements, meal combinations, and so on. That's flexibility that'll make keeping your nutrition plan and lifestyle blend very well.

However, as you will find out later on, there is a lot of value in setting aside the time to create your own set meal ideas based on your tastes and macro goals that you can always go back to and keep constant in your life. You enjoy them and they are in line with the nutritional goals.

This will take all of the guesswork and tediousness out of constantly having to plug in your numbers and manipulate foods to try to hit your macros spot on. As always, have a stable base and allow the rest to fall as it may without stress. We're looking for direction not perfection. Consistency and satisfying sustainability rules all.

27

MEAL SPLIT

ITH YOUR CALORIES AND MACROS SET UP, now you have to divide them up into your meal split. When do you want to spend them throughout the day and how much at each time?

Meal factors such as the size of your meals and when you have them often take care of themselves and are best left to **individual preference** outside of *broad* general recommendations with regards to the span of hours Pre/Post workout.

Simplicity reigns supreme.

Overall calorie intake and *macro split* will determine the vast majority of your physique results. With mixed meals containing protein, carbohydrates, fat, and fiber, everything else simply becomes *secondary*.

There is negligible – if any – benefit to higher meal frequency from a physical standpoint, in terms of making gains, burning fat, or heightened metabolism [1,2,3]. The world is not going to end, and the only potential benefit is appetite regulation, but that is also heavily dependent on your meal composition which we'll get to and optimize later.

With that in mind, the main objective of meal splits are to ensure you are satisfied, adherent, and set yourself up for training success and recovery. Here are some general guidelines that are helpful to follow when coming up with a meal split to follow.

- CALORIC BUDGET
- SCHEDULE
- PREPARATION
- PERI-WORKOUT NUTRITION

Let's look at each and then follow that up with my recommendations and some examples of meal splits.

CALORIE BUDGET

How many calories do you have to work with for the day? This will impact your decision in how best to split up your "budget to spend."

If you have a ton, you'll probably want smaller, more frequent meals. If you don't have many, you'll want larger, less frequent meals that fill you up [4]. Trying to push a person to have 6 small meals a day when their daily intake is a mere 1500 calories is dietary torment 6 times a day.

If you don't have a lot of calories to work with and aren't satisfied, you may be a good candidate for intermittent fasting.

INTERMITTENT FASTING

Intermittent Fasting (I.F) is a meal setup where you have no meals for an extended period of time followed by a shorter period in which you train and get all of your nutrition in for the day. Though it sounds counterintuitive, it is still a very viable nutritional strategy [5,6,7] and allows for many lifters to adhere to their program and achieve lifestyle balance, especially while cutting.

There are several ways it's done, but I find a 14-18 hour fast followed by a 6-12 hour meal period to be best [7]. Any less is just a late breakfast, and any longer is pushing it for serious lifters looking to provide proper pre and post workout nutrition while living a balanced lifestyle. This means you will have your last meal at 9pm and then not have your next meal until 1pm the next day. You will see how you plan your meal split based on this in the examples section later on.

Intermittent fasting works best for those with busy mornings and/or smaller caloric intakes (cutting). Most of the specifics of this book will not change for those who do I.F. The exception is in the pre-workout period if you train fasted, where you should consume 5-10g of BCAAs or a scoop of whey.

SCHEDULE

Are you busy sunrise to sunset? 6 meals a day would be a headache and have the potential to kill the momentum of your day and make eating a chore. A reduced frequency would be a better bet here.

Are your mornings fast-paced and you don't get a real break until lunch time? Having to cook and sit down to a large breakfast could be working against the current rather than with it. A nonexistent or smaller breakfast and bigger lunch and dinner would be a more logical option.

After lunch time, is it another 8 hours before dinner? It would be a wise choice to add a smaller meal in between that time to avoid hunger.

NIGHT TIME

When the sun goes down and the stars come up, fitness folk run in fear of the Carb Monster who comes out to terrorize souls and transform anything you eat into fat. Yeah right. If you have the calories available, go for it. As late as you want.

Night times are when people wind down and relax or go out and live life. Having a larger meal in the evening and decent amount of carbs is better for social reasons, diet satisfaction, sleep, and mood.

If you train in the evenings, you'll be doing this by default. There's nothing quite like hitting the iron, feasting, and then knocking out into a deep, recuperative slumber.

MEAL PREPARATION

How is the meal prepared? Unless you have access to your kitchen throughout the day or a hoard of sexy chefs to cater to your nutritional needs around the clock, this can be a big determining factor that can discourage a higher meal frequency and the lifestyle of meal prep or carrying protein bars or other foods around with you. If joining the ranks of the plastic container warriors isn't appealing to you, consider having larger, less frequent meals.

PRE AND POST WORKOUT

Pop quiz. What is the single-most important event in terms of physique construction?

LIFTING. WEIGHTS.

You take the weights out of the equation, and the muscles vanish. Why would they stay?

Battling the barbells is the stimulus that will trigger the favorable responses to muscle growth that will sculpt our body when we provide the proper nutrition.

With our peri-workout (around the workout) nutrition, we want to give our bodies what it needs to perform at its best and optimize growth and recovery. Given that training is the most important factor in determining your aesthetic state, how can plan our nutrition to take advantage of this across the board?

PRE WORKOUT

On training days, workouts should fall between two meals with 1-3 hours on either side, comprised of a decent sized mixed meal of protein, carbs (and fiber), some fat, and adequate hydration. The further from training, the larger the meal should be, and vice versa.

Pre-workout, the meal should be large enough to satisfy but light enough to not interfere with training. Post workout is when you can throw down.

Consume ~0.4-0.5g/kg bodyweight in protein on either side of the workout [8]. For simplicity, another way to put this is to consume ~20% of your daily protein needs during these periods. This can be as simple as one of your normal meals, a sandwich and an apple, or a protein shake and a banana if you're on the go and hit the gym right after conquering your work day.

WEIGHT	PROTEIN PRE-WORKOUT
120lbs	25g
150lbs	30g
180lbs	35g

At least

Lastly, a dose of a stimulant can be taken shortly before the workout to provide a boost. A cup of coffee or a scoop of pre-workout 20-30 minutes before your first set gets the job done just fine, although if you work out in the evenings, you want to watch how this affects you. Sleep is key for peak performance and recovery, and you don't want to disrupt your natural patterns.

POST WORKOUT

In the period after a workout, you are primed for muscle repair and growth. However, as I mentioned in my recommendations for training frequency, this is not a perpetual process. It trails off the further in time you go from when you trained before returning to baseline, so you want to ensure that you are providing your body with what it needs when it's in its best state to do something with it.

After training, the timing of the post-workout meal is not immediately necessary, despite popular claims promoting rapid refueling for enhanced muscle growth [8]. If you did you pre-workout meal right, you'll still be releasing amino acids into the bloodstream 4-5 hours later to assist in growth and recovery [9]. Get back to the castle. Take a shower. Chef it up. In other words, *you do not need a post-workout shake* assuming you have meals before and after training and meet your daily protein intake.

For the post workout meal and span of time afterwards, don't go weak on the caloric content. You want to ensure that you set aside plenty of calories for post-workout, and this should continue into the next day, tapering down the further in time you go. Remember that calories are key for recovery and a surplus is the biggest weapon in your fight for gains, so whether cutting, maintaining, or gaining, you want to put a good amount here.

This is to be done within reason and not at the expense of the dietary enjoyment for the rest of the day. This is done based on a blend of performance, post-training growth, and psychological reasons. Train like a beast and then feast and bask in the post workout state of bliss.

You'll see examples of this in the meal split examples I provide later in the chapter.

<u>OTHER CONSIDERATIONS</u>

Fiber in the pre-workout case can be lower to none if it causes discomfort during training, provided it's sufficient in the rest of the day.

MEAL SPLIT RECOMMENDATION

All things considered, 3-5 well rounded meals total is optimal for the majority of individuals and the sizes/timing thereof should be chosen based on your individual factors, routine, and preferences.

- Meal setups with less meals than this can create problems for hunger, flexibility, and peri-workout optimization.
- Having more meals than this can be cumbersome, disruptive, and less satisfying.

Therefore, meal totals less than 3 and more than 5 are reserved for individuals with very low or high calorie intakes for whom this would be a more favorable option, all things considered.

This chosen number of meals and time they are eaten should stay relatively constant from day to day, rain or shine, cutting/gaining/maintaining and follow sound nutritional concepts as discussed in the rest of this book.

EXAMPLES OF MEAL SCHEDULES

Now let's look at some examples of how you could split up your meal timing and size. These values are based on maintaining at 2400 calories per day, but you could easily add or subtract from the listed values to get to the total calorie intake requirement based on your individual needs.

These are by no means the only way to do it, but they will point you in the right direction. When in doubt, remember the basics and use common sense as your guide.

EVENING TRAINING

	Meal 1	Meal 2	Meal 3 Pre-WO	Training	Meal 4	Meal 5	Total
5 meals	500	500	300	-	700	400	2400 cal
4 meals	600	600	400	-	800	-	2400 cal
I.F	-	600	400	-	1400	-	2400 cal

As you can see, meals are kept fairly constant with the pre-workout meal being a bit lighter and the post workout period containing a relatively larger meal size for the day.

This type of setup would be best for those who are busy during the day and train afterwards at about 6-8P.M.

AFTERNOON TRAINING

	Meal 1	Meal 2	Training	Meal 3	Meal 4	Total
4 meals	600	600	-	800	400	2400 cal
4 meals B	600	300	-	1000	500	2400 cal
I.F	-	500	-	1200	700	2400 cal

Afternoon training (1-4PM) is more workable because it allows for training to fit snugly between good pre/post workout meals (lunch/dinner).

For this reason, reduced meal quantity is often more of an attractive option, although you can certainly still work in 5+ meals in if required. This is mostly dependent on how late in the afternoon you train. Earlier afternoon training may work better for more meals following.

MORNING TRAINING

	Meal 1	Training	Meal 2	Meal 3	Meal 4	Meal 5	Total
5 meals	500	-	700	300	500	400	2400 cal
4 meals	500	-	800	400	700	-	2400 cal
I.F	50-100*	-	950	750	600	-	2400 cal
Early morning	50-100*	-	800	700	500	350	2400 cal

preworkout BCAA or whey is desirable here if training fasted

Morning training is often a good bet on weekends or those who work and have a busy evening schedule. Which option is best is largely dependent on when you train in the morning. The early morning option is for those who train shortly after waking and don't necessarily perform intermittent fasting.

You can see how calories are tapered after training, however meal 4 and so on -typically around dinner time here - has a good amount of calories for a satisfying dinner.

OFF DAYS

Off days allow for a much more flexible setup because there is no need for a heightened awareness of pre/post workout nutrition, nor is there a workout to schedule around. The key here is moreso to split your calories up in a way that is enjoyable and satisfying and meshes well with your daily schedule.

The values here take into account the reduced calorie requirements brought about by not training.

	Meal 1	Meal 2	Meal 3	Meal 4	Meal 5	Total
5 meals	500	500	300	500	300	2200 cal
4 meals	600	600	-	700	300	2200 cal
I.F	-	900	-	900	400	2200 cal

In the first option, more calories are allowed for lunch and dinner (Meals 2 and 4) as this fits most people's schedules best.

In option 2, you see a large lunch and more calories towards the evening for dinner/dessert.

In all of these options, you can see that the first meal of the day is not skimped on with a mere 100 or 200 calories such a shake or small snack. This is to continue the post workout recovery of the day before. If you are having more than one day off in a row, this becomes less important or not important at all, but maintaining constant meal patterns is helpful no matter what, so stick close to it.

WRAPPING UP

When it comes to creating your meal split, collect the hard factors and then use your creativity to determine the best way to weave them together harmoniously.

At the end of the day, adopt the meal schedule that suits you best that you enjoy and can stick to long term while accomplishing your goals. Those will outweigh any potential other benefits every time.

Once you have determined the best set-up for you, keep it fairly constant. Habit is powerful, and having a pretty consistent timing schedule will help with adherence, consistency, prep, and tracking, and so on.

28

FOOD AND MEAL CHOICES

$\mathcal{A}$FTER PLENTY OF HEAVY LIFTING, we're finally to the fun part: Picking your foods. How do you want to execute your calorie/macro spending plan?

Building a healthy, aesthetic physique often comes with the idea that you must have a strict diet of 'clean' foods or else you will be haunted by a posse of poltergeists and get no results. Don't fall for this madness.

Food isn't good or bad - clean or dirty – magical or murderous.

Even the claimed superiority of organic foods is unfounded [1-3], and weight loss, metabolism, and blood lipids with a diet of 43% sucrose are similar to those of a diet of 4% sucrose [4].

Foods are all just *tools* that we can use to accomplish our goals - and our goals include enjoyment, flexibility, and satisfaction.

You have to look at the calories, macronutrient composition, how filling and nutritious it is, and your personal preferences. Based on that, some foods will be a better choice than others *in the context of the diet as a whole.*

FOOD CHOICE GUIDELINE

My rule is this:

> Your diet should consist of at least **85-90%** wholesome, nutritional foods with the rest coming from other sources of your choice.

This is not to be understood in absolute terms, but rather based on *the underlying principle.* Some may opt for lower. Some higher.

That means that if you have 2000 calories, at least 1800 of them should be 'clean' sources, including lots of colorful fruits, vegetables, and things of that nature. 200 can be flexed to your liking.

Do not take this to the weekly level and eat 'clean' all week and 'dirty' on the weekend. This generates a bad dynamic and unhealthy relationship with nutrition. The specifics of how you choose to do this is up to you.

MAXIM OF AESTHETICS: YOUR PROGRAM SHOULD BE ENJOYABLE EVERY DAY NO MATTER WHAT YOUR CURRENT GOAL IS.

CHOOSING FOODS

So you've got your caloric needs, macros, and meal split. Now what...

> You've got to create your meals.

Looking at the multitude of food options out there can be overwhelming and intimidating when trying to work them into your macros and fit your plan.

Meal tracking applications have made this easier, but it's far too often a tedious guessing game of tossing different foods into the calculator to see if it fits the bill, and this leads to some suboptimal meal combinations, time wasted, and people getting fed up and saying "fuck this shit" far too often than not. Let's fix that.

THE MACRO SPLIT DIAGRAM

When you start checking out nutrition labels and looking up the nutrition facts on online databases for foods to fit in your 'budget', you will find that different foods contain the 3 macronutrients in varying degrees, but as it turns out, most foods are primarily ONE main macronutrient with smaller amounts of others.

Fewer foods combine 2 macronutrients on a significant level, and even fewer combine all 3 macros to a meaningful extent relevant for our nutrition set-up.

By segregating our food options based on this idea of looking at food choices based on their primary macros, we are able to create a diagram that looks like so:

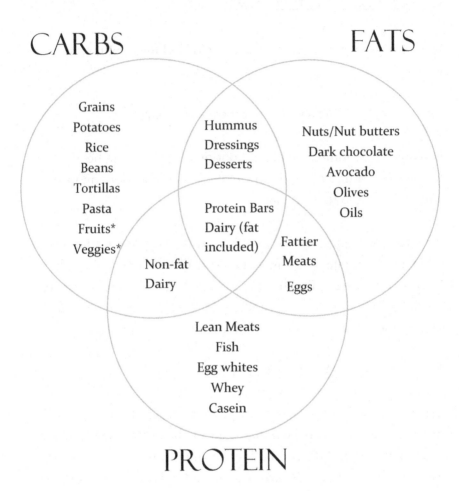

CARBS

FATS

Grains
Potatoes
Rice
Beans
Tortillas
Pasta
Fruits*
Veggies*

Hummus
Dressings
Desserts

Nuts/Nut butters
Dark chocolate
Avocado
Olives
Oils

Protein Bars
Dairy (fat
included)

Fattier
Meats

Non-fat
Dairy

Eggs

Lean Meats
Fish
Egg whites
Whey
Casein

PROTEIN

Beautiful, isn't it.

As you can see, many common foods split apart into their own spots and make visualizing your meal options simple and smooth. We will be using this diagram to devise our meals that fit into the meal split we came up with in a previous chapter. Simply follow the guidelines outlined below and you'll be well on your way.

UNO: LIGHT 'EM ALL UP

A proper, well rounded meal should highlight some portion of
every major macronutrient circle. That means you'll need a protein,
carb, and fat source.

You can either highlight the entire circle through selecting the
primary macro alone or through an area where it overlaps with
another. That's a well-rounded **meal**. Anything else is just a snack
and doesn't count. You'd be better off making better meals.

Protein?	Carb?	Fat?	Rating
Egg Whites	Oatmeal and Fruit	Cheese	Good
Steak	Vegetables	Steak	Good
Chicken Breast	Rice	-	Bad
-	Apple	Nuts	Bad

The exact quantities of each food and the macronutrient
composition of the meal as a whole that you dial up will be
dependent on your goals. You can have more than one if it fits in
your plan, and you can work it throughout the day for various
meals.

Use food labels and reliable information from nutritional databases
to provide the accurate nutritional information on the foods listed
that you want to incorporate. Ensure you weigh them the right way
as you'll see later on in another chapter.

2. FIRE UP THE FIBER THROUGH FRUITS AND VEGGIES

On top of lighting up all of the circles, you also want to include fiber into the meal. This can be accomplished through grains and legumes, but preferentially, this should also be supported through a serving of fibrous fruits or vegetables, which I've put asterisks by on the diagram. Remember, you want about 10-15g per 1000 calories you eat, and one 30 calorie serving of fruits of veggies will give you 2-3g.

Vegetables are easily workable in your main sit-down meals, and fruits are convenient for when you're on the go. Add that zap of color and variety to your plate. They're nature's gems.

BENEFITS

By dialing up your meals in this way you will:

1. Cover all your macros at every meal to give your body what it needs across the board
2. Enjoy a varied plate with different tastes and textures
3. Have a satisfying meal every time
4. Provide vitamins and minerals for healthy function
5. Stay fuller longer
6. Simplicity of meal planning
7. Easy scaling of serving sizes to adjust calories/macros
8. Flexibility - the ability to make simple swaps*

Needless to say, it's an excellent tool and will serve as the foundation for our meal setup.

*see meal examples to see this in action

ADDITIONAL CONSIDERATIONS

Geared with the Macro Split Diagram, let's look at some other factors in food selection that can sway your decision on which foods to include in your meals based on the principles of the diagram.

Picking the foods you enjoy is obviously a given, but here are some other things you may want to consider:

KEEP MEASURING IN MIND

Some foods can make measurements and consistent tracking a difficult task because there are no standardized options and each item varies by default. This can come into play if you're being precise with your nutrition to reach a certain goal.

For example, fattier cuts of meat can vary in their marbling and fat content. The given nutritional info may be a standard number, but it can sway largely in each direction depending on the cut selected.

Additionally, you may like potatoes and want to include it in your plan to the tune of 200 calories, but depending on the size at the store, this can make measuring a more tricky task than it would be otherwise. Do you cut off the extra and throw it away or eat it anyway and juggle your macros somewhere else? Let the existential crisis begin.

Most foods are pretty immune to this phenomenon, but when measuring precisely is critical for your goals (lean muscle gain, getting shredded), this can be a very important factor to consider if they're eaten very frequently.

ENERGY DENSITY

Calories may tell the whole story for energy balance, but they certainly don't tell the whole story with regards to how satisfying or filling a meal is.

Check out the examples below with similar calorie/macronutrient totals.

OPTION 1	OPTION 2	TOTAL CALORIES
1lb strawberries	1 bagel	250
Veggie omelette with cheese, oatmeal, and fresh fruit	Protein powder + 3 cookies	400

The differences are astronomical when you view things side by side in real life. Clearly, one will fill you up way more than another, and that's important when it comes to staying away from overconsumption or hunger. This is due to fiber content, weight, and volume of the food.

For this reason, depending on your goal and individual factors, keeping energy density in mind will help you plan better meals that better suit your nutritional requirements and tolerances. This goes hand in hand with the next point on satiety.

SATIETY

Satiety is simply a measure of how filling or satisfying a particular food is. It often goes hand in hand with energy density. Common sense would indicate that a larger amount of food would be more filling, and satiety is very important for a sound diet that you enjoy and can stick to.

Here, let's focus more on calorie equated foods of the same type:

OPTION 1	OPTION 2
8 oz milk	8 oz greek yogurt
32g peanut butter	32g peanuts
1 scoop whey	4oz chicken breast
8 oz apple juice	1 apple

In general, unless you have problems getting down enough calories, chewing your food is the best bet for the majority of your food options.

TRAINING/OFF DAYS

Lastly, based on what we've seen over calories and meal timing for nutrition, we know that the body is most receptive to nutrition around and especially after training. We also know that calorie requirements and effective utilization are going to be higher in these periods.

Therefore, on training days and after training, more energy dense carb sources will be useful because calorie intakes can be higher and lower energy density, more fibrous sources will leave you incredibly full and looking at your off days like second class citizens.

On off days, carb sources should be more fibrous, less energy dense, and more satiating to make up for the lower calorie intakes for these days.

By doing this, you will effectively smooth out those perceived large fluctuations in diet between training and off days and ensure that your diet will be satisfying and enjoyable no matter what day it is.

MEAL CREATION

Now that you're acquainted with the Macro Split Diagram, it's time to whip up some examples so that you can see it in action for creating meals based on macronutrient needs.

There are no magical meal combinations in existence, so feel free to mix and match your food choices however you want so long as you stay within your dietary plan and enjoy a satisfying meal.

MEAL EXAMPLES

Let's take another look at our warrior, Achilles.

With a dietary goal of 2400 calories with requirements of 170g protein, he has decided upon a certain meal split that sets aside 600 calories for breakfast. He has decided to take the simpler route as explained in the chapter over Macronutrients regarding setting up your macros and is letting carbs and fat fall into personal preference by using this diagram.

Realizing that he needs a protein, carb, fat, and fibrous fruit or vegetable based on the diagram, he decides to create the following meal composed of the foods he loves that get him in line with his nutritional targets.

BREAKFAST OF CHAMPIONS

FOOD	CALORIES	PROTEIN
1.25 cup egg whites	120 calories	25
1 oz cheese	90	5
2 tbsp salsa	10	1
3 oz veggies	30	1
½ cup oatmeal	150	5
1 banana (100g)	100	1
1 tbsp PB	100	4
TOTALS:	600	42

As you can see, he's nailed all of the categories and done well in staying close to his target macros. Remember that hitting them perfectly is not required, and if you want to be a minimalist about it, stay true to calories and overall protein intake while letting preference dictate the rest in regards to carbs and fats.

If he was cutting, he may just simply remove the banana, swap the cheese for nonfat, and add an extra 1/2 cup of egg whites. If he was gaining, he may just add a large apple. It really can be just that simple.

Now let's look at lunch.

SIMPLE SWAPS

Because of the meal requirements of 600 calories with roughly the same amounts for protein, carbs, and fat that means that simple swaps of serving sizes can bring about the same results.

For example, let's turn that breakfast into lunch by simply making simple swaps within the macro category:

Meal 1	Swap to Meal 2
1 cup Egg Whites	4 oz Chicken Breast
Vegetables	Vegetables (no change)
Oatmeal + Banana	Medium sized potato
Cheese	Cheese on Potato
Salsa	Ketchup
1 tbsp Peanut butter	2 squares dark chocolate

Look at how quickly you can completely transform a meal by breaking it down into its components and making simple changes. Although the meals are entirely different, they are both tallying up to roughly the same macros.

This is what I call "macro splitting" and it's very helpful for going freestyle on meals. It's less helpful on foods with lots of overlap (the intersections of the diagram), but it's incredibly powerful for foods with more isolated macronutrient distributions.

This same process can be applied across the board to all of the various meals. Now it's your turn to dial up some ideas for both training and off days.

CREATE YOUR OWN COMBINATIONS

Based on the Macro Split diagram, think about what meal creations can you concoct that fit in line with your nutritional goals.

Look at the macro split diagram versus your nutritional requirements we calculated, and start to put your creativity to use to find what you love the most.

LOOK UP RECIPES

If you're new to whipping up your own meals, look up recipes to give you some ideas as to where to begin.

The internet is crawling with healthy recipe options for the fitness crowd, and they're good places to start so long as the nutritional info matches up with your plan.

HAVE GO-TO EATING OUT MEALS

Unless you live like a hermit or carry a stock of food around you wherever you go (don't be that person), chances are you'll find yourself eating out every now and then - either out with friends, being busy, or whatever else. Because of this, you'll want to have a game plan and ideas in mind for when it's meal time and you're out.

Think of the restaurants in your area that you frequent the most. What do you order from there? Do they fit in line with your goals and/or can you make them fit? Scan the menu and look for food items that fall close to your calorie and protein goals.

KEEP YOUR FOODS CONSTANT

Once you've got your basic food selection and meals down, stick to them and keep them constant. This will accomplish a variety of good things.

COOKING

When you've got a select pool of foods that you keep stocked in the fridge and pantry, you will learn them well over time. You'll get better at cooking with them, and your meals will taste better and better to match.

TRACKING

When it comes to weighing foods, the more you see what 4oz of chicken or 100g of berries looks like on the scale, the better you will be at sizing them up when they're not on the scale.

For tracking your own body composition changes, eating the same foods regularly forms a more stable variable. There are less big fluctuations in body weight, and any food tracking errors will be magnified and apparent.

TRANSITIONS

Keeping your foods constant makes swapping between cutting, gaining, and maintaining a breeze.

The foods themselves aren't changing - the quantities are. You can enjoy the same foods no matter what phase you're in - all year round. If you don't like them, then why do you have them? Plug these in different amounts to tailor to your nutritional needs. This right here is the secret to long-term fitness success and maintaining your physique year round.

There are no cutting diets or gaining diets. There are only diets.

ENJOYMENT

You will always enjoy your diet.

Always pick the things you enjoy that can accomplish your nutritional objectives. Every day and every meal of your life should be enjoyed. The benefits far outweigh the cons.

EASE OF SHOPPING/FINANCIALS

Lastly, a simple trip the grocery store is hardly ever simple. That is, unless you have a pretty standard list.

Sticking to the same foods will allow you to keep track of your inventory at home and avoid lots of time making lists or forgetting items, make grocery store trips a simpler, quicker task because you know exactly what you need and where it's at, you'll get to save on bulk wherever applicable, and you'll minimize waste, to boot.

If you know you have an apple a day, you wouldn't buy 10 "just to be safe" and let the extra 3 go to waste. You would buy 7 and nail it every time.

Simple and efficient.

INCORPORATE VARIETY?

Staying consistent doesn't mean that the diet you pick today must stay that way forever. That'd be ridiculous. Certain foods are seasonal and sometimes you want to switch things up and try new items and recipes.

The idea is to have a steady, standard base diet and then rotate items in and out in blocks. This highlights the efficacy of the Macro Split Diagram once more.

For example:

- 100g of broccoli is roughly the same as 100g of bell peppers, cauliflower, snap peas, and many other vegetables.
- 100g of strawberries is comparable to 100g of blueberries, 100g of blackberries, and so on.

The comparisons aren't always perfect and there are some outliers (fruit-wise, a 100g banana can have 2x the calories of the same weight of berries), but simple swaps like these are everywhere, and portions can easily be dialed in to account for differences amongst the exceptions. (Have twice as many berries)

It may be unpractical or unfeasible to have all of those components in your fridge all the time, but alternating week to week or season to season is surely feasible, and it makes for a more enjoyable, varied diet.

Don't ever let your diet be a rigid, limiting factor.

MEAL REFERENCE SHEET

Having to pick out meals, calculate macros, figure out weights, and so on makes for a big hurdle and time sink when it comes to nutrition. Even with a tool like the Macro Split Diagram, it creates a lot of duplicate effort, wastes mental energy, and is inconvenient and tedious.

Given that a solid nutrition plan is a paramount for any training program, wouldn't it be nice if there was an easier way? There is:

Never eat again.

If you don't like that solution, then here's what else you can do:

Do it all beforehand once and then create a reference sheet.

Here's how:

Step 1: List all the foods you enjoy and eat the most along with their nutritional information for their serving size that you use.

Step 2: List the meal combinations that you enjoy the most that you've created using the Macro Split Diagram and falling in line with your nutritional goals. Record the quantities of each food used in the meal and the nutritional information it contains.

Create 2-3 meal combinations that fit your dietary budget for every meal. If the meals are the same content, you can overlap and use the same ones.

Step 3: Get your Sheet Together

Now go forth and create your sheet.

You can plug in all of the information on a notes app on your phone, a food tracking application, or even an actual physical sheet so you don't have to have your phone with you.

If you make a physical sheet, put it where it's easy to see and read in your chef space - by your scale and where you slice and dice is ideal. You can also consider laminating it to be longer lasting and endure the heat and mess you make in the kitchen. Go as all out as you so desire.

APPLICATION

By having a consistent meal plan based on your goals and preferences, you always have something to reference when its meal time that takes all the confusion and calculation out of the picture based on what YOU like - not a cookie cutter template.

When it's meal time and you don't know what to whip up, look at your sheet that *you* created with everything already done.

If you're shifting gears from gaining to cutting or maintaining, you will go through this process again, but because you're smart and are going to do what I say, you'll mostly only be adjusting the *quantities* – not the food choices themselves.

29

MEASURING
NUTRITION

WHEN YOUR DIET IS SET UP to hit a specific goal
(i.e muscle gain, fat loss), tracking and knowing what
you're eating to some degree of accuracy becomes *vital* in
order to know if you're on the right track or way out of whack.

If you don't have a way to keep track of what you're putting in your
body, you'll just end up spinning your wheels in frustration. We
didn't go over several chapters of nutritional guidelines for no
reason.

However, if there were one factor that holds people back from
optimizing their nutrition to fine tune their physique and
performance, it'd have to be tracking. With that in mind, let's clear
things up and get you right.

MEASUREMENT LEVELS

First and foremost, you need to determine just how precise you need to be with your nutritional tracking. The reluctance to track dietary intake often comes from having the wrong view of what is necessary for them, so read the below options and determine where you fit best.

1. OPTIMAL (HIGH)

Optimal nutrition means that you will be tracking and measuring everything meticulously to ensure that no stone is left unturned in your plan. You will be measuring calories, macros, and the foods that contain them to a high degree of accuracy. For this reason, eating out often is not recommended.

This level of detail is the best choice for peak performance, physique competitors, and trial periods to pinpoint your personal responses to nutrition before descending into the lower levels.

2. FLEXIBLE (MEDIUM)

The flexible level is just a step down from optimal and will focus exclusively on the major players in the nutritional ball game, calories, protein, and EFAs. Foods are measured accurately, but utmost accuracy on all of them is often not necessary. Here, eating out can be done 1-2x/week.

This level is best suited for lifestyle purposes, broad goals, and flexibility. It is my recommended level for everyone to be on.

3. CRUISE CONTROL (LOW)

Lastly, we have cruise control. The least strict of them all, cruise control abandons the notion of concrete counting altogether and instead focuses on making choices based on broad, overarching principles rather than refined, precise decision-making. It instead looks at general trends over time through the scale, mirror, and performance in the gym.

This level is for best suited for long-term maintenance phases, vacation periods, and other times when nailing nutritional numbers isn't a key component of success.

WHICH ONE?

As you'll soon see, tracking your nutrition is very simple and accessible, so the gaps between the levels is much smaller than you'd expect and only requires 5-10 minutes per day with slight habitual modifications.

Read each of the options and determine which one of them best suits your currently goals and lifestyle.

Regardless of which level you reside in, I recommend that everyone spend at least 2 weeks-1 month in the Flexible level or above to gain a solid glimpse as to what their nutrition needs look like both on the dinner plate and weight plates. After this, you can make your own judgement call as to where you want to spend your time.

If you decide to track at Cruise Control, at least 4x per year, spend time in one of the higher levels for a week to calibrate your dietary habits and make broad adjustments as necessary.

WHAT YOU'LL NEED

Measuring your intake is simple and easy. You only need 3 things:

1. MEASUREMENT TOOLS (DIGITAL SCALE)
2. NUTRITIONAL INFORMATION
3. PLACE TO RECORD YOUR INTAKE

MEASUREMENT TOOLS (DIGITAL SCALE)

First, you'll need the tools to measure properly.

A dependable digital scale is a necessary investment to make for every aesthetic architect's kitchen. Some come with a nice plate or bowl. Some don't. If it doesn't, you can put one on there to put the foods you want to weight and then zero-set it to calibrate the scale for weighing. These come cheap these days and can be found all over.

Keep it where you do your cooking, so it's always in easy access. A simple push of a button and a minute or two are all that's required to guarantee your nutrition efforts are on point and setting up your success.

In addition to this, some measurement cups ranging from tablespoons to 1 full cup can also be in use when the scale is less practical.

NUTRITIONAL INFORMATION

A scale will do you no good if you don't know the values of what you're weighing. Many foods that you buy will have the nutrition facts on the packaging that will provide the information you need to know to factor the value into your daily intake. It will tell you the calories and macronutrient content that you will fit into your plan. This is my preferred method.

For foods that don't such as fresh fruits or vegetables, there are several online databases and smartphone applications that can provide information on the nutrition facts for those items. For these, be very careful. They can be unreliable, so check multiple listings and reliable sources only.

Here, you want to pay attention the serving size listed for the nutritional information. If it says 3oz and you want to use 6oz in your meal, you'll have to multiply everything by 2. If the serving size is 100g and you only want 50g, you will have to divide everything by 2.

PLACE TO RECORD YOUR INTAKE

Lastly, you need a place to record the values of what you're consuming. This will enable you to track your numbers to stay in line with your nutritional goals and compare your food intake to your results in pictures, the gym, and scale to optimize your program.

A notes app on your phone can work, but there are tons of sites/applications that have built in tools to do this where you can input your info and even save templates. Many even have a nutrition info database, so you can carry out your goals all in one fell swoop and view all of the relevant parameters of your nutrition.

HOW TO MEASURE

Once you've got the tools for the job, let's look at how to use them properly. The 4 rules of nutritional measurement are as follows:

1. OBEY THE LABEL
2. USE WEIGHT WHENEVER POSSIBLE
3. KEEP DENSITY IN MIND
4. KNOW YOUR GOAL

OBEY THE LABEL

When it comes to measuring, we want objective numbers to go by. Measure each food as it is listed on the nutritional information. Dry and uncooked is the common standard. If you don't follow the label, you will either be over or under what you have planned.

USE WEIGHT WHENEVER POSSIBLE

The point of the scale is so we can measure weight. Depending on the food, either grams or ounces will be easier. For reference, 3oz is about 85g.

Although many foods are listed in terms of many forms of measurement, sticking to a scale weight is the best way. Let's look at why.

❧ SIZE

Who exactly is the judge of a "medium sized apple?" Everything is bigger in Texas, and they might have a different opinion on "medium" than another state.

➤ VOLUME

If the label for a particular food says ¼ cup/28g, you may fill a ¼ cup measuring cup and think you're golden, when in reality, if you were to measure the ¼ cup that you just filled up on the digital scale, you would get 35g.

That may seem like a trivial amount, and in most cases it is (think leafy greens), but surprise. In the example I just used, the food was almonds, and that 7g difference is 40 calories. If you eat a lot of almonds, that will add up over time and throw you off your game.

What about liquids?

You can't just toss everything on the scale. Some foods - like liquids - are going to have to get measured via volume measurements. What do you do?

➤ WEIGH IT ANYWAYS

Some liquids actually provide a weight value alongside a volume value, so put it on the scale and see where it stands. Calibrate a large measuring cup or the cup you'll be using, and then pour it in.

Having to measure things out like egg whites every time on a scale can get tedious, so test it once, see where it's at on the measuring cup for the true value, and use the measuring cup in the future to avoid having to repeat the process every time you cook. You can repeat this process every once in a while to make sure your freestyle skills are still on point.

&ep; BE CONSERVATIVE

If there is no way to weigh it, just be a little conservative and don't fill things to the brim to where you have to get in the zone like an expert sniper because another heartbeat will cause things to spill.

ENERGY DENSITY

The more calories per unit of measurement (energy dense), the more important accuracy is. Small mismeasurements can erase your progress and cause you to think that you've hit a plateau. Put your attention towards these. This is the case for fats and more starchy carbs.

For fibrous fruits, vegetables, and things of that nature, you'll be able to use wider measuring ranges and your visual estimation experience to judge it.

KNOW YOUR GOAL

Lastly, always keep in mind where you are at in terms of your tracking level. The fate of the Universe does not rest upon how accurate your measurements are, so use the knowledge from the other rules of measurement and determine how detailed you need to be based on your current goals.

VISUAL ESTIMATION EXPERIENCE

If you've followed my suggestions in getting a good scale and measuring your common core base of foods you love, you'll begin to learn exactly what 8oz of chicken breast, a 100g apple, or a 200g potato looks like in real life

When this happens, you'll be able to look at certain quantities of food and be within good shooting distance of the actual value by guesstimating. You'll get scary good at this and can make some good side change by joining a traveling circus guessing nutritional info. This comes in handy when you're being flexible with your nutrition or out at a restaurant and want a rough idea of what you're eating. All royalty checks can be mailed to me personally.

MEASURING FOR EATING OUT

Any decent plan will have a plan for you to eat out. Great moments happen out there, and you're going to live them. What do you do?

VISIT THE WEBSITE'S NUTRITIONAL INFO

Most restaurants in this day and age offer nutritional info online or in apps for their dishes, so use these whenever possible and log them in your tracker. If not, you can still use some visual estimations to at least guide you in the right direction.

EYEBALL IT

As I mentioned in the Chapter on tracking your food intake, you'll soon get very good at looking at a plate of food and estimating the values of what you're eating. When in doubt, err on the side of caution. We have the tendency to underestimate how much we're eating, and a chef's job is to make your food delicious, not hit your macros. Building in a little safety net and being conservative is your best bet.

SET ASIDE THE CALORIES

If you know you're going to be eating out, set aside some space in your calorie budget to allow for the extra intake and any estimation errors. We went over this in the section over calorie cycling and meal splits, so give those a run through once more and tune up your nutrition to follow suit. It's easier than you think. Simply shave off 100 calories here or there for the day and allow a little more calories on this day in the weekly scheme of things. No big deal.

LOOK AT LIFESTYLE

To wrap this up, a point about lifestyle needs to be made. We know that by eating out more, knowing what your real nutrition looks like is going to be off to some degree or another. In general, you will be eating more than you think, so don't underestimate things

Learn how to cook and try out good recipes you love. Find ways to carry your favorite culinary creations with you to work or school so you don't have to run off for lunch because you're starving. Invite people over to cook together. Keep snacks on hand so you don't have to rush out somewhere for a meal.

Make eating out more of the exception than the norm. You'll enjoy it more and have better control in your fitness ascent.

30

MEAL TIME

*A*N OFTEN OVERLOOKED FACTOR when it comes to nutrition is - lamentably- where and how the meals are prepared and eaten. In modern times, people live a life of excess work, obligations, and business that delegates the role of food to simple sustenance to shove into the fire. Tragic.

And in the fitness world, the tendency is strong to get so wrapped up in the numbers that we lose sight of the extreme value of nutrition in other areas.

Meal times are times to relax, re-center your mind, and fuel up. They're a time to get together with friends and fam. Make meals an experience to be enjoyed that anchor your day.

MEAL PREPARATION

For at least some of your meals, it's likely that you will be making them in advance. No matter how they're being prepared, enjoy the process and don't delegate it to a simple chore.

Throw on some music, listen to your favorite podcast or audiobook, or invite someone over to chef it up with you.

Put energy and attention into what you do always. Be mindful throughout the entire process. Cooking is an art.

MEAL SETTING

Your meals should be centered around a calm, comfortable environment you enjoy, either alone or with the people of your choice, free of distractions and with ample time so that you aren't rushing or feeling any external pressures or pending commitments and things left undone.

If you're working on a project, reach a stopping point. Put your phone on silent or better yet: put it away. Optimize your workflow and agenda so that you can have time for your meals in peace.

If you've got a lot going on in your head, clear your mind and unwind a bit beforehand. Bring yourself back into the present moment and a state of calm. Relax. Gain awareness of your body.

Check your posture. Relieve the tension. Re-center your attention on the here and the now. What good is it to put a stop on your work and eating somewhere else if your mind is working and somewhere else?

CHANGE LOCATIONS

If you spend most of your day in one location, have your meals in another. The change in setting is refreshing.

- Pick a place that's calm and comfortable. Your environment impacts your inner state.
- Avoid bright, cold artificial lights. Seek out dim, warmer light or natural lights.
- Stay away from blinding white walls and lots of visual or auditory noise
- Find where you feel at home. The colors, the textures, and the ambience all interplay into creating your mood.

A bit of music, a good book, or a stimulating documentary or conversation with those you're sharing your meal with are great additions. Feed your mind.

THE MEAL ITSELF

During the meal itself, focus on the experience. Take your time and focus on enjoying each and every bite. Note the flavors, aromas, and sensations at play.

A large, yet frequently unrecognized reason people tend to overeat or feel that their diet isn't satisfying is because they aren't mentally there while they eat [1-3]. They're time traveling all over the place from what happened in the past to what they need to do in the future and thinking of things that have nothing to do with meal time. Meal time is important. You should enjoy it and take it as an opportunity to disconnect and regain mental clarity.

FOOD ORDER

The foods you pick may determine your satiety from the meal, but the order in which you eat them can determine your satiety during the meal.

Eating the fibrous fruits/greens and proteins first can be more filling and satisfying. This is good if you're cutting but may not be good for everyone during gaining phases.

PLATE TRICKS

A subconscious trick to use is to alter your plate size. If you are cutting, make your plate sizes smaller so that it looks like there is more food on the plate.

You can also experiment with the shapes and colors of your plates and silverware to see the effect that this has on your meal experience. Rest assured, meals are an *experience* that must account for several variables.

31

VITAMINS, MINERALS, AND FLUIDS

OUTSIDE OF MEETING A CERTAIN base level of protein and EFA intake, there are some other things our body simply must obtain through the diet for optimal functioning purposes. Those would be vitamins, minerals, and fluid intake.

VITAMIN/MINERAL INTAKE

Although most of the nutritional attention is given to the larger, more attractive macronutrients like Protein, Carbs, and Fats, the micronutrients such as vitamins and minerals are vital components of any healthy diet.

- ❧ Minerals include calcium, sodium, potassium, magnesium, and so forth.
- ❧ Vitamins come in two forms – fat soluble and water soluble. The fat-soluble vitamins are A, D, E, and K, and the water soluble are the B vitamins and vitamin C.

Together, they carry out a wide array of functions in the body, and the list could very well fill up an entire page. From healthy bones and connective tissue to aiding in processes everywhere you can look, the simple fact is that you can't afford not to get them.

FOOD CHOICE

With a diet made up of a wide array of whole, nutritious sources that I've supported, we can be sure that we will be packing in a solid amount of the essential vitamins and minerals that our bodies need to function optimally.

Plenty of fruits, vegetables, and wholesome sources should form the backbone of any sound nutritional program, and this is one of the reasons why that's the case.

Counting micronutrients meticulously simply isn't a huge concern unless you know you are deficient due to particular allergies, regional food availability, or personal preferences, and as you'll see next, the addition of supplementation can put any worries to bed.

If you do desire a higher degree of accuracy in looking at your micronutrient intake, track your daily food intake over the course of a week in a reliable nutritional database that provides micronutrient information. Then, you can see how you stack up to the RDAs and fine tune your food choices.

CONSIDER SUPPLEMENTATION

A low level, daily multivitamin is an economical, sound addition to your diet - with meals since there are fat and water-soluble vitamins, so consumption with a meal ensures it gets absorbed properly. Consider it your insurance policy. For only ~20USD/year, it's not a tough decision to make.

My recommendations of meal composition all have fat included to ensure absorption, fullness, and meal enjoyment.

NOTE ON SODIUM

Specific to fitness, many people run in terror from sodium. Many others try to manipulate it to extreme degrees to "dry out", shed water, and look lean. This is all idiotic on a whole 'nother level.

Higher sodium *than usual* will cause you to bloat and gain water weight, and lower sodium *than usual* will cause you to look slightly leaner and lose water weight, but here's the kicker: this is temporary and the body will adjust and compensate accordingly.

The body regulates all of this very precisely or else you would be dead, and it's an exercise in futility that can actually do much more harm than good. Don't try to outsmart the system. You will lose and probably get worse results than you planned for.

If you are a healthy individual, don't be afraid of a little sodium and seasoning your food. It'll taste better, and you'll be just fine.

And if you're doing it to look leaner, how about this: just get leaner. You're not holding water, you just need more fat loss.

FLUID INTAKE

Water is essential for proper physical function and performance. This should come as no surprise to you. You're made of it!

We can discuss the concrete amounts you should intake, but fluid balance is so variable due to climate, training conditions, and individual differences that I advocate you follow this one simple rule: ensure that your trips to the restroom are always clear or close to it. For most people, 3/4-1 gallon daily is right on the money.

6-8oz per waking hour is a general guideline that will help you meet this amount and also get up more often to combat poor posture and mental haze. It will also assist in boosting your caloric expenditure a bit, a useful tactic when cutting and facing lethargy and inactivity.

Additionally, ensure that you are drinking enough water around your training sessions. This is when it's most important.

FLUID SOURCES

Water is your number one, but coffee, tea, sodas, juices, and other liquids count towards this amount. Alcohol, however, does not.

For drinks that contain calories, this will have to be taken into account towards your calorie/macro goals. For some, it's a huge help. For others, it is an issue and leads to hunger or overeating.

32

SUPPLEMENTS

ALK INTO ANY SUPPLEMENT STORE and you'll be greeted by a maze of aisles resembling a magic potion shop overflowing unusual concoctions of every type, shape, and color. The magazines and advertisements are jam-packed with flashy claims and supposed success stories, and to the untrained eye, it's hard to resist the temptation of an extra edge or shortcut to climb to the top.

Many have fallen victim to the enchanting allure of supplement magic, but when all is said and done, supplements account for the *smallest amount of your results.*

When the rest of your diet is setup right like we just did, there are only a few supplements worth your hard-earned cash that will consistently give you a solid return on your investment. Don't waste your money or fall for the hype.

MULTIVITAMIN

By adopting the diet composed of mainly healthy, wholesome foods with fruits and vegetables at every meal I've recommended in the book, you'll be packing in loads of beneficial vitamins and minerals that will keep you running in pristine condition.

Nevertheless, we don't always have the best days, and due to individual preferences or medical restraints such as allergies, we might not eat enough of certain foods to get the optimal amount of certain vitamins and minerals.

To keep our bases covered, a low level, daily multivitamin is a solid insurance policy in regards to any potential deficiencies, particularly during periods of lower calories such as cutting phases [1]. There is no need to get fancy here, and a one year supply is only ~20USD.

Take one every day with a meal to ensure proper absorption.

FISH OIL

The fabled idea of a "magic pill" is nothing but fantasy at this point, but if ever there were a close contender, it'd have to be fish oil capsules [2]. They provide EPA/DHA, two essential fatty acids that must come from diet. The body cannot manufacture them on its own.

The demonstrated benefits of fish oil supplementation are widely documented and range from improved insulin sensitivity to joint health to better overall health markers. Fatty fish like salmon are excellent naturally-occurring sources, so if you like sushi, you're in luck. However, due to the fact that most diets in this day and age are low in EPA/DHA content and frequency, I strongly recommend daily fish oil supplementation if you don't consume fatty fish often. Economically, they are the best option as well, as the regular dietary sources can be quite pricey for the given fish oil amounts.

Aim for about ~2g combined EPA/DHA a day. Check the label to see the actual quantities of EPA/DHA provided – not just what the label calls "fish oil". They must be factored into your daily calorie intake (60-100 cals per day max) and should be taken alongside your meals, split up when able and practical. Some companies sell this in flavored liquid form, and that is acceptable. However, flax oil is not, for the conversion is not as efficient.

CREATINE

Most of the training supplements out there on the market are just fluff, but one has consistently been proven to deliver the goods: Creatine. It can provide a small boost in performance and muscle growth, and it's the only white powder I'll ever tell you to take [1,3].

Despite unfounded health concerns, creatine is safe, effective, and cheap. Buy creatine monohydrate. There is no need for the fancy kinds. It's all absorbed very well and does the same thing.

3-5g per day will give you all the benefit you need. There is conflicting evidence as to whether loading creatine with high doses (20g/day) for 2 weeks initially is of benefit to work faster, but the effects of creatine are small, so it is a moot point. Timing of daily intake does not matter.

CAFFEINE

Caffeine is a common stimulant that can increase your energy and performance, reduce the perception of fatigue, improve moods, and improve mental functioning [4,5].

❧ PREWORKOUT

Pre-workouts are the most common source of caffeine before lifting, and there are several on the market to choose from, but they are often loaded with other unnecessary additives to make them more marketable. Caffeine pills or coffee do the trick just fine. 100-200mg twenty to thirty minutes pre-workout is more than enough, and only take them if you need them. 1-2x/week is just fine.

❧ TOLERANCE

If you decide to take them, test your tolerance, temper your intake, and don't get dependent on them. It's easy to get hooked and start increasing your doses [6], but the withdrawal will come to bite you.

❧ SLEEP QUALITY

For any stimulant, be aware that they can lead to sleep issues if taken later in the day. This is important for those of you who lift late. Past 4-5pm, and you may run into trouble.

DAILY INTAKE

Caffeine is pretty awesome, but that's also its downfall. Keep your daily intake to ~400mg. For comparison, a cup of coffee has ~100mg and a diet soda has ~50mg. If you need more, check your sleep.

PROTEIN SUPPS

Not everyone finds it easy to get in enough protein through their
regular diets, so protein supplementation may be necessary or even
preferred. It is also a convenient option for many due to schedules.

If you're simply needing to meet your protein target, stick to
protein powder. You can buy huge tubs of it and it's a very
economical option. There is whey and casein, with the difference
being that casein is a slow-digesting protein, so taking it at bedtime
or when anticipating long periods between meals is its practical
use. Typically, you will get ~100-130 cals/25g protein per scoop.

If you're using it more as a meal replacement for pre-workout and
so on, then protein bars are a good idea to be a bit more filling and
provide a more well-rounded 'meal'. Watch out with these. They
can become glorified candy bars, overload you on calories, and get
on the pricey end. 200-300 cals/25g protein per bar is a good bet.

OTHER

In addition to these, depending on your multivitamin, Vitamin D
(D3) supplementation can be useful if you do not get much
exposure to the sun due to lifestyle, seasonal, or geographical
reasons. This is how your body produces it, and although some
cereals and dairy are fortified with small amounts, dietary intake is
usually insufficient. Aim for at least 1000 IU daily.

If you do not consume much dairy, a calcium supplement may be
necessary to ensure that you get enough. 1000mg per day is a good,
conservative dose, and many of them also come with Vitamin D3.

SUPPLEMENT QUALITY

Lastly, with any and all supplements that you take, buy only quality. Always ensure that you check the label and go with trusted, time tested companies who take pride in their product, tell you exactly what is in them and the quantities thereof.

Supplements often use lots of fillers, throw things you don't even need in there to make them sound more effective, and make shaky claims that are unfounded by research. Therefore, keep it simple to just what I have listed here, and seek to use supplements that come in isolation without unnecessary added ingredients. Avoid proprietary blends, and stick to the boring stuff. That's what works.

SUPPLEMENTS SUMMARY

SUPPLEMENT	DOSAGE
Multivitamin	1 per day with meals
Fish Oil	2g combined EPA/DHA per day – check label
Creatine monohydrate	3-5g/day
Caffeine	100-200mg Pre-WO 1-2x/wk 400mg max/day Start low and assess tolerance
Protein Powders	Only if you need it for convenience or to hit daily protein intake

- ❧ Keep your supplements in a place that makes taking them an easy, accessible habit.
- ❧ Only go for high quality, reputable sources

33

ALCOHOL

ANY PEOPLE SAY THAT ALCOHOL isn't necessary to have a good time. Maybe not, but if a great night out is up for grabs, you won't find me sipping lemon water.

Alcohol has been cast into a negative light and harshly demonized in the fitness community, but is it truly an evil inebriating monster?

THE FACTS BEHIND ALCOHOL

People have been getting hammered for thousands of years. Alcohol consumption dates back to the oldest civilizations, and it's a common social sipper in the present day from parties to nights out and everything in between. In addition, a nice glass of wine is an excellent way to end your day.

At 7 calories a gram, alcohol is the second most energy-packing macronutrient behind fat, and this is important to take into account before champagne showers and partying for hours.

Its large energy content is in large part why it's gained such a bad reputation amongst the fitness crowd, however the fact that alcohol is treated as a toxin to the body also tends to create a conniption in the minds of those who hear that.

In reality, this 7 calories is actually a bit under 6 due to its thermic effect, but since most alcoholic drinks don't come with nutrition facts slapped on the label, it's much easier to use general numbers or look up the values of your favorite drinks.

For a frame of reference, these are some average calorie contents on drinks out there.

DRINK	CALORIES
12 oz light beer	100
12 oz regular beer	150
12 oz dark beer	175+
Draft pint (reg.)	200
Wines	125-150
Shot	100
Mixed Drinks	Beware

As you can see, these figures are nothing to have nightmares over unless you have the energy expenditure of a rock.

If calories are an issue, you'll want to stick to light beers, dry wines, and spirits in lieu of dark beers and mixers.

HURTING THE GAINS?

Cool, so you know the calorie situation, but does drinking hurt your gains? Not likely [1,2]. 1-2 drinks daily will have a negligible effect on your gains, but going *hard on the drinks will* start to impair muscle protein synthesis after training [3], so keeping heavy drinking away from your workouts and recovery is good practice if optimal gains is what you're after.

Additionally, not only do moderate doses of drinking not hurt your gains, but moderate amounts of alcohol consumption are actually *beneficial* from a health standpoint [4-8].

BOTTOM LINE

With a solid diet, it's easy to fit in a couple drinks here and there. Life is meant for living, and if you are shutting yourself off socially because of a fear of alcohol hampering your fitness progress, you are only doing yourself a disservice for no good reason.

DRINKING WHILE STAYING ON FIT GOALS

With those facts laid out before you, how do you fit drinking in with your fitness goals? Let's see.

HIT YOUR ESSENTIALS

We've already established that calories followed by macronutrient content - with protein being the most important - are the most important factors when crafting a diet. We also know that we need EFAs, fiber, and micronutrients from the diet on top of that.

Therefore, on days you want to enjoy a couple drinks, ensure you hit your protein goals and EFA content while dropping carbs and fat to free up your caloric budget. If you plan your meals based on macros, simply swap out the quantities and make sure you account for the calorie differences (alcohol has 7 cals/g, carbs have 4, and fats have 9). To get your fiber, stick to more fibrous vegetables to fill you up because alcohol will not fill you up like a regular meal would.

TIME APPROPRIATELY

Based on your diet from hitting those essentials, you're going to have to create your daily meal split to plan your drinking times and nights out. This is important, because the amount of food in your system will impact your response to alcohol [9,10], and alcohol intake can also increase your hunger levels and inhibit your decision-making which can lead to poor choices during your drinking or after when you get back home [11]. Because of this:

- If you want to have several drinks, leave yourself lots of dietary room and before you go out, have a high protein, high fiber meal of a good size with enough dietary space for another meal when you get home.
- If you just want the effect of alcohol in and of itself, then only have a small meal before drinking and consider saving more dietary room for after you get home. It'll take less alcohol to get the same effect on a lighter stomach.

This will ensure that you tailor the diet based on your goal.

During the drinking itself, keep away from the common foods out there. This is what will do the damage to your diet and progress. The meal beforehand will make sure that you're satisfied and less likely to mess up here.

No matter what you do, ensure that you are safe and handle your business and transportation arrangements appropriately. Go have your fun, but make sure that you set yourself up to keep having it in the future and look out for others.

APPLY TO OTHER TIMES

This same strategy can be used around holidays and other events where you want to indulge a bit.

Cycling them properly with a plan you love can allow you to do just that and maintain your physique easily, and we'll talk about that because it's a great tool that's often overlooked for maintaining. This is a good technique to use consciously, but if you're coming from the mentality of "restricting" yourself so that you can splurge later, you have a problem.

IN SUM

Alcohol is far from necessary, and if you're not a drinker, don't feel the need, but if it floats your boat, my practical recommendation is to limit your daily intake to 1-2 drinks and if you go out and drink several drinks, keep it to a maximum of one time per week. This will allow you to live a little and still have solid nutrition and training.

PART V
RECOVERY

34

THE TEMPLE AND
THE SAMURAI

THE SAMURAI OF JAPAN were some of the most elite
and esteemed warriors of history. They were highly skilled,
highly respected, and highly driven to their mission. Their
weapon of choice? The sword.

The samurai treated their sword with great honor. Their very
SPIRIT was said to be contained in that sword. It was to be honored
and valued, and swords were meticulously crafted and finely made.

This is how the most elite warriors treat their weapons, yet look at
how the world treats their own bodies.

MAXIM OF AESTHETICS: WORKING OUT IS A PRIVILEGE. TAKE CARE OF YOUR BODY SO THAT IT CAN TAKE CARE OF YOU.

Before you slap on tons of muscle mass and start loading up the bar, your body needs to be healthy and ready to do so. And being able to move and function in daily life comes before making gains in the weight room. Don't let the latter disrupt the former.

Your body is your temple. It's a magnificent temple, but even the greatest temples and architectural constructs need to be properly maintained to ensure integrity and continuance of the structure and beauty.

We can do this primarily through nutrition, sleep, our posture, and tissue quality - soft-tissue work, stretching, and so on.

THE FUNDAMENTALS

A well-rounded diet based primarily on whole, nutritious foods will always serve you well. In the nutrition section of the book, you will learn in further detail how to set up the optimal diet for your needs.

In addition to this, your mental states will impact your recovery efforts. In a later part of the book, you will discover how to use your mind to your advantage and eliminate negativity, stress, and other undesirable things.

Lastly, don't smoke, do drugs, or any of that other nonsense. It should go without saying. Life is your drug now.

SLEEP

> *"Sleep is for the weak."*
> *"I'll sleep when I'm dead."*
> *"You have to sacrifice sleep for success."*

Sound familiar? Forget all of that.

Sleep is *absolutely critical*, and you need to be getting as much as your body needs *each and every* night. This is when you repair, recharge, and grow from a day well spent.

Mental function, mood, recovery, and physical performance are all directly impacted by your sleep levels [1-4], so don't cut yourself short here. When you're sleeping like a beast, you're going to be able to train like one and maximize your results.

HOW MUCH SLEEP

Every night, aim to get at least 7-9 hours of quality sleep. Not laying around in bed thinking about ghosts and aliens. *Actual sleep.*

Some can feel great off of 7 hours, and some may need 9. Don't marry the number. Observe, see how you feel in the morning, and adjust accordingly. Track it in your logs, and you may be able to catch some trends between how much shuteye you're getting and the quality of your day and workouts.

If you're woken up by your alarm every morning, then at least once per week, allow yourself to be woken up naturally when you're good & ready. You should feel refreshed, recharged, and ready to tackle the day. If that means 9, 10, or 11 hours, then so be it.

Listen to your body. It's wiser than you give it credit for. We humans are the only creatures on the planet who need an alarm clock to wake up in the morning. THAT's the reason for alarm. Let nature take its course every once in a while (if not often).

SLEEP ROUTINE

The key to a great night's sleep is in the pre-bed routine.

Put these tips in play with a consistent sleep schedule, and you'll be well on your way to recharging and getting ready to tackle the day.

∂ BIT OF EXERCISE

Your workouts and regular daily exercise will make it easier to slip into a deep, recuperative slumber later on at night [5,6]. If you work out late in the evenings, watch out for your pre-workout stimulants. They'll keep you awake at the time when you most need to rest up.

∂ FEAST UP

All of my programs make sure that you're getting solid meals in on the last leg of your day. Cutting, gaining, maintaining – it doesn't matter.

Evening time is a time to relax and unwind. Throw on some chill music, cook yourself a delicious, well-rounded meal to feed your body what it needs, and enjoy that dinner time drowsiness.

❧ SOFT LIGHT AND AROMAS

Rather than keep a bunch of big lights on, light up some candles or wax melts and get your place smelling divine. Less bright lights will allow you to adjust better, and the aromas are relaxing. Whenever you have company, you'll be drowning in compliments. Mix it up for the seasons, and you'll instantly spruce up your house.

❧ HOT SHOWER/BATH

Before you hit the sheets, hop in the shower or tub and wash away that tension. This will relax your muscles and your mind and diminish any lingering soreness built up from your training. Take this as a time to de-stress and shake your mind from any negative thoughts.

❧ FOAM ROLL

After you get out of the shower or bath, you'll be feeling refreshed and limber. This is the perfect opportunity to work on a bit of self-myofascial release. Use your foam roller, small ball, or massage cane to gently work on any nagging areas that are tight on your frame.

You will learn more about self-myofascial release later in the chapter.

❧ CUT OUT ELECTRONICS

Create a cut-off time at least 30 minutes before you hop in bed for any visual entertainment, phone use, or work you've got on your plate. The only media or electronics allowed after this time is chill music – no lyrics even better.

Late night texts from a hottie? Too bad. You're catching Zs. After X
o' clock, your phone is off your radar entirely.

Don't be afraid of missing out. You're playing into their frame if you
do. Remember: you make the rules of your own life and live how
you see fit. And when you do, more often than not people will bend
theirs to accommodate it. Build yourself up to where you don't
need to rely on out of the blue texts to hang out with people.

Extra tip: Blue light filters

If the sun sets much earlier than when you knock out, put a blue
light filter on your monitors or devices. This makes it easier on your
eyes and doesn't give your body mixed signals about what time it is
out there [7-9]. There are lots of applications out there to put this
on your computer, and most TVs and smartphones these days have
that option in the settings. Do some digging and you'll find it.

❧ BLACK OUT

When it comes to sound sleep, your bedroom needs to be Dracula's
lair level dark. Go get yourself thick, heavy curtains and keep all the
remaining sunlight out or else the rays will zap all your gains.
When you hop in bed, blow out any candles still going with the
shadows dancing around the room.

❧ TURN ON THE FAN

You want your bedroom to be a little bit cold. If it's hot and stuffy
in there, you're going to have a hard time getting comfortable and
drifting away. Turn the fan on and check the thermostat to keep
the heat down. A touch above 'too cold' is just right.

⮞ MEDITATION

It's impossible to sleep when you're staring up at the ceiling drowning in thoughts.

Your mind will run all over you day and night if you let it, so before bed, meditate to clear your head, relax your body, and gain that peace you need before you sleep. See the next point to drive this home. You will learn more about meditation in the next part of the book.

⮞ RECAP YOUR DAY

Tracking progress is vitally important. You do it for your nutrition and workouts, so why wouldn't you do it for other things -- like *your life*. As the day comes to an end and you are winding down, take a moment to reflect upon your day.

What went well?
What could be better?
What did you learn?
What are you thankful for?
What did you contribute to the world?

Jotting down your thoughts and gaining clarity will help you to mentally tie up any loose ends and gain closure so that you can learn from your day and sleep in peace.

The day is over. Accept today. Tomorrow is a new day with new opportunities.

&v EXTRA COMFORTABLE

Make your bed a paradise. 1/3rd of your life is devoted to sleep, so invest in an amazing mattress, soft, silky sheets, cozy blankets, and great pillows.

In addition to your head pillow, a body pillow and a couple smaller pillows will do wonders for getting in a good sleeping posture. That brings us to our next point:

&v PERFECT POSTURE

The posture you sleep in is going to be an important factor in how you feel in the morning. We've all woken up with a crick in our neck from an awkward sleeping position the night before. Imagine a lower level intensity of this over years.

Sleep in a natural, neutral position whenever possible. On your back with your hands straight at your sides and a pillow under your knees or on your side with your arms and legs supported with a body pillow or bae are two great go-to options.

SLEEP SUMMARY

Put these sleeping tips into play by adopting a regular sleep time schedule, and the quality of your sleep and the life that follows when you wake up will surge upwards.

Not every night is going to be perfect. Go have your wild nights. But even so – this is your standard target to shoot for.

BUILD THOSE HABITS.

POSTURE

Picture-perfect posture is essential for both lifting and life success, but these days, it's a diamond in the rough.

Strong posture will make you look and feel mighty, and that's going to translate into better gains in and out of the weight room. If you roll your eyes and keep up your bad posture ways, here's what you've got coming full-speed your way:

1. ACHES, PAINS, AND INJURY
2. INHIBITED PERFORMANCE
3. UNBALANCED PHYSIQUE
4. SOCIAL SUCKAGE
5. LACKLUSTER MOODS

Therefore, we need to cut that mess out and get you in line.

MAJOR PROBLEMS

The main problems spots for posture are kyphosis, lordosis, and forward head posture. The body works as a full-functional unit, so these are all related, and they lead to 50 other negative things you don't want in your life. The biggest culprit of them all is lots of sitting, something the population does far too much of these days.

ぞ KYPHOSIS

This is the classic hunchback posture where your thoracic spine curves over your midline. This leads to a stiff, cramped upper body, screwy scapulae, and internally rotated shoulders that throws off your biomechanics and will cause shoulder pain sooner or later.

• LORDOSIS

This one is a bit harder to describe, so if you want to know what lordosis looks like, check out the posture of girls making their squat gains look better on social media. This is excessive anterior tilting of the pelvis and is caused by tight hip flexors and weak glutes.

• FORWARD HEAD POSTURE

Forward head posture is where the neck and head jut outwards from the body, and it's also heavily linked to riding a desk all day. This will only lead to headaches and people thinking you can't hear.

POSTURE REPAIR

To get around these, you'll be doing several important things:

1. BE AWARE AT ALL TIMES OF HOW YOUR POSTURE IS.

How's your posture right now reading this? I caught you, didn't I. Sit and stand up straight. If you catch yourself slipping, adjust. Relax and keep a neutral posture. This will soon be second nature to you. Practice in a mirror – both standing and sitting.

2. KEEP YOUR TRAINING BALANCED

Everyone loves to build up those mirror muscles. The chest and quads get all the love, but that only exacerbates your postural problems, and it's those muscles on your backside that will take your physique to the next level. When's the last time you saw someone with a juicy set of hamstrings or rear delts? Never huh.

Training needs to be balanced out to put the body in its best position and avoid postural issues from popping up. The programs I've laid out in the book already take that into account, however if posture is a large issue, training needs to *be unbalanced* in the opposite direction, and specific movements are indicated, however due to the biomechanical complexities, they are beyond the scope of this book and are needed on a case by case basis per individual.

3. MOVE MORE TO AVOID STATIC POSTURES

The biggest enemy to great posture is not bad posture – *it's not moving.*

The more you put yourself in one position, the more your body will adjust to that position, and if it's a bad one, then bad posture is what you're gonna get. The best posture is the one that's always changing, so don't sit still. Get up and move around often. Make it a habit not to sit for more than 30 minutes at a time.

4. INCORPORATE MOBILITY DRILLS, STRETCHING, AND SOFT-TISSUE WORK

Poor posture causes your body to realign negatively and get sluggish where it needs to be sharp. To get around this, you'll be using some simple tools and techniques like these to move more towards your ideal state.

LET'S MOVE ON

If you nail all of these, you'll be standing tall and mighty, feeling great, and pushing better weights in the gym in no time. Let's look at how to do that all in further detail in the following sections.

GET MOVING

The human body was made to move, and if you don't use it, you lose it.

Specificity goes further than just how you train. The body will adapt specifically to whatever you throw at it, so if you throw sitting at it all day, it's going to follow suit, and the results are not pretty for your athletic and aesthetic endeavors.

You're sitting around all day then want to go throw around some heavy iron for an hour? Send me a postcard from Snap City. *I* will send my condolences.

FREQUENT MOVEMENT

The longer you stay still in the same spot, the more the negative effects pop up. Your muscles get tight, your joints get stiff, and your energy levels fizzle out.

To combat this, make it a habit to get up periodically and move. Shoot for 5 minutes standing, stretching, and moving around for every 30 minutes seated. An hour seated is *the maximum*, and it needs to be complemented with a 10 minute break afterwards.

- Set an alert on your phone, computer, or watch to let you know the time has come.
- Aim to drink 8oz of fluids every hour on the hour to get up and refill

It'll help with moods and productivity as well by giving your mind a chance to get fresh, so get up and get moving.

DAILY ACTIVITY

I know you love that workout sesh, but doing some sort of regular daily activity outside of training is *just* as important. This is fantastic for helping with any lingering soreness, boosting your mood, and getting some fresh air in your day.

For example, go on two 15 minute walks mid-morning and mid-afternoon. Use this as an opportunity to stretch, shake loose and disconnect your mind from your work day and all the other happenings of the world. An evening walk is also an excellent way to end your day and destress before hitting the sheets for a great night's sleep.

Alternatively, you can ride a bike, swim, skate, or play some pick up games. No matter what you do, keep it light and do no more than 30 minutes to a 1 hour per day total. You've read the section on cardio, so you know my thoughts on these matters.

Lastly, stay out of the gym on these days. No treadmills or machines. Go do real life things.

STRETCHING

Our muscles work across a range of motion to perform the work that we ask of it. As is often the case, we lose that range of motion that is necessary to be able to perform at the optimal level. The body will adapt. Positively or negatively.

To get around this, do a little bit of light daily stretching alongside all of the other tips I'm dishing out. Here are a few of the spots that typically need more attention:

- HIP FLEXORS
- PECS
- LATS
- FOREARMS
- CALVES
- NECK

For any area you stretch, watch the rest of your body and keep a neutral spine and head position.

Frequency is more important than incredible lengths of time. A few times throughout the day for a hold of 5-10 seconds works just fine to start. You are simply tossing nudging reminders at your body throughout the day of how it's supposed to be so that it's always fresh and in sync.

Under no circumstances force your muscle into pain or further than it wants to go. You are only restoring motion, not trying out for the contortionist Olympics.

MOBILITY DRILLS

Mobility drills are great for training your body to move in its functional patterns the *correct* way and maintain great posture.

Just like not moving a muscle through its functional range of motion can cause the muscle feel stiff, not activating certain muscles across their movement patterns will cause them to get dull and forget how to fire off the right way.

Here are a few favorites that will work your whole body. Perform them circuit style 1-2x a day and/or before your workouts:

❧ T-SPINE MOBILITY

The thoracic spine is the key to proper upper body movement. To get it into a more natural position and allow for better motion through the shoulder, you'll be doing some T-spine mobility drills.

1. Lay with your upper back on a foam roller on the ground. Do not – under any circumstances – ever do this with your lower back. Keep your chin tucked by cradling your head.
2. While keeping your core braced nice and tight, rock back onto the foam roller to extend your upper back and then return to the starting position. Repeat for 2-3 repetitions.
3. Slide a couple of vertebrae upwards and repeat the process. Stop once you get to where your upper back meets your neck.

❧ GLUTE BRIDGES (+ BANDED)

The glutes are the powerhouse of the lower body and a key core component of any aesthetic physique. Too bad they're so underdeveloped and neglected in most of the world. Not anymore.

1. Lay with your head, back, and feet flat on the ground and your arms straight at your side. Your knees should be up and forming a nice triangle with the floor.
2. Contract your glutes to bring your hips up off the floor to form a nice straight line from your knees to your head. Don't hyperextend your lower back, and squeeze for a count of 1.
3. Lower your hips back down and repeat for 8-10 repetitions.

To add to this drill, place resistance bands around your thighs and push your legs outwards for a little hip abduction action. This will get your glutes firing the right way and prep you for a productive leg day session.

❧ LUNGES WITH ROTATIONS

Now it's time to get up. Some lunges and rotations will put your legs, ankles, hips, and upper back into some good motion.

1. Step out in front of you to a 45 angle and sink into a nice lunge. Feel the stretch across your entire legs.
2. Place the hand of your lunge leg on the ground to form a steady base and then rotate your upper torso away from your lead leg to point your arm to the ceiling. All of the motion should come from your upper back. Keep the core and head stable and use your *eyes* to follow your hand.

3. Rotate back and stand back up into starting position. Do this for 5 repetitions each leg.

❧ WALL SLIDES

Wall slides will get your shoulder blades moving the right way, and you'll even get a little thoracic extension, serratus/ rotator cuff activation, and lat stretch tacked on for the cherry on top.

1. Face the wall with the karate chop portion of your hands and forearms touching the wall at around chest height, shoulder width apart. You can stagger your feet with one slightly ahead of the other to resist the temptation to slip into lumbar hyperextension for the drill.
2. Slide your arms and hands directly up the wall and out to a slight angle. Keep your core tight, a neutral back position, and your chin tucked as your shoulder blades rotate smoothly.
3. Slowly lower back down and repeat for 8-10 repetitions.

To add to the drill, you can place a resistance band around your forearms to increase rotator cuff activation.

❧ CHIN TUCKS

Chin tucks will straighten out that forward head posture you've got going on and round out the circuit.

1. Put your back flat on a wall so that your head is touching
2. Flex your neck so that you make a double chin. Hold for a count of 1 and then release back into the starting position
3. Repeat for 8-10 repetitions.

WHEN TO GO MOBILE

Incorporate a quick circuit of these drills at least 1-2x per day.

You can do this first thing in the morning, before bed in the evening, or at daily breaks. If you're really jacked up, quick flashes of these posture fixes will work wonders for getting you back to postural perfection. You'll be done in just a couple minutes tops.

Perform them in your warmups as well to ensure you're moving and grooving as you should be before handling the iron.

MOBILITY CIRCUIT

T-Spine Extensions	2-3 reps each section
Glute bridges (banded)	8-10 repetitions
Walking Lunges w/ Rotation	5 reps each side
Wall Slides	8-10 repetitions
Chin Tucks	8-10 repetitions

If you're doing in a spot where you don't have a foam roller and can't lay on the ground, make these simple swaps:

1. For T-Spine extensions, find a chair with a backing that isn't high up on your upper back and perform the same motion.
2. For glute bridges, stand up and perform some glute kickbacks and abductions for 8-10 each repetitions each leg. Feel the glutes contract and watch the posture of the rest of your body.

Good to go.

SOFT-TISSUE WORK

Have you ever seen those big columns of foam on the ground in the matted area of corner of the gym? No, they're not for the kids people bring to the gym to beat the hell out of each other. They're used for foam rolling, also known as self-massage/self-myofascial release.

They're not limited to those hunks of foam either - there are also small balls, massage canes, and so on, but for simplicity's sake, I'll be referring to them as foam rolling or SMR.

Foam rolling will:

- ૐ Permit optimal workout performance [1-3]
- ૐ Help improve flexibility [4-6]
- ૐ Aid in recovery and alleviate soreness [7,8]

And therefore:

- ૐ De-stress and remove muscular tension
- ૐ Assist in restoring proper posture
- ૐ Serve as a prehab measure

WHAT YOU'LL NEED:

- ૐ SMALL BALL

Get a lacrosse ball, tennis ball, or a dedicated rubber rolling ball that's sold online or in stores. The key here is to find something firm. If it is too flimsy, you won't get that bittersweet pressure you're after.

This will be used for smaller muscle groups or areas that you want to give more targeted pressure. Most of the upper body tends to work better with a small ball than our next option, the foam roller.

ଇ FOAM ROLLER

You will also need a foam roller. This is a large, cylindrical section of foam that you'll roll on. The hardness will vary on these. There are softer ones and ones that are hard and solid like a brick. I recommend you start in the middle and work your way up as needed for more pressure. A PVC pipe is another alternative that's been used by many as well as a worthy substitute.

The foam roller works best for the lower body and other big muscle groups. It's also good for performing thoracic extensions to open up the upper back's range of motion as you saw in the previous section.

For smaller areas or more targeted pressure, opt for the ball or the tools below:

- ଇ SMALLER BALL (for more pressure)
- ଇ CANE MASSAGER
- ଇ HANDHELD ROLLER/MASSAGE KNOB - for rolling more precise portions without your bodyweight.

The two mandatory materials for foam rolling can be secured for less than $10-$20 bucks. That's a solid investment for years of benefit that'll pay dividends time and time again for your workout performance, health, posture, and nagging aches and pains.

If you go the premium route and secure more foam rolling items, you will still sit comfortably under $50.

For contrast, an hour-long session of massage can cost upwards of $50, and unless you have a very open and attentive or tenured massage therapist, often times you'll get a better session working into your target spots yourself. You know yourself and the ins and outs of your body the best.

That's not to say massage and manual techniques can't be useful - see the end of the section.

HOW TO FOAM ROLL

So you're sold on the benefits of getting your roll on and have the tools to carry it out. How do you do it?

❧ ROLL OVER THE MUSCLE

No matter whether you're using the ball, a large roller, or a cane, you're going to want to position yourself to work on the targeted muscle by applying pressure on it with room to roll back and forth. This can either be on the floor or on an empty wall. Certain body parts play better for the wall or floor than others.

For example, if you're targeting your chest, you'll face the wall, place the ball in between yourself and the wall on your chest, and then apply pressure by leaning into the ball and rolling back and forth over the muscle. For your back or shoulder, simply turn your body accordingly and do the same.

For the quads, you'll face the floor and place the roller between the floor and your quads. Let gravity apply the pressure and roll out your quads by sliding up and down, using the support of your arms on the floor as a stable base to move from. For hamstrings, calves, and IT bands, you simply turn accordingly.

You're only limited by your imagination here, and you'll find what works best for you. If you're using a knobber or rolling pin, you can do these either standing or sitting to get yourself into the best position.

࿇ WORK THE AREA

You can roll out the entire area of the muscle from top to bottom or break it up into smaller segments for more targeted work, or any combination thereof.

Do a few light passes over the entire muscle and then apply a little more pressure in individual segments followed by a harder few passes over the entire muscle before moving on to the next muscle group you want to roll.

࿇ LOVE THOSE TENDER SPOTS

Foam rolling can be like when you were younger and had a loose tooth. It hurts a little, but it's also pleasurable in a weird, twisted way.

In some areas, you will roll over them and just feel good, but in key areas, you'll notice a little burst of tenderness. If you're new to SMR, this might be your whole entire body.

Take extra care on these areas. Start lightly and do a few extra passes over them. These are trigger points, places of hyperactivity or previous workload. They're often very tight and dense, and you'll notice a huge increase in how you feel and move after targeting them. Over time, you'll see a definite improvement.

❧ WATCH YOUR WHOLE BODY

During your SMR, don't end up in any odd or biomechanically awkward positions. This can actually *reinforce* bad posture and spur *new* bad habits in addition to putting strain on your body in ways that should be avoided.

Keep a neutral spine and head position as you roll, and don't put too much weight or stress on any body parts in particular for support outside of what's necessary to get the job done.

YOU SHOULD BE FOAM ROLLING:

1. BEFORE WORKOUTS

Foam rolling before workouts will prepare your body for the workout ahead. Your muscles will be loose and more pliable, so you'll get better flexibility and performance out of your workout, and any postural deficiencies that crept up won't block your workout performance. No proper warm up in my books is done without a little SMR.

Focus most of your attention on the areas involved in what you'll be doing. If it's an upper body day, give special attention to the chest, back, shoulder & rotator cuff regions, and arms. For legs, give attention to the various parts of the quad, the hamstring, IT band, and calves.

That's not all, however. You'll want to use the big foam roller to do some thoracic extensions, and it's a good idea to at least touch briefly on your whole body. Why?

- Proper movement is a body-wide affair
- You could benefit from doing so as a check in case you skip your other sessions (daily session, see below), and to help iron out your posture (almost surely in need of an upgrade).

This is to be done at the beginning of the warm-up before any weights are touched. It's a crucial part of every warm up, but not the end all be all. Don't forget movement drills, light stretches, and a proper weight warm up, too.

Foam rolling is only a couple minutes of a warm up that's less than 10 minutes, and it's a valuable investment of your time that should not go skipped over.

2. A DEDICATED SESSION DAILY (EX: MORNING/EVENING)

I start every day off with a light bound of foam rolling after a nice, hot shower alongside some bomb coffee and the airwaves drenched in uplifting music or audio content. It gets me loose and feeling excellent before tackling the day. Any lingering workout soreness is smoothly ironed out a bit as well. It's a daily routine.

In the evenings before bed, I usually take a shower or soak in a good bath to read a bit, meditate, or enjoy some music. During or after this, I'll take a few minutes to roll out and get rid of any of the tension of the day to slip into a solid slumber.

Morning or evening? Both. It's only a couple of minutes that's well worth your time.

3.   THROUGHOUT THE DAY AS NEEDED

If spending a lot of time in one position throughout the day is your reality or making changes to your improve your posture is something of interest to you, you will get a lot of benefit from doing mini sessions with your foam rolling tools.

You can use a massage knob to work through spots while you work, are on conference calls (stand up if possible), or during break times. While you sit, you can roll your feet out with a small ball. You'll be surprised at how good you feel after doing these - and not just on your feet. The feet are where a lot of problems higher up in the body originate. Everything is connected.

KEEP IT ON HAND

To ensure this goes down, make your SMR tools readily accessible. Your environment and accessibility are often-overlooked aspects of forming solid habits, so keep your rollers and other SMR tools in your bedroom, in a gym bag, or wherever else you need to put them so that you see them all the time and be reminded of what you've got to do.

Wipe the rug out from your excuses.

OUTSOURCE

Foam rolling is a great thing all on its own, but if you need more attention than this, I'd also recommend that you outsource it periodically as well. They can hit areas that are hard for you to reach properly, and you get the boost of being able to relax a bit.

- Schedule a good massage with a great massage therapist once a month/2 months/quarter
- Have your bf/gf/loyal servant hook you up. Alternate. Make In a relationship, this is a way to create more connection and learn each other more on a physical level. Try it out.
- Consider a chiropractor for more targeted techniques (ART, Graston, etc.)

No matter what you do, ensure solid communication and make it known where your tender spots are and any restrictions you may have. Through trips over time, you'll see the improvement in quality of treatment and your results that stem from it.

	ROLLER	BALL	CANE
Neck	-	X	X
Chest	-	X	X
Shoulders	-	X	X
Rotator Cuff	-	X	X
Arms	-	X	X
Lats	X	-	-
Midback/Traps	X	X	X
Glutes	X	X	-
Quads	X	-	-
Hamstrings	X	-	-
IT Band	X	-	-
Calves	X	-	-
Feet	-	X	-

PART VI
PROGRESS

35

TRACKING
PROGRESS

WHAT DOESN'T GET MEASURED doesn't get improved. This is true in the business world, your personal habits, and *especially so* in fitness & nutrition.

MAXIM OF AESTHETICS: TRACK YOUR PROGRESS OR YOU ARE ON THE TRACK TO NOWHERE

Here we'll go over tracking your workouts, nutrition, body composition, other factors, and the various ways you can carry this out to put you on the path towards optimal progress.

TRACKING WORKOUT PROGRESS

Your objective lifting weights is to continually progress by increasing the weight on the bar, the repetitions you do with it, or the number of sets done of them.

That is a patient, methodical progression, so you will need some way to capture your results and monitor your progress to see where you stand up over time. If you don't know what your workouts looked like in the past, you are setting yourself up for failure.

Off the top of your head, do you remember what you did 3 Sundays ago at 3pm? I bet you don't.

Recording your workouts will give you a good standard to go off of and provide you with the valuable information you need to analyze how you are doing and what changes - if any - need to be made to the program to achieve the results you are after. It's essential to seeing how you're doing over time - and also highly motivating.

THE WORKOUT LOG

The important variables to record in terms of workouts here are:

- Exercise selection
- Weight used
- Repetitions Performed
- RITTS (Repetitions in the Tank)
- Sets performed
- Rest times
- Date, Day of week, and time of day
- Any additional notes impacting training

Record these DURING your work out sessions. Waiting until after can blur your memory of what you did or how things felt.

Before every workout, open up your log and look at the last workout and what you're aiming to beat. This will allow you to capture focus and gives you a place to reach for. You know before that first set EXACTLY what is on the menu for your gym session today and what you need to beat.

If WHEN - you do, it's a great feeling. Celebrate the mini victories. They'll lead you to the ultimate prize.

NUTRITION TRACKING:

Proper nutrition is absolutely, positively, definitely, certainly, and whatever other synonyms you want to throw in the mix, NECESSARY for progress in our journey. You've simply got to track it in one way or another to be sure of your efforts. Through the combination of a digital food scale and accurate nutritional information, record your daily:

- Calories
- Macronutrients - at minimum calories and protein
- Meals/Meal times
- Supplements
- Feeling or additional notes and thoughts

Several free applications make this a breeze and is easily achievable with less than 5-10 minutes a day, so there is absolutely zero excuse not to. It's best to record your meal intake before you even eat your meal so that you don't worry about it or forget.

Even for more broad goals, tracking your nutrition precisely should be done at least for a week or two so that you can see how you're eating and make changes to put you better in line with your goals.

After this, you can use visual estimations and intuition while having periods of tracking every once in a while to calibrate your diet. However, if you're not getting the results you want, you know what you need to do. Tracking is the way to go.

You can find more information on the simple act of tracking in its section in the Nutrition section of the book.

TRACKING BODY COMPOSITION

What is your goal? AESTHETICS. What does this involve? Our body composition. Therefore, tracking it is vital to our efforts.

There are several ways to track your body composition, and incorporating all of them is the best bet, as each gives you a different perspective on how you're progressing.

THEORETICAL TRACKING

Theoretical tracking refers to the supposed rates of change that you would expect to see based on your calculations and estimations. For example, you set your nutrition up to lose a theoretical 0.75lbs per week or gain 0.5lbs per week.

Having a firm, objective target that you've arrived at will allow you to have yourself firmly rooted and see what is working and what isn't so that you can make changes accordingly. This can later be compared to what is going on with the other methods of tracking like the scale, mirror, and photos.

If the theoretical values show that you should be gaining 0.5lbs per week but over the course of time you see that you are gaining 1lb per week on average, you know that a change should be made to better calibrate your nutritional efforts by reducing your caloric intake.

BODY WEIGHT

Body weight is a major input into the calorie formula, determines the rough levels of macronutrients for your diet, and is an important thing to track in terms of progress itself to see whether you are marching forward towards muscle growth, shredding fat in a cutting phase, or remaining constant in a maintenance period.

Most people get their idea of results based on the scale alone. This is silly stuff. Weight is like a politician. It only tells you part of the story. Your body weight can fluctuate by several pounds overnight, and clearly this isn't explicable by caloric intake alone. Body weight is impacted by:

- The amount of fuel in the tank
- Carb intake
- Sodium intake
- Time of day
- Hydration levels
- Supplementation (creatine, etc.)
- Stress and hormonal levels
- Mother Nature
- etc

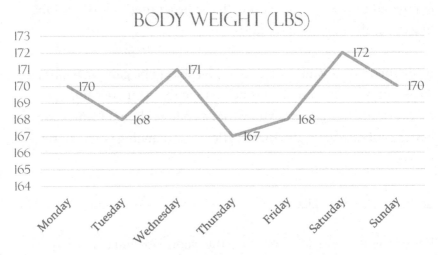

If you judge your progress by the scale alone, you'll be on a rollercoaster of emotions. Look at how it moves up and down.

Trying to masterfully manipulate all of these variables is extra effort that's not worth the mental gymnastics. You will lose. Weight moves up and down. That's just how it goes. With that in mind:

1. Weigh yourself every morning upon waking after a trip to the restroom and before consuming anything
2. Record your weights
3. Track the averages over time on a spreadsheet

By doing this, you'll be able to see how things flow over time. Combined with your other tools of tracking body composition, you'll be able to compare and see what works and what doesn't so that you can make any necessary changes. I recommend that you keep your calories side by side with body weight for this reason. The scale is a helpful tool for tracking progress and setting up our plans, but let's not forget that you have other tools in your arsenal.

THE MIRROR

Common knowledge says that you should use the mirror and not the scale, and in a sense this is true, but the mirror should not be used as an objective standard either.

What you see in the mirror also changes day to day, and you only see your reflection in the *present moment,* so your perception of how you look is limited *to that moment.* It isn't good for tracking long term progress, so pictures should be used for that.

The mirror can be useful for seeing how you react to different things nutritionally, however. Your muscles may look more full one day. You may be more lean another. This can be big in seeing your reactions to training and nutrition, but this doesn't tell the whole story either, so look for trends over time.

PICTURES

The scale may be playing mind games with you, the mirror may not be so generous lately, and the theoretical results of your plan indicate that you should be making progress, but you're simply not so sure. This is why pictures are the king of them all.

Having a series of pictures to compare from this week and a month ago can be the winning ticket when it comes to objectively analyzing the progress you're after.

Make it a habit to take pictures on a series of days periodically to store and use as a comparison of how you look through TIME. This is what the mirror alone can't do. You will do this 3 days in a row every 2 weeks to a month to see the progress that has been made.

Take pictures from different angles in good, neutral lighting. That means lighting that doesn't wash you out or make you look spectacular on purpose for stunting on social media. This makes it harder to see true progress. Sticking to the same picture location at the same times works best. Either you or someone else can take it.

At times, you may feel disappointed by what the picture reveals, but rest easy. When you see the fruits of your labor over time, you will be overjoyed.

BODY FAT MEASURES?

The rage in the fitness world is to fixate on and brag about their body fat percentage. Guys will say "I'm 4%!" and girls will make claims of being in the single digits. No you're not. If you really were, you'd either be dead or hanging in a Halloween store.

Typically, they were measured by a trainer at their local gym with a set of calipers or a handheld electrical device to come up with that figure. Both are notoriously inaccurate, and such low levels are not healthy in any form or fashion.

Quite honestly, I see no point in chasing specific body-fat percentages. This is yet another flaw in using numerical values to conclude success.

What do we care about? Visual appearance.

For planning purposes, we can "estimate" what body fat a person is at instead based on the mirror and series of pictures and leave it at that. The best relevant indicators are the abs. This is what most want, and having abs brings definition elsewhere along with it. Men will get them around 10%, and women ~17%. This will be useful for setting rates of fat loss and upper/lower limits for when to gain or diet down as I outlined in the Chapter on Calories.

Staying between 8 and 12% for men and 16 and 20% are good general guidelines for aesthetics and working ranges for gaining and cutting phases. Much less than this would start to get into murky physiological territory and intrude upon the aesthetic ideals.

TRACKING MEDIUMS

Legend has it that back in the day, warriors used to record their workouts and macros by candlelight at dusk on parchment with a quill pen. It took precise scribesmanship and was an affair that lasted several hours.

In modern times, we have upgraded quite a bit, and tracking our workouts, nutrition, and body composition is a much simpler task.

APPLICATIONS/WEBSITES

There are tons of free applications readily available for download on smart phones that also have accessibility via their website. Use them.

They have a database that you can use to look up the foods in your program (be cautious) and plug in the amounts of them you eat to calculate the calories, macros, and micronutrients.

This is great not only for your grocery items, but also for when you go out to eat and need to look something up to plug into your plan.

    ⮞ SIDE BY SIDE

You can also plug in workouts, your daily weights, and so forth. Some apps even have the ability to track your intake over time through graphs, store progress pictures, and determine how things are progressing over time.

If and when possible, track your nutrition info and your training info in the same place. The link between our nutrition and the results we get in the weight room is strong. By seeing how your nutrition plays along with our performance, you'll be able to reach conclusions and make better decisions as a result.

DIARY

Keep a diary for your own personal life reflections. This should be done independently solely for your own personal growth, but nevertheless, you can see some parallels between the gym and your life as well that may shed light on your results.

CHECK-IN PERIODS

Tracking would be useless if you didn't check your progress. With the various methods and tools out of the way and in play, make it a habit to check your progress once per week to see how you're trending. Nothing more. Nothing less.

Brew up some java, fire up your favorite playlist, check out your results, and see how you're moving in relation to your goals. See what's working and what isn't. See how things relate to each other to improve maximally on the tactical day to day side.

Once per month, look at the month in its entirety to see how you've done. Look at your pictures, check out the monthly totals, and examine the trends. This will give you a much better idea of what's truly going on, and it is a true joy to see how far you've come. Strategize and plan like a general rolling out into foreign lands to accomplish his mission.

I've given you all the tools. Make adjustments as you need to. If you've hit a plateau, check the next chapter. This type of periodic check-ins should be done regularly for all areas of your life.

CELEBRATE

You will be doing check-ins weekly and on a larger scale, monthly. When you see that you are making progress, reward yourself. CELEBRATE your victories and achieving your goals.

We live in a world where everyone is afraid to be proud of themselves and celebrate their success at risk of being braggarts or show-offs. Nonsense.

- Grab dinner after you hit a PR with the gym gang.
- Schedule yourself a massage after a hard, successful training cycle.
- Buy yourself something cool. Some kicks for the gym you've been wanting, a new outfit to accentuate your physique, etc.
- Get a fresh cut/new hairstyle.
- Go see a movie with bae.
- Get yourself tickets to a concert or festival
- Take a vacation and explore uncharted territory
- Roll out on a Saturday night and turn up

Go feel good and live life.

Your body is your vehicle. Don't be afraid to take it out for a spin. Let the top down and feel the breeze. You've earned it.

When you achieve great progress from this book, send me the results and I'll celebrate with you.

36

PLATEAUS

Whosoever desires constant success must change his conduct with the times.
Niccolo Machiavelli

HOW NICE IT WOULD BE if everything worked predictably forever with no stalls or bumps in the road. In practice, plateaus rear their ugly head and must be dealt with. Have no fear. These plateaus are only signals of how you can further improve. They will be handled appropriately.

MAXIM OF AESTHETICS: EMBRACE THE ERRORS AND PITFALLS. THEY ARE THE FIRST STEP TO FURTHER IMPROVEMENT

TAKE A CHILL PILL

When people hit a plateau, their first response is to enter panic mode & assume that the training program isn't working because they're really an extraterrestrial who has different physiology.

Doubt creeps in and consumes their every waking thought.

Am I working hard enough?
This doesn't work for me.
I have to do something now!

This feeling of despair will drive them to kamikaze themselves into the ground, completely revamp their program, or fiddle with it haphazardly. Consequently, they screw themselves over and erase their standard of progress.

Don't be one of them.

Here we will take a true look at what's really going on and what to do about it to keep you pushing forward and gaining ground towards your aesthetic goals. Don't worry. We got this.

GAINING PHASE PLATEAUS

We've all been there. Workout after workout goes by and no matter what you do, the weight just won't go up. Progression has reached a standstill, and even blasting battalions of heavy metal and a scoop of potent pre-workout won't save you anymore.

There are few things more frustrating than grinding it out in the iron dungeon for little to no result. Let's shed some light on this & get you back on track.

<u>NUTRITION</u>

Training is *the stimulus*, but your nutrition is what enables you to fuel, grow, and recover from your training.

You can crush your workouts with class, but if your nutrition isn't dialed in, you will never achieve the results you seek. The main culprits for lack of gaining progression due to nutrition are insufficient caloric intake and protein consumption.

I.   DIAL IN YOUR CALORIES

First, ensure that you are truly gaining. Is your scale weight trending upwards similar to the theoretical rate you planned for (0.25-0.5% per week and half for women)? You may not be consuming as many calories as you thought you needed to get to gaining.

Ensure accuracy of your food measurements and nutrition tracking. If you've got this under control, then slowly start bumping up your daily food intake by 100-200 calories to get things moving in the right direction again.

Some people simply tend to burn more calories when they are in a surplus because of NEAT. They eat more and then subconsciously start moving around more that burns up calories. If things don't get moving again, add in more. Eventually, you will hit your required intake and find a new sweet spot for your caloric intake.

2. ENSURE ADEQUATE PROTEIN

In addition to having enough calories to go around to support muscle growth, you need to make sure you're consuming enough protein to give your body what it needs to grow.

Past 0.8-1.2g/lb bodyweight, there is no more additional benefit in going higher for either muscle building or satiation on a gaining diet if you're a natural, so do not go overboard here. Protein isn't hard to get for most, so this isn't usually a major issue, but every now and then, it does make a difference.

RECOVERY

Besides nutrition, proper recovery is also essential in making progress in the gym. How do you feel? If you are feeling worn down and lethargic, it is a sign that recovery is the cause.

1. PULL BACK

It's tempting to train all out and crank up your volume with the thought that more is better, but this will only wear you down and cause you to plateau and backslide.

Failure is only a tool to be used wisely, and volume will only do you good *if you can recover from it*. Assess your training and be honest with how hard you're working yourself. Adjust down if needed.

Additionally, deloads are a must, so consider taking them more often. If you drag your cycles out for 8 weeks, move to 6. If you are at 6, go to 4. If you are in the gym every day, reduce your frequency. Provided you're putting in quality work, remember *less is more.*

2. LIFESTYLE

Outside of the actual training variables, look at your lifestyle. You can push yourself for one hour in the gym, but it's what you do for the remaining 23 *hours* of the day that marks the difference.

- ઌ Sleep more.
- ઌ Clear your mind and eliminate the stress.
- ઌ Organize your workload and priorities more efficiently
- ઌ Take care of yourself and utilize preventative and recuperative measures like foam rolling, stretching, massages, hot baths, and so on.
- ઌ If you're doing a lot of hard daily activity, trim it down.

TRAINING

After the issues of nutrition and recovery have been addressed, THEN we can start to look at some of the other things that we can do to sidestep the plateau.

I. UTILIZE DIFFERENT REP RANGES

The rep range of 6-15 offers a wide range to choose from. If you've been training to much on one side of the spectrum, spend some time in the other end for your main lifts before switching back. Often times, this will get things jiving once more. This was discussed in the section on periodization.

2. INCREASE VOLUME

We know that volume is the biggest driver of hypertrophy there is, so if you're stalled out, then you could be prime for adding more.

If you are still feeling fresh, not in need of a deload or more rest, and aren't progressing, then you may need more volume to grow. 4-6 sets per workout per muscle group 2-3x/week was just a *starting point,* and you may require more as an individual or simply due to your training status.

You can only increase weight and reps to a certain extent, and progressive overload is achievable by more than just weight.

Therefore, to add more of a stimulus to grow, you can look at increasing the total volume side of the muscle building equation. Add in an extra set for your exercise per workout and build from there to see how you progress.

3. SWITCH OUT EXERCISES

Lastly, sometimes a change of exercise pace is just the ticket.

If you've been back squatting your whole life, give front squats a shot. If you consistently use the barbell, perform a cycle with some dumbbells. Muscle confusion is vastly overrated, but slight alterations in the exercise can target the muscles to varying degrees that can develop you further so that when you return to the original, you are more apt to battle it stronger than ever.

You can then cycle back to the previous exercise to get gains going again. These can be alternated back and forth as time goes along. For more on this, visit the Chapter on Periodization.

CUTTING PHASE PLATEAUS

Dieting plateaus suck. Hard.

When you're stranded in a gaining phase, you've got more delicious food to comfort you, but when you're cutting, the presumption is that you're wanting to reach the goal as soon as possible with as little damage done as you can so you can get the hell outta there.

When a cutting plateau strikes, follow these steps *in order:*

1. RULE OUT WATER RETENTION
2. CHECK CALORIC INTAKE
3. INCREASE DAILY ACTIVITY
4. REDUCE CALORIES
5. INCORPORATE REFEEDS
6. DEPLOY A DIET BREAK

Don't skip around at will. This is a *step-by-step* plateau busting process.

RULE OUT WATER RETENTION

Before anything else - make sure it's truly a plateau.

The scale may not budge, but for the 2 millionth time, the scale isn't the only measure of progress.

Water retention will skew your results and you may see no changes on the scale for 2 weeks or more. This is normal while dieting - especially for women. Trust in the program, stay on your grind, and instead lean on your *picture updates* every 2-4 weeks to check your progress. Stay away from relying on the mirror here. Continue recording your weights every morning to check the averages.

If weight stays constant and you're not seeing any visible differences in pictures, THEN you can move to the next steps.

CHECK CALORIE INTAKE

Secondly, ensure that the caloric deficit that you think you're creating is actually there. Mismeasurements in food intake will wipe out your theoretical deficit in the blink of an eye.

Check to see how everything racks up on the scale. Poll over your diet to identify any potential problem areas. A little bit here. A little bit there. It all adds up.

People tend to greatly underestimate their caloric intake, and tightening things up here will qualify you to move to step 3:

INCREASE DAILY ACTIVITY

After dieting for an extended period of time, you will burn less calories than predicted by your original calculations. Don't trip. This is completely normal. This occurs due to:

- ❧ Reduction in basal metabolic rate
- ❧ Reduction in subconscious activity (NEAT)
- ❧ Decrease in daily activity
- ❧ Reduction in exercise intensity

All of this combined can lead to decreases in your daily caloric burn of 200 calories or more.

When you get lower in body fat and are eating less, you won't be as high energy and torching calories like you were. This isn't the fabled starvation mode fairytale; it just comes with the territory [1,2].

As you get leaner, you're already running a smaller caloric deficit, so after you combine a reduction in energy output with mismeasurements in food intake, you can quickly see why you've stalled out.

HOW TO FIX IT

To remedy these adaptations, there are 2 easy ways:

1.   CONSCIOUSLY MOVE MORE THROUGHOUT THE DAY

If your NEAT is bringing you down and your energy is low, you can artificially make up for it. Remember, NEAT is subconscious, so if your body is bringing it down, you can *consciously* bring it back up by doing the things your body isn't doing on its own anymore [3].

Set an alert on your phone or watch to go off every 20-30 minutes to get up and walk around for a couple minutes to clear your head and get fresh. Park further away. Do all the little soccer mom tips and tricks like walking the stairs and drinking more water to get up more. If you have a smart watch or pedometer, track your movements to determine how often you are getting up and moving and how much. Make it a game.

5 minutes of moving around for every half hour of your work day is 40 minutes of extra moving.

Plus, you'll be keeping your body healthier by avoiding tissue creep that drives poor posture, mental haze, and other things that knock you off your prime. This is my preferred method.

Don't overdo it and pretend the chair is hot lava, but it is a sure-fire way to pull you from a diet plateau.

2. INCORPORATE CARDIO

Then of course, you can reach into your bag of tricks and start implementing dedicated cardio sessions.

Cardio should be released into battle *strategically* during a cut, and generally speaking, you should do as little formal cardio as you need. When the tide of the war is turning against you, you can unchain the cardio beast and allow it to go kick some ass on the frontlines and get fat burn going again.

2-3 sessions a week of low intensity cardio of 45 minutes is more than enough. Make it productive. Don't watch some brainwashing TV or broadcasted gossip about someone's life that isn't your own. (Even if it was, it doesn't matter). Get up, get outside, and listen to audiobooks or podcasts that develop your mind instead.

And voila. After this step, you're golden again.

Understand these two things and you'll see why figure athletes always say cardio or fat-burners are a must to get lean. It's not that deficits stop working or the energy balance equation is busted. It's that adding in a bunch of caffeine and cardio replaces the deficit that was lost from a downregulation in factors influencing calorie burn. But that's none of my business.

REDUCE CALORIES

Cutting calories or cutting veins? Notice how far reducing calories further is on the list. This is where people aggressively hack away from the get-go, but this is actually one of the LAST things to tighten up.

During a dieting phase, you want to keep food intake as high as you can while being satisfied with your diet. Making simple changes in your daily habits to make up for the drop in calories burned during the day can get things moving again, but you can only move so much. Sometimes, the calories simply have to drop.

To do this, start small. 100 calories a day combined with the above methods is a good place to start.

INCORPORATE REFEEDS

Refeeds are periods in the diet where you raise calories - primarily from carbohydrates - to maintenance levels or slightly above (100-200 calories). Going higher is where people get into problems mentally and develop bad habits.

Refeeds are excellent for psychological reasons, can help boost your performance and get you training harder and moving around a bit more, and it gives you a chance to test-drive how your diet will be once you've hit your goal. You should do this with everything in your life. Preview the future you wish to see. Don't wait.

You should be refeeding at least once per week when you get into the lean trenches. If not, start. You can see how to seamlessly incorporate them into your nutritional program in the section on calorie cycling in the nutritional part of the book.

These are not cheat meals. Losers cheat. You're a winner.

DEPLOY A DIET BREAK

Lastly, if you've been dieting for 2-3 months or more, you are in prime condition to take a diet break. No one ever wants to do it, but once they do, they'll wonder why they never did this before. During a diet break:

1. Raise your caloric intake back to your new maintenance levels -10% or so to factor in the different adaptations we just talked about.
2. Ensure sufficient carbohydrates as outlined in the Nutrition section in the book. More than 1g/lb bodyweight. Minimum.
3. Cut back on all your extra cardio.

Then, *relax.* Don't go psycho over the scale. Don't check the mirror every 5 minutes. You will gain weight, but this will be water and stuffing your muscles with more firepower.

Enjoy the physical and mental break from the grind of dieting down, and watch as the magic happens. Start your diet earlier so that you can take advantage of these periods and make the cutting process more enjoyable and sustainable. It's ALL about the process.

You'll come back fresh, energetic, and training hard once more. Don't be surprised if you fill out, look even leaner, and start dropping body fat like a charm upon your return. What plateau?

37

PROGRESS
PITFALLS

The path to the top is far from straight. There are all sorts of bumps and bends along the way. This chapter is all about common issues that people face in making progress and what to do about them to continue on your path to success. We'll discuss staying consistent, perfection, injury, and social issues.

CONSISTENCY AND F.A.T.E

What's the first thing people think when they see a world class physique?

All genetics. All cheaters. All people who drive themselves into the ground and don't have a life.

Nothing but victim mentalities and excuses. What a pity. Success isn't a roll of the dice. Accomplishing great things isn't because the wind blew the right way that day.

Your success is all about consistency.

How can stay consistent and make success an inevitability? You've just got to make it F.A.T.E.

I'll put you in the right direction, but don't limit yourself. Think of what other ways you can expand upon these concepts in life.

FUN

If you want to get somewhere good in life, you better make it fun. Common custom is to say work now, play later. I say do both right now. Provided you are meeting your requirements for success, inject as much fun as possible into your processes.

- Train with a training partner
- Dress like a champ for the gym
- Custom pick fire workout playlists
- Set mini goals for yourself and celebrate or reward yourself when you achieve them
- Mix up your training (within limits - see Chapter on periodization)
- Give yourself a change of gym scenery

ACCESSIBLE

To ensure consistency, accessibility is incredibly important. Your tools must always be within reach. For example:

- Place your bodyweight scale right there next to your sink with a notepad of dates and records of your bodyweight for tracking purposes.
- Keep your kitchen scale right by the stove and cutting board
- Keep your supplements in plain view where you know you will take them
- Keep your gym bag locked and loaded so you don't have to look all over the place for your workout threads and equipment
- Put your nutrition tracking app right on your home screen and bookmark the desktop site
- Find a gym close by to where you live and/or work

TIMELY

Time is our most valuable asset in life. Intuitively, we all know this and are always seeking to maximize our investments here. Therefore, you should aim to reduce that feeling of large scale commitment to keep things flowing smoothly.

- If you begin to view the gym as a time sink, cut your workouts short and spread your volume out more.
- Reduce your workout frequency
- Incorporate supersets that do not impede your performance
- Find meals that are quick to create or cook in advance

EASY

Although going great places will require hard work, whenever possible, you must aim to work smarter, not harder. There are no bonus prizes for making your path more difficult than it needs to be to achieve the same result. Make things easy.

- ❧ If precise measurements and tracking macros are becoming tedious, stick to calories and protein alone for a while.
- ❧ If manipulation of variables are becoming overwhelming, remember your roots and stick to the basics I've given you
- ❧ If figuring out your daily intakes is difficult, use a nutrition app instead
- ❧ If looking up nutrition facts or creating your meals is a time sink every time, look up the values, create a few that fit your goals, and save it as a template (see Meal chapter)

THE MYTH OF PERFECTION

Take time to deliberate, but when the time for action has arrived, stop thinking and go in.
Napoleon Bonaparte

The most common trap that people fall into is believing that they must achieve perfection in order to make progress by meticulously fine-tuning every last variable. If one little thing is off or goes wrong, all progress is lost. This form of thinking is incredibly detrimental to sustained success and productive mental attitudes.

- ❧ If you miss your workout, hit it tomorrow. Or the next day. Your muscles aren't going anywhere, and the extra time off will ensure that you crush it when you *do* go.
- ❧ If you go off of your nutrition plan, get right back on it. One bad meal is nothing, but one bad day sure can be.
- ❧ If you don't know what to do, remember the basics I gave!

Don't let one bad day turn into a whole bad week. Don't let one bad week turn into a whole bad month. Don't get paralysis by analysis. And if you notice a trend, identify the root cause. This will allow you to better refine your process for the future.

INJURIES

Make no mistake about it. Training hard is a risk, and every time you battle the barbells there's a chance for injury. Throughout the book, I've been adamant about safety, form, and pushing forward only when you have firm ground to stand upon, but every now and then, small aches and pains can arise that knock you off your game.

These are injuries such as minor strains and tendonitis. Severe injuries will not be discussed, and it is up to you to see a medical professional no matter what your situation is.

REST UP AND REPAIR

First and foremost, you must slam the brakes and address the situation at hand. Discontinue any activity or style of training that instigates the issue and begin to implement the PRICE protocol (Protect, Rest, Ice, Compress, Elevate). Use of NSAIDs are also of use here. This will help with the pain, inflammation, and allow the recovery cycle to begin.

If there is legitimate cause for concern outside of minor discomfort, see your healthcare provider as soon as possible to seek proper diagnosis and treatment. In addition, be a proactive patient and do your own research. However, know yourself and do not allow this to become a compulsion. It will not help you heal faster.

IDENTIFY THE ROOT CAUSE

If your injury is training related, look back through your training logs to see what you were doing to cause such a thing to occur. Every effect has a cause. Oftentimes, they are a result of:

- RAMPING UP VOLUME AND/OR FREQUENCY TOO FAST
- IGNORING PRE-PLANNED DELOADS
- IMPROPER FORM
- CONTRAINDICATED EXERCISE/MODE FOR YOU
- EGO LIFTING
- NOT PERFORMING A GENERAL WARMUP

In these cases, once you pinpoint where you strayed, you will be able to correct that for the future once you are healed and back in action. Use them as a learning tool to further fine tune your program and understanding of the body and how it works.

DO WHAT YOU CAN

When you are injured, you need to treat yourself like a warrior and not a victim. Focus on what you *can* do and not on your limitations. You may very well be able to train unaffected body parts provided they aren't included or at potential risk for the exercises.

- EXERCISE SELECTION

For upper body injuries, machines for the legs will still allow you to get a training effect. Lower body injuries can be more tricky to work around, however most upper body should still be doable barring any severe restrictions. In this case, machines are better, and if set-up is an issue, hire an attractive gym assistant to do it for you.

- LIGHT LOADS FOR GROWTH

As you learned in an earlier chapter, muscle growth can take place even in very high rep ranges, so do not think you must train heavy.

In fact, see this as a good opportunity to mix up your training in that regard. So long as you keep effort high, you will be fine.

In addition, occlusion training (also known as blood flow restriction or KAATSU) can produce comparable growth even at 20-30% 1RM and can help you to maintain your gains if even light weights (~60% 1RM) prove to be problematic [1,2,3].

This is training performed with a moderate pressure cuff or wrap around the limb that restricts venous – not arterial - blood flow and leads to an increased metabolic stress buildup within the muscle. For this reason, it can generate an intense pump and mild discomfort, so start slow.

Knee wraps or dedicated blood flow restriction bands can be used and should be placed at the top of the limb with a moderate pressure of 7/10 or so. Perform 3-5 sets at 20-30% 1RM with 30 reps on the first set and 15-20 on subsequent sets with ~30 seconds in between. This appears to give the best responses, and isolations tend to be better for these by virtue of band placement, although growth has been observed in neighboring areas as well.

Although it looks intuitively dangerous, it has proven quite safe in research across various populations [3]. This style of training may also be of use to you as you transition back into proper training to accustom yourself to lifting again and during regular training to mitigate the need for heavy loads.

OTHER CONSIDERATIONS

When you are healing up and transitioning back into regular lifting, ensure that you are warming up properly and conscious of how you feel at every stage, as you do not want to reaggravate anything. Here, sleeves can be of assistance to provide warmth and stability. Start light and make small steps.

Nutritionally, bump your calories back up and stick to sound nutrition as you've learned about in the book. Caloric restriction is only adding insult to injury (get it), and there's no need to torment yourself. For tendon injuries, 15mg gelatin and >50mg vitamin C an hour pre-workout shows much promise for repair [4].

WATCH YOURSELF

Lastly, do not be stubborn or stupid when training around injuries. They are nothing to fool around with, so when in doubt, stay conservative and pay close attention to your body. I have included this section to let you know that you have options, but it is always your job to stay safe and use your best judgment.

Your gains will be sustained for up to 3 weeks [5,6,7], muscle memory is a very real phenomenon, and even if you must maintain, you can do so off of very little volume [8], so rejoice. Stay smart.

SOCIAL

As cool as it'd be to train hard excluded from the outside world in a hyperbolic time chamber, the reality is that you've got a social life to sustain outside of the weight room. This is one of the biggest causes for failed fitness progress, but there is much you can do to get around this:

1. PLAN AROUND IT

There are very few social situations that you can't work into your program without a little forethought. Throughout the book, I have provided you with the knowledge and understanding of the material to be in prime position to make choices that do not make fitness a limiting factor for living your life.

For diet, you now know the importance of the various factors in regards to one another. You can rearrange your caloric intake for the day to give you a little extra budget for the occasion. Alternatively, you can implement a bit of calorie cycling to allow you a higher intake for that day that is offset by a lower intake on another day. Keep this mild and within reason.

Training wise, there is no harm done in waiting an extra day to train. There are no hard, rigid schedules for getting your workouts in. The gym will be there tomorrow, but that moment may not be.

2. LET THEM KNOW

If you've been in the iron game for any meaningful amount of time, chances are you've heard the following more than you can tolerate:

"You already look great."
"One ___ isn't going to kill you."

It is human nature for people to desire others to behave as they do for comfort, and it is also human nature to seek power and influence others to do as you wish. However, your decisions are not determined by the desires of others.

In many cases, these statements are true and are easily taken care of by the previous step. However, depending on your goals, you may not wish to partake in that activity or eat that food. Of course you could work that into your plan, but that may detract from your enjoyment in other areas.

In times like these, simply say thank you and let them know that you would not like to. You don't have to give reasons.
If they persist, openly let them know that this is part of your personal fitness goals. Whenever you meet resistance for your fitness goals, do so in a way that is nonjudgmental or implicative of your superiority for being more health-conscious. Done in this way with honest and open communication, most people will get and respect it by understanding your position. If not:

3. SEE YOU LATER

As a last resort, sometimes you've simply got to do what it takes and separate yourself from the pack to head where *you* want to go. You can't expect everyone to understand your goals and what it takes to achieve them. As nice as it would be to live in a world in which success is attainable with the snap of your fingers, the fact of the matter is that there are several constraints that have to be met to accomplish your goals. Provided you have exhausted your other options and are at peace with your decision, do not stress it.

MENTAL

But of course, we've saved the best for last. The biggest obstacle to sustainable progress is none other than that person looking back at you in the mirror. For that, we have to enter the world of the mind.

PART VII
MINDSET

38

MIND OVER MUSCLE

You have power over your mind - not outside events. Realize this, and you will find
strength.
Marcus Aurelius, Emperor of Rome

𝕿HE PEARLY PALACE OF MOUNT OLYMPUS is
rather empty. Many strive to reach the golden summit high
in the sky, but only a select few succeed - no matter how
great their plans or process. Why is this the case? Simple.

You are both the sculptor *and* the sculpted.

YOU'RE the work of art, and you're biased and blinded by your own
perspective.

To accomplish your goals in the gym or in life, you've got to push past the pain. You've got to get past the fatigue and hunger. You've got to overcome your temptations and desires. The negative beliefs. The critics. The fears. The stress. The memories. The doubts. The distractions. The worries. The uncertainties. The pressure. *Yourself.*

Achieving greatness doesn't come without a price. That's a weight that's too heavy for most to handle, and they drop off, give up, or accept being average as their fate.

But I am not here to build average. I am here to build you into the BEST that you can be. And that's exactly what I'll do.

Now how do you solve this dilemma?

The answer lies in the separation of the sculptor and the sculpted by training and forming *your mind.* Your job as a sculptor doesn't stop at the body.

Mental fortitude is the key to your success. To build a beautiful physique with no regard to the mind and person within is a disgrace. The body is just an extension of the mind, and your mind will either be a prize or a prison. Your decision.

IMMENSE IMPORTANCE

FITNESS

Despite living an active, 'healthy' lifestyle, eating disorders, body dysmorphic disorder, and compulsive behavior are all very common in the fitness community [1-4].

This is in large part due to many of the piss poor processes undertaken in training and nutritional programs, which is why I've gone to great lengths to make the approaches in this book flexible and in your best interest. I refuse to put your mental health and well-being at stake.

However, much of this also just comes with the territory. Muscle gain and fat loss are slow, methodical processes that involve consistency, dedication, and a solid dose of mental, physical, and life investment. Not enough is done to assist lifters in this area.

BIGGER PROBLEMS

Additionally, mental afflictions such as depression, anxiety, addictions, and substance abuse are at all-time highs all around the world. Depression alone is suffered by over 300 million worldwide, and suicide is the 10th leading cause of death and the 2nd amongst the age group of 15-24 reading this book [5,6]. This is inexcusable.

Outside of these, the day to day demands of life bring their own challenges. Academic pressures, work, and personal life all play a role and have the potential to create emotionally corrosive and stressful situations damaging to health and life outcomes.

Furthermore, there is a component of the mind that is primed for maximizing benefit and minimizing harm to ensure survival. This is a normal trait for any organism, but it works through mechanisms that create negative behavioral traits and mental states.

As I revealed earlier in the book in the discussion of biological bias, you can see the connection between survival benefit and mental states:

BASE DESIRES	EGO OPERATING SYSTEM
Pleasure	Selfishness
Control	Binary Scales and Labeling
Abundance	Greed/Hedonism
Power	Jealousy
Security	Identification with the Self
Safety	Seeking of Meaning in External Things
Importance	Living in the Past/Future
Respect	Attention Seeking
Ease	Impulsiveness
Time (Speed, duration, etc.)	Irrationality
	Self-rationalization
Permanence	Reactive/Defensive
Maximize benefit	Attachment
Reduce harm	

As you may have guessed, lack of control and misunderstanding over these mental processes will lead to disaster. Indeed, I have demonstrated that this is the source of human-based suffering.

BENEFITS OF MENTAL TRAINING

Needless to say, these truths do not speak well for achieving your physique or an elevated life of freedom, happiness, and success. There is a strong, but unfulfilled need for more awareness and implementation of mental training techniques to address this.

Therefore, I have answered the call and wrote this part of the book for you to forge a strong mind, regulate your thoughts, emotions, and behavior, and give you the tools to maximize your success and the journey along the way. I will not let you fail or else I would have failed you, and that is something I cannot do.

Mindfulness training practices are beneficial for:

-   PHYSICAL PERFORMANCE [7-10]
-   STRESS MANAGEMENT [11-17]
-   RECOVERY [17]
-   DIETARY REGULATION [18-21]
-   HAPPINESS [22,23]
-   MENTAL HEALTH [11-17]
-   SOCIAL OUTCOMES [24,25]
-   PAIN TOLERANCE [26-28]
-   MENTAL FUNCTION [29,30]

And is largely the result of and supports further:

-   UNDERSTANDING OF YOURSELF
-   HEIGHTENED MIND/BODY AWARENESS

In other words, you can't afford not to do it. But best of all, it's 100% free and accessible anytime, anywhere.

GOALS

In the sections and chapters that my follow, I will equip you with the tools to understand, develop, and regulate your mind to elevate your results and experience in and out of the gym, no matter where you may roam.

First, we will look at the mind and how it works. Then, I will show you how to position yourself to manage your thought flows and reality. Finally, I will reveal how you can transform the foundations of your mind and feed it the fuel for growth. This is where we separate the good from the great. This is where your glory resides.

THE MIND

At the beginning of the book, I gave you the keys to your dream ride. Pristinely polished, turbo-charged, exquisite. A lady at the light, but a beast in the streets.

Think back to that car. Picture yourself driving it. Imagine winding and weaving through the roadways in any exotic location you desire. It's all yours. Got it? Good.

Your body is that car.

Your mind is the steering wheel, pedals, and dashboard.

...and YOU are the driver.

You're right there behind the wheel. Observing traffic. Checking the dash. Taking the ride to wherever you want to go.

When you feel intense emotions...when you feel that fatigue kicking in...when you feel hurt and anger...when you're hit by your memories...when you're met with temptation...those are nothing more than the little signals on your dashboard going off.

Check-engine light appeared. The gas-light just came on.

Anger light just came on. Hungry and drained just appeared. Same thing.

Sometimes you get a dent or a crack in the windshield. You've got to flip the tires or get an oil change. You rack up thousands of miles and pass by lots of cities as your adventures unfold. The scenery, song on the radio, and parts are always changing, but you are always the driver.

I know that a whip like this is pretty damn sweet, but I'd sure as hell hope that you don't run around thinking that YOU are the car. You're not.

---

*You are not your body or mind. You are much more than that. They are at **your** service, not the other way around.*

You are more than just your make and model. You are more than just where you born. You are more than just your beliefs. You are more than just where you have been and what has happened to you. *And so is everybody else.*

When the driver is strong and skilled, they can hop in any car and make magic happen. THAT'S putting the **PERSON** in the 4Ps of Success.

Extra tip: Next time you are on the roadways, observe the actions of others driving and how you view the things that appear on the roads and in the driver's seat. You will learn much about human nature and understand this analogy even more this way.

THE AUTOPILOT

In that fine whip of yours, you've got a cruise control and an auto-park. Any lavish luxury vehicle does. And once you've got your money right, you can upgrade to a private jet that has a fully functional auto-pilot so that you can pop bottles with the models a mile high in the cabin on your way to Tokyo. It handles what you need to so that you can chill.

Well guess what, your mind and body does too. But it's selfish, narrow-minded, and outdated.

It will try to steer you all over the place and take you where *it* wants to go, so you've got to grab the wheel and take control before you crash into a wall, hit someone, or end up in a place you don't want to be in.

You must make the distinction between you, your mind, and your body.

You must learn to view everything that happens in you and the world you're driving in as external to you and *under your control*.

That's step #1.

MASKED VIGILANTE

Once you've made that distinction, you start to view things a little bit differently. The mind, body, and all that they're capable of are simply *tools at your service.* Now you've got to learn how to use them the right way at the right time.

Think of it like this:

You're a superhero with a utility belt and all sorts of high-tech armored vehicles. In that utility belt, you've got a bunch of weapons and gadgets at your disposal. They do all sorts of incredible and amazing things, but you don't just pull them out at random. You use them for their *specific purpose* based on the *specific task* at hand.

> *You are the superhero and the mind is your utility belt.*

In that belt of yours, you've got:

-   ATTENTION
-   KNOWLEDGE
-   MEMORIES
-   THOUGHTS
-   BELIEFS
-   DESIRES
-   CHOICE
-   WILLPOWER
-   IMAGINATION
-   CREATIVITY

And much more. In that general order.

My question to you is, are you using these weapons of yours at the right time, at the right place, and to the right extent?

Learn how to use them for the task at hand, and learn how to put them away when they're no longer necessary so that you can sit atop the skyscraper and enjoy the city lights below you.

Here, we will look at the 3 biggest tools you've got: Attention, thoughts, and choice. These will drive the rest. Then we will apply them by training your mind and renovating your mental building blocks.

FOCUS AND ATTENTION

Where you place your attention is where you will place your life. It's the most valuable thing you've got, and nothing can ever affect or 'exist' to you unless you put your attention there in this present moment. Let that marinate for a few.

What you focus on will expand and set the gears in motion for the rest of your mental activity and the reality it creates, so let's get it right.

DARK ROOMS

Imagine that you are in a pitch-black room with nothing but a bunch of orbs floating around you. Each one of these orbs is its own little world made up of either a memory, a thought, a desire, an area of your life, or something outside of you like what someone says, something you hear, a song, or a show. Some pop in and out, and some are permanent.

The present moment is the biggest orb and right in front of your eyes.

Your attention is a flashlight cutting through the darkness and the only way you can see anything is if the light shines on it. By default, it's stuck on the present moment, but your mind is a rebel and likes to shine it all around the room. When it shines on one of those floating worlds, the light beams create a bridge, you travel to that world, and it becomes your reality. Your *only* reality.

The more it shines on one, the bigger it grows and because the room is only so big, the more likely it is that you'll shine on it again.

The less your flashlight shines on it, the smaller it gets and the less likely it is that you will shine on it again.

Here's the catch: your flashlight only has so much battery life every day.

Where are you going to shine it?

SHINE YOUR LIGHT

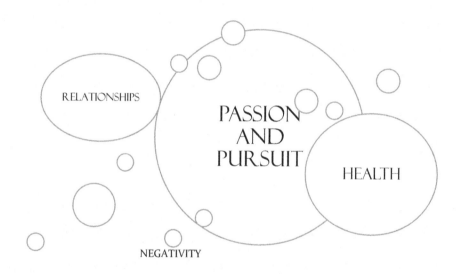

Guard your mind by keeping your attention occupied by your passions, positive thoughts, and the present moment. Do not put your attention anywhere unless it is beneficial, necessary, or you have a concrete action to carry out. It is too valuable to let loose.

Eliminate any and all distractions from your life that knock you off course, contribute little, or bring you down. That's most things. *You* give them life, and they can't touch you unless you allow them to. I will show you how to wield your attention better later in the book.

THE THOUGHT SEQUENCE

Our life always expresses the result of our dominant thoughts.
Soren Kierkegaard

Look around you, wherever you are. Now tell me: What does it all have in common? Think long and hard.

The answer is that everything you see was once nothing but a thought. This sentence, what you're wearing, even you. Everything begins in the mind. The mental creates the physical. The invisible creates the visible. Reality gets created in this order:

THOUGHT → EMOTION → ACTION → EFFECT

To break things down and get practical, you're going to need the expanded version I've developed, so here you go:

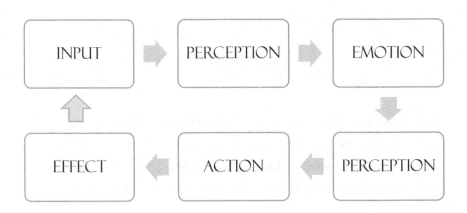

We'll take it one by one so you know exactly what's going on in your mind and can fine tune things to forge your path to greatness.

STEP ONE: INPUT

To kick off the thought sequence, you need input. This input can either be internal or external to you.

→ INTERNAL INPUT

Internal input can either be a thought you have, self-talk, a memory, a physical feeling, or a desire. You have thousands of thoughts per day, and most of them are the same as yesterday. If we took the time to list them all out and plot them on a graph, what would we find? Good things or bad things? Would you be proud of what you see? Proud or not, that's going to be the basis of your reality.

→ EXTERNAL INPUT

External input is just like the name implies and is made up of media, an event, or something someone does or says. You may think you have no control over this, but think again. You can choose what you expose yourself to in order to drive desired results. See the chapter on Mental Input Material (MIM).

STEP TWO: PERCEPTION

In order for that input to make its way to the land of emotion, it's go to pass through the sea of perception. Nothing inherently has any value until you accept that power. Nothing truly even 'exists' to you unless you are there to experience it. The way you see the world is more important than the world itself, so in a way, the world is nothing more than a mirror showing you who you are based on your values, beliefs, and experiences.

✎ AUTOMATIC

Most of your responses are going to be automatic. This comes from a variety of areas, including basic biological responses and conditioned, habitual responses.

A biological response would be feeling fear upon seeing a dangerous creature about to attack, and a conditioned response would be things such as prejudice, jumping to conclusions, and the divide between pessimism and optimism. This can come from your upbringing and idea of reality based on your current environment. The good news is that you can bend and mold your responses to what you encounter, especially those formed by your surroundings.

✎ PERCEPTION FIXES

You are limited by your singular position in understanding what happens all around you. You only have a sliver of the truth, so always remain open and humble.

Therefore, for every source of input you encounter, seek to see it from every angle and regardless of what it is, make the *choice* to use it for your benefit. I've termed this the Midas Mindset. Just like King Midas, *turn everything that touches your life into gold.*

STEP THREE: EMOTION

Based on how you view your input, you're going to generate an emotional response. Emotions are the physical response to the input based on your personal perception of it. Feelings of euphoria. Feelings of fright. Feelings of sadness. Anger. Excitement. Worry. You know the names in the game.

Life would be bland and mundane if there weren't emotions. It's not a matter of getting rid of them, but rather *understanding them* and *managing them appropriately.*

Emotions are powerful and multiply the same thoughts that created them, leading to a cycle that then forms habits. Use them wisely.

STEP FOUR: PERCEPTION

So you're sitting there behind the wheel and come across an emotion. You feel it, and depending on the emotion, it can be quite intense. This will influence you to take action, so you must be aware of what you're feeling and why before progressing into the next step, action. How you view that emotion is critical.

STEP FIVE: ACTION AND EFFECT

Fueled by your emotion, you make that decision to act on it. This can either be congruent with how you feel or against it, but this action will generate an effect that brings you to the last step:

STEP SIX: PERCEPTION AND FEEDBACK

Based on the result your actions generate, you've got to perceive them again and add value to the outcome. This will create a feedback loop and influence either a reinforcement of behavior or a change in behavior.

Here again, you must be aware of the consequences of your actions, understand why things have occurred the way they have, and always seek to use the outcome to your advantage by seeking a higher perspective.

IMPLICATIONS

The thought sequence is a powerful weapon in your arsenal. The thought sequence serves as a mental map that you can use to track down your mental activity and fine tune your results.

- When you are thinking certain thoughts, ask why.
- When you feel a certain way or are stuck in a certain mood, look for the cause it's coming from. What thought created it? What perception did you have of that thought?
- When you find yourself stuck in habits, look at which thoughts and emotions caused that action to take place that later got reinforced to cement itself as a habit.
- When you find yourself unhappy with your results in life, look back at what led to them. Dig deep, and you'll find your answers.

With this simple tool, you have the power to redesign your mind and consequently, your entire life.

- Can you change your input/environment? Yeah.
- Can you change your perception of things? Yep.
- Can you change your course of action in response to this all? Of course you can.

So therefore, you can control your reality to get the effects you want out of it. *And only you.*

The mind is like a factory. Put good in, have a good team, and you'll get a solid ROI.

CHOICE

Lastly, we come to choice.

Choice is what makes you human. Choice is what separates the robots from the royalty. Choice is what guides your life down whichever path you choose.

Your life is the result of all of the decisions you make or don't make, so for everything you do in life, ask yourself:

Am I doing this by choice or by conditioning?

If you do 100 things a day, then ask yourself 100 times. Hone your habits and never act on impulse. You are in control.

Disconnect the autopilot and live how *you* choose to live.

FLEX YOUR FREE WILL

You're tossing around that iron in the gym like no tomorrow, but how about you flex in your daily life on top of that. Learn how to exercise *your choice*. Flex your free will. For example:

- Set your alarm clock to 6:27 instead of 6:30.
- Take a different route to work...to the gym...to the store
- Eat with your opposite hand or try out different utensils
- Listen to music from an entirely different language
- Cut or comb your hair a different way
- Walk on the left instead of the right
- Ride your skateboard instead of walking
- Party on a Wednesday

- ❧ Pick up the phone and call instead of text
- ❧ Have dinner for breakfast
- ❧ Have breakfast for dinner
- ❧ Send a voice note instead of a text
- ❧ Honk and wave at randoms
- ❧ Change careers
- ❧ Change cities
- ❧ Pay with cash instead of cards when you're out
- ❧ Schedule date night for a Tuesday
- ❧ Jam heavy metal and trap music at 6am
- ❧ Then answer the door in a pimp robe and Halloween mask when your disgruntled neighbors knock on your door for waking them up
- ❧ Spark up conversations with strangers
- ❧ Hit legs on a Monday. The Chest-day police won't come for you
- ❧ Take a spontaneous trip
- ❧ Howl like a wolf
- ❧ Do surprises for others
- ❧ Try out new styles – trendy or not. You make them trendy
- ❧ You're a bar type? Go to the club instead
- ❧ Say no. Don't succumb to and appease others

Life is full of options and opportunity. Don't limit yourself.

Cultivate the habit of venturing outside of the norm. Just for the hell of it. Just 'cuz you can.

CHOOSE NOT TO CHOOSE

What's the best way to make a good decision? Simple. Don't make it.

AVOIDANCE

Out of sight, out of mind. You can't make a bad decision if there is no option to do so in the first place. Therefore, don't put yourself in places that will affect your judgment, and don't surround yourself with things that will do so either. This alone is most of the battle.

PRE-PROGRAMMED DECISIONS

Next, you pre-program your decision making so that you already have your answers for determined situations ahead of time.

In your daily life, organize your habits, scheduling, and so on to take any guesswork out of the equation. This structure will fine tune your process flow and eliminate the psychological stress or potential for erroneous decisions being made.

Secondly, if you come across situations frequently or have seen that you have acted negatively in a particular situation and don't want to repeat it, take the time to note what the best route to take is should it happen again. This one simple move will save you a tremendous amount of time and effort.

SUMMARY

Attention, Thoughts, and Choice. Fine tune those and watch your life and success grow. With those basics laid out, you've got your mind, body, and how it operates down pat, so let's bundle that up and give you the tools you need to put this in motion. Application is everything.

39

MENTAL TRAINING

*N*OW THAT YOU'VE GOT THE MIND and how it works figured out, it's time to dial up the mental training. The process of training the mind is very simple. You're a stronger driver than you think. I am going to give you a mental R.O.A.D map to put in play so that you will be able to drive that speedy stallion wherever you want to go.

Here it is:

1. RECOGNIZE
2. OBSERVE
3. ADJUST
4. DRIVE

You will use this mental R.O.A.D map and apply it in 2 golden ways each and every day from this point forward to optimize and refine your mind and your results in the gym and life. They are:

- ❧ MEDITATION
- ❧ DAILY MINDFULNESS PRACTICE

We will look at both. They are both important. Let's take it from the top and start with the R.O.A.D map itself.

THE MENTAL R.O.A.D MAP

1. RECOGNIZE

Number one. You now know that you are not your car, the cockpit, or anything that pops up on the street. When you come across something as you drive or autopilot kicks in and brings up a thought, desire, or sensation, recognize that it has appeared and recognize that you are separate from that.

2. OBSERVE

Once you're aware and disconnected from that thought, sensation, or input from the outside world, step back and observe it. Hover above it and see it from every angle to truly see it for what it is.

Identify:

- ❧ WHAT IT IS
- ❧ WHERE IT CAME FROM
- ❧ HOW YOU FEEL ABOUT IT
- ❧ WHY
- ❧ IS IT EVEN RELEVANT
- ❧ IS THIS OF HELP OR HARM

Don't cut corners here. Don't make assumptions. Don't jump to conclusions. Face it and understand it.

You will be tempted to react, but resist that instinct. You must view it as external to you. *You* are in control here.

3. ADJUST

After you see things for what they are and have all the info laid out in front of you, you have a decision to make. You must decide what –if anything - to do with it.

DO NOTHING

Most things in life do not need any action. Redirect your attention and let them drift away and disintegrate or handle themselves. Your time and attention are sacred, and you don't give it away to just anything or anyone. Reserve your right to do nothing.

DO NOW

On the other hand, it could be that it does require action. Because you've understood it for what it is, you are in a better position to make the right decision and follow the right course of action. Trust in yourself, and make every action you take excellent.

DO LATER

The mind constantly produces, and oftentimes you will come across things in your life that are valuable to you – just not in that moment. Therefore, I recommend keeping a note app to record all of the thoughts you want to keep for the future so that you can review it later and plug it into your life. This will supercharge your productivity and assist you in pooling information to make better decisions and adjustments to your schedule and processes.

For example, in your notes you can list:

- ✺ Things you have to do
- ✺ Information you need to remember
- ✺ Books, movies, places, podcasts, etc. you want to check out

At least once per week – such as during your aesthetic progress reviews – fire this up and then allocate your schedule accordingly, plug in items into your MIM or wish lists, or file away for your personal reference.

4. DRIVE

Once you've done all that, keep driving and enjoying your journey. More things will pop up along the way, and when they do, run through the process again. As you go along, your skills as a driver will skyrocket and you'll develop a sixth sense for every feel of the road and shake of your engine. You will master your vehicle and be free to take it anywhere you want in the world.

TEST DRIVE

To help you in your journey, think of how you'd use the R.O.A.D map to respond to pain, hunger in a cut, tiredness in the gym, a rude remark, a great idea you have, a bad memory from your past, and so on. The possibilities are endless. This method works for all.

Now let's take that mental R.O.A.D map and put it into your daily habits and way of life to further engrain this way of thinking.

MEDITATION

I say meditation, you say _____.

Lame? Weird?

All wrong.

Meditation is often seen as a useless, silly spiritual method that is reserved for monks, hippies, or religious practices. Nothing could be further from the truth.

Meditation is *neutral*. It is a simple, powerful daily practice with thousands of years of history behind it that is done to calm your mind, 'know thyself', and get in touch with the present moment and the world around you. It will train your focus and you will achieve an elevated mind/body awareness, mental clarity, and understanding that will benefit you in every area of your life.

Medi-tation is medi-cine for the mind, and if there one single thing that I would recommend to every human being on the face of the earth from children to the old and grey, it would be to start the simple daily habit of meditation. It is never too late to start. You will start today.

HOW TO MEDITATE

Meditation is very simple. You can do it virtually anytime, anywhere.

Here's how:

1. Seek out a comfortable, tranquil location free of distractions.

This can be at home or outdoors. You can light up some scented candles and get some instrumental music playing in the background to help you relax. No words.

The time of day does not matter. You can do it first thing in the morning, before bed to unwind, any time in between, or all of the above. Find what works best for you and your schedule.

2. Clear your mind by bringing your attention to the rhythm of your breath and the sensations of your body.

Close your eyes or fix them on a neutral point in front of you. As you breathe in and out, focus on the feeling of the air entering and leaving as your chest rises and falls. If you enjoy visualizations, picture the air coming in clean and pure, revitalizing you down to the very last cell, and then leaving like smoke that carries with it all the stress and problems within your system.

Once you've locked into that rhythm, scan your body from the bottom up. Note how it feels at every point. Note what's tense or tight and then relax it. You'd be surprised at how much you never noticed before. This will enhance your mind/body awareness.

3. Maintain your focus here, following the natural rhythm of your breathing as you inhale and exhale.

If your mind wanders and you lose focus by latching onto a thought or memory, gently shift your attention back to the rise and fall of your breathing.

I'll tell you right now: you will think. That's normal. The important thing here is to *recognize* that you are thinking, *what* you are thinking and *why*, that *you are not that thought*, and that you have the ability to let it pass without being affected by it.

Your mind is like a yo-yo. It can travel away and do all sorts of tricks, but it always comes back to the master.

4. Continue this for 10 minutes.

You can set a timer to alert you when time is up. There is no limit to how long you can go, so experiment with what works best for you to find your groove. Some days, it'll take longer than others. This is to be expected. Don't stress it. Simply stay consistent.

When time is up, slowly open your eyes and adjust to your surroundings. Then go about your day like normal with a heightened sense of awareness in everything you do.
That's all there is to it.

MEDITATION SUMMARY

Meditation is deceptively simple, but a small investment in this practice every day will take your life to a whole new level.

Over time, you will gain dominion over your mind. You will be able to see things for what they truly are. You will see what thoughts and feelings run through your mind and how you react to them. You will be able to redirect them, let them pass, and replace them with better thoughts that do you good. You will be able to slip into the present moment naturally with ease. You will have more compassion for others. You will live a life worth living.

DAILY MINDFULNESS

The unexamined life is not worth living.
Socrates

Mindfulness doesn't stop at meditation. That's just practice. Mindfulness is a *way of life.* You've got to learn to view life as a whole in an entirely different way.

Take what you've learned from meditation and inject awareness and attention into everything you do. Live directly in the present moment without your mind distorting the picture. Focus on the activity of your senses and the experience that generates. Without judgement. Without filters.

- When you're tearing up the weights, focus intensely on the movement and the feeling. Fine tune your form. Concentrate on the mind/muscle connection. Feel the burn. Enter that burn. Make it yours. Because no matter how much it burns, it'll never burn You.
- When you feast after a furious training session, focus on the meal at hand. Savor every bite. Savor those flavors and aromas.
- When you walk, walk. Feel the weight in your steps and the sensations in your legs and feet.
- When you're talking to someone, don't get caught up thinking about what you're going to say next. Focus on the person and the entire communication process - verbal and nonverbal.
- When you're outside walking somewhere, don't start daydreaming or thinking about what you have to do later. Feel the sun, feel the breeze, listen to the birds.

- ☙ When you find yourself affected by a negative thought, action from someone, or memory, let it pass by, put a positive thought in its place, and retune your attention to the present moment.
- ☙ When you're out having a good time, don't think about how others view it. Don't lose that present moment by caring more about posting it up all over the place.
- ☙ When you are stuck on a belief, step back and look at that belief. Your beliefs will blind you from the bigger picture. Always question and seek full understanding.
- ☙ When you have a desire to do something, observe that desire. Then decide. Don't react on impulse. I could care less if that's how the world acts. You're better than that.

Use your mind *exactly* for what it needs to do for the task at hand. Nothing less, nothing more. When you put this into play, life itself will transform right before your very eyes.

You will appreciate the little things you ignored and took for granted. You will enjoy every moment much more because you're fully there and in living that moment full of all of the details that you glossed over in the past. You will live on a clean burn of happiness, peace, and inner power. You will drive that car right to the top of the mountain.

The world is yours.

It always was.

40

MENTAL INPUT MATERIAL

*I*F I TOLD YOU TO bake a cake with nothing but a bunch of bricks and cement, could you do it? What about if I told you to build a castle with nothing but eggs, flour, and sugar?

Of course not. You would need *the right materials.*

Now where do you think *your mind* gets the material it uses to think, remember, desire, imagine, and create? Everything has to come from somewhere, and nothing can be created that is more than the different pieces that went into creating it.

The answer is: From everything you put and allow into your mind. This is what I call **Mental Input Material (MIM).**

BASICS OF MIM

Your mind is a big supercomputer, and the way you see the world is going to be heavily determined by all of the information that has come in through your senses and been stored over the years.

As you saw earlier, this big 'database' is key in my aesthetic theory, and it's a key driver for the first perception stage in the thought sequence by generating automatic responses and belief systems.

SOURCES OF MIM

MIM comes in many forms and flavors, and by definition, it is everything that you input into your mind, either internal or external as I've demonstrated with the thought sequence. This includes people, places, media, and the thoughts you've formed in relation to your experiences with all of this.

ও TROJANS AND IMPs

Before digging into MIM, you must look at where you are now. Much of your MIM 'database' has come from your upbringing or times when you simply didn't know any better. This can either be good or bad and highlights the importance of forming young minds the right way to set people up for success instead of distress. Based on this, you've formed a worldview and beliefs about yourself and the things around you.

Society, media, and social institutions all play a role, but these usually come in the form of Trojan horses or are thrust upon you by IMPs (Installed Mental Programs). Trojan horses are sources of input that package themselves as being useful or good for you but are truly only hurting you silently. IMPs are belief systems installed in you through authority or outside influence. This will blind you from truth and alter your perception of what you believe to be important. The world taught you *what* to think, not *how* to think.

But it's all good. Once you've recognized your current situation, it's up to you to remodel your mental mansion how **you** choose by giving your mind the fuel it needs to achieve your goals. You may even have to completely demolish it. But it's all good because: *Sometimes you've got to break down the mess to get to true success.*

BENEFITS OF MIM

You now know that nutrition is vital for giving your body what it needs to grow and function at its best. MIM is the same thing to your mind. By fine tuning your mental input material, you will:

- Give yourself the building blocks for your reality
- Grow and develop into the person of your choice
- Destroy any negativity
- Stay on the right track to success
- Live clean, happy, and efficient

THE BIGGEST RULE

The #1 rule when it comes to MIM is this:

*Everything that you expose yourself to is **your choice** and for a **purpose** that takes you further and lifts you higher.*

That means no negativity. Nothing holding you back. Only things that help you grow. No exceptions.

VISUALIZATIONS

Your thoughts can be diamonds or daggers, so here you are going
to use your mind productively to dial up thoughts that take you
places. The first place that reality is created is in your mind.
Remember the Maxim:

MAXIM OF AESTHETICS: SUCCESS BEGINS WITHIN. BEFORE YOU CAN BE IT, FIRST YOU MUST SEE IT.

VISUALIZE

Put your mind to use and visualize what you want to see in your
life. Your dreams. Your goals. Visualize it in vivid detail. Leave no
stone left unturned. Make it stimulate each and every sense you
have. Transport there. Do this every morning, every night, before
and during your workouts, and whenever else you need to
recapture focus.

CREATE VISION PORTALS

Visualizations are good, but surrounding yourself with them is even
better. Take that vision you have and go hunt for pictures, quotes,
and snippets from magazines or books that demonstrate that
vision. Post them everywhere you frequent. Everywhere. In your
bedroom, on the fridge, on the bathroom mirror, and in your office.

Make your goals and motivation visible no matter where you look.
If you ever need a dose of inspiration, all you have to do is take a
quick glance at your surroundings. By surrounding yourself with

these things, you'll be surrounding yourselves with targets. Always knowing what to aim for. Always able to focus in and stay on track.

ᕂ GO DIGITAL

Apply this same concept in the digital realm. Your phone and desktop background can be a picture of someone you look up to, a beautiful place you wish to live at, or anything else you truly desire. It's not your phone background. Your phone screen just so happens to be a portal to see your future. It's simply a matter of time.

Create a folder on your phone and/or computer with pictures and quotes that inspire and motivate you. Pull these up whenever you need a dose of greatness.

SELF-TALK

Within just a minute of speaking with someone, you can tell exactly whether you're dealing with a go-getter or a no-getter. Language has an incredible impact on the way that you see the world and yourself. Every word has a series of feelings and memories tied to it, so you need to choose your ingredients carefully.

LANGUAGE

Because of the power of language, you will now start using language that opens doors for you and builds you up. You will no longer use words that imply negativity. Slowly but surely, this will change the way you view things, and you know how important your perceptions are for generating emotions and results now. Look at these simple swaps to explain:

This is hard → This is a nice challenge.
That's weird → That is interesting and unique.
They don't like me → They don't realize my worth yet.
I feel bad → I don't feel my best.

To be a winner, you've got to act and speak like it.

AFFIRMATIONS

To expand upon this idea, begin implementing affirmations into your daily life. Any time you doubt yourself, rip that shit out by the root and replace it with a **positive** affirmation instead.

I can do this.
I will find a way.
I will not be broken.

To make this more powerful, say it out loud. But don't just say it. That's not good enough. You need to **believe** deep down to very core of your soul that this is true. Then, it will be.

On top of this, give yourself some positive self-talk every single day. In the morning with a good cup of coffee and music drenching the airwaves as you get ready in the mirror is a great place to start.

Today is going to be a great day.
I'm going to crush this workout.
I'm a winner.

Lots of people will try to tell you this is conceited, but if you speak the truth, they'll learn to shut up sooner or later. Do not ever let others drag you down. Set the example, and let them be.

MEDIA

We're living in the greatest time in history. Information and entertainment are abundant, inexpensive, and incredibly accessible. If you're smart, you'll combine the two and get even smarter.

❧ BOOKS

As you can see by now, books are an excellent source of information. Within the palm of your hands, you have unified, coherent information on the topic of your choosing. Hardly anyone reads anymore, but you're one step ahead for being here.

Aim to read at least 1 book per month. 15-30 minutes per day will take you to another level, and with e-books being available on your smart phones, tablets, or e-readers, you have no excuses.

❧ MUSIC/RADIO

You already know that music is essential to great gym sessions, but it will also assist in your moods and productivity throughout the day as well.

With regards to the radio, you're better off without. You're at the mercy of what they play, and there's too much filler that's unproductive and unnecessary. Hook your phone up with an aux cord or wireless sync and you're good to go.

❧ PODCASTS

Podcasts are excellent ways to enrich your mind on various topics that stimulate your interest. You can listen to them in the background while you work, drive, cook up your meals, and so on. Consider how much time you spend doing these things daily. Now consider how much you have to benefit by dialing up good MIM at these times over the course of a year.

❧ TV AND MOVIES

As you'll see later, TV and movies are ways that you can simulate your real-world environment and reap the benefits digitally. On top of being enjoyable ways to spend your down time, you can use these as teaching tools to fine tune your mannerisms, behavior, and language choices. Of them all, these should be the most minimal.

❧ THINGS TO AVOID

Of course, you must also avoid bad sources of media MIM. These sources are particularly sneaky sources of Trojan horses, so you've got to be conscious here.

For example, it is common custom to watch the news every day, but I can assure you there is nothing new about it. There is nothing psychologically healthy or more corrosive to your mental states than exposing yourself to cherry-picked death and destruction every day. Surprisingly, this is how people begin and end their day.

Get your weather and traffic off of an application instead. Focus on your life, what's relevant to you, and what's in your sphere of control. There's a beautiful world out there, but you'll never see it on the screen.

MEDIA TRICKS

୭ SECRET AGENTS

A hallmark component of the tools of the trade for secret agents is the earbud. This gives them valuable intel unbeknownst to others while they're on their mission. Now you're going to do the same.

Invest a solid set of discreet wireless earbuds and carry them with you wherever you go. Ensure that they are comfortable and have excellent battery life. If your budget allows, go for two pairs so that you can switch into your second pair for prolonged sessions. Doing so will enable you to:

1. WORK IN QUALITY MIM IN THE BACKGROUND
2. SEAL YOURSELF OUT FROM BAD MIM

These will also come in handy for the next tip:

୭ PREMADE PLAYLISTS

A little preparation goes a long way. You will often find yourself with time to kill throughout your daily life, and because of the power of MIM, you can specially select it to achieve a designated outcome. For example, if you are feeling sad, you can select a song that makes you feel great.

Because of this, take the time to create playlists of the best of the best for different occasions for the different sources of MIM. A gym playlist, a chill playlist, a list of books to read, podcasts you want to listen to, and movies to watch on a rainy day.

Whenever you come across a song, movie, book, article, website, or any other source of MIM you want to work into your life or check out later, toss it in your notes app for later. Go through that list periodically and create your playlists to keep on hand, so you're left with no excuses why you don't have meaningful MIM with you.

PEOPLE

Tell me who you hang around, and I'll tell you who you are. The people you surround yourself with will either lift you to great heights or break you down and bury you. Many greats throughout history have been destroyed by terrible relationships, and many potential greats in the modern day are limited by them.

- ONLY surround yourself with like-minded people who share and/or support your goals. Feed off each other's energy and positivity. This is your success network.
- Cut ties or limit your exposure as much as possible to those who lead you astray or try to bring you down and knock you off course, whether they mean to or not. These are energy vampires who will do you no good.

MAXIM OF AESTHETICS: THE ONLY NEGATIVITY IN YOUR LIFE SHOULD COME FROM THE ECCENTRIC PORTION OF YOUR LIFTS

Do not judge or resent them for this. Everyone is on their own journey, and they are acting in line with where they are at this point in their life. Respect them. Love them. But don't adjust your life to accommodate theirs.

SOCIAL MEDIA

This also extends into the digital world. Social media has made a huge surge in the past few years, and this has been revolutionary in helping people connect and share with each other, however as with all power, it must be used wisely.

Surround your online space with nothing but the best. Positive, helpful information only. Social media is a place where people go to complain, spread distractions, and seek attention for their ego. None of these are good for you, so avoid them.

Lastly, if you are checking social media all day, every day, it's a sign that you need to get your life in order and get your mind right. Focus on your real life – not how it appears in a picture on the internet. 10 minutes a day is more than enough. Check yourself.

ENVIRONMENT

Lastly, you've got to fine tune your environment for success. No matter where you are, it's right there staring you in the face, so it's a source of MIM that's very important for your internal state.

- ❧ Keep your spaces clean, simple, and organized. A dose of minimalism works wonders aesthetically-speaking. The main focus in every room should be the people in it who give it life.
- ❧ Follow my earlier recommendations and place vision portals wherever you frequent.
- ❧ Lastly, enhance your surroundings by manipulating the various sensory channels around you. Pleasing fragrances,

lighting, textures, colors, and designs all contribute to an optimal environment.

OUT AND ABOUT

These same factors also play a role in places you go such as stores, gyms, restaurants, cafés, and so on. Surround yourself with quality. Frequent the places you enjoy the most with people who exude positivity and enjoy what they do.

You will get better service, spend your money in support of them, and by becoming a regular, you will forge better relationships and establish go-to spots for dates, business meetings, and other occasions.

WHEN YOU HAVE NO SAY

In situations where you can't have optimal input, there is no reason to worry. Simply be aware and observe, knowing full well that this is not the way things should be. That is all that you need to do, and that is all that separates you from those who live it blindly every day.

SUMMARY

Your MIM renovation will not happen overnight. It is an ongoing process, but I have given you the tools to understand your own mind and have pointed you in the right direction to begin making changes in your life for the better. Begin today, and enjoy the results coming your way.

BONUS: STYLE AND MOVEMENT

41

FASHION AND STYLE

𝕿HE HUMAN BODY IS AN AESTHETIC MASTERPIECE on its own, but adding in clothes can actually enhance the body by breaking up space, drawing the eye, accentuating certain parts over others, and expressing your personality to create a more powerful, intriguing image.

Do this correctly, and your aesthetic efforts will be sustained into the world. Do this incorrectly, and your efforts will be buried and forgotten in the folds of the fabric.

The seasons fade in and out and fads come and go, but from the gym grind to a solid night out, don't worry; I've got you covered to keep you looking stylish and fresh-dressed at your best.

STEP ZERO: GET AESTHETIC

Right off the bat, the absolute best thing you can do for your style is to build a fine physique.

Aesthetics are the best fashion statement there is, and having a great physique will make everything look better on you by default. On the other hand, if you don't have it and let yourself slip, hardly anything can save you.

When you've got aesthetics on your side, style game is more about *accentuating* your frame and expressing your personality and image than anything else.

You've read the book and know how to make that happen.

So make it happen.

Its impact can't be spoken for enough.

1. IT'S ALL IN THE FIT

You can have two identical articles of clothing with different sizes and create two completely different visual results. Baggy or ill-fitting clothes will bury that physique you've forged and detract from the natural flow and beauty of the body.

Therefore, when you're fueling your body right and hitting the iron like the beast you are, you've got to shoot for having an excellent fit on all of your clothes. This will showcase the positive proportions, attributes, and overall aesthetics of your physique on center stage.

Hunt for slim fits that taper and contour to the natural dimensions of the body from top to bottom. You want to show that figure and silhouette that you've built without distortion or detraction, and excess fabric will clutter that up in a heartbeat.

From your tanks and your tees to your jackets and jeans, always get the fit right on the money. Make it a concrete habit to try everything on and factor in any potential shrinking.

Not all articles of clothing are built to be 100% fitted, and a little flare can be a nice touch, so for those cases, remember the accent and detractive points of an aesthetic physique that we went over earlier in the book. This will highlight your proportions favorably no matter what you wear and set the standard for all of your fashion choices:

A E S T H E T I C   S T Y L E

POINTS TO HIGHLIGHT	POINTS TO MINIMIZE
Shoulders	
Lats	Joints
Forearms	Waist
Glutes	Muscle groups directly adjacent to the accent
Calves	points
Hips (girls)	

In other words, don't rock shirts that make your waist look wide. Make sure your pants contour from the glutes to the hams to strut your squats. Straight leg fits will crush your calves, so watch out. Don't have flappy long sleeves, and dresses and skirts for the ladies should always fit snug around the waist and hips.

If you knock it out of the park here, the rest of your fashion fiddling will be a walk in the park.

2. MATCH YOU

Have you ever seen someone rocking a great style, but something just didn't quite feel right? That's likely because although *the outfit* was great, it didn't go with *the person* who was wearing it.

This can either come from a mismatch with their:

- Personality
- Build
- Natural tones (skin, eyes, hair)
- Hairstyles

Everyone is naturally going to have certain styles and colors that work best for them based on who they are. This is highly variable, but highly critical.

Clothes are just ONE part of the entire work of art that is you, so they need to work into the piece as a whole and gel well with who you are as a person and all that you are.

Fashion makes a SPEECH, not a statement.

In some cases, a little clash can be a good thing - when done tastefully. See the point on contrast.

3. <u>MATCH THE REST</u>

If you start to develop a tribe of leprechaun nomads following you in hopes of reaching the pot of gold, then it's likely you're going overboard on the color scheme. Walking around like a rainbow or mismatched colors that clash is ugly to the eye.

As a general rule of thumb, 2-3 main colors is about where you want to be. Another one or two mixed in can be okay when done tastefully as accents. This doesn't include accessories per se, so you can spice things up with some silver and gold.

Whatever you've got going on in your outfit should revolve around these main colors.

4. <u>CONTRAST IS KING</u>

If you want something to pop and incorporate variety, then contrast is the way to go.

Colors will look more vivid when displayed against another for contrast. An outfit with contrast incorporated will be more visually interesting and appealing to the eye.

Even if you are rocking one color throughout, you want to make sure that at least some contrast is involved.

Let's look at an example.

Say you're going murdered out today (to match your soul?). You can have a black shirt, black pants, and black shoes, but make sure that either the textures, tones, or material differs on those blacks. In other words, matte black, glossy, faded, and pitch black should be mixed around rather than going all one direction.

The contrast doesn't have to be for everything though. As long as the items touching each other have contrast, you should be good to go. For example, the shirt can match the shoes but not the pants. Got it?

As a final point: Contrast can oftentimes come from something outside of the outfit itself. How? Your hair color, eye color, skin tone, personality, and so on.

- If you have darker skin or hair, a brilliant white will make you pop more than someone who has a lighter complexion.
- If you are a rugged type, a simple, sharp outfit can offer contrast that adds complexity to your character and image. Or vice versa.

Work the palette and manipulate your variables. There is no one size fits all solution when it comes to fashion.

5. HAVE A CENTERPIECE

In most great works of art, there is a crucial element that the artist wants to draw your attention to. The same is true of fashion.

You can have relatively neutral colors for your clothing accented by an article that is bright and pops to add that spark to your attire. As stated above, there are components of contrast to take into account.

- ❧ SHOES
- ❧ ACCESSORIES
- ❧ SPECIFIC GARMENT

Get creative here. The context will change depending on all of the other variables of your outfit, but always look to have one item that stands out above the rest and draws the eye near.

6. ACCESSORIZE

Accessories are what really make an outfit shine. Necklaces, bracelets, rings, watches, sunglasses, scarves, anklets, earrings, and hats add that extra dimension of flare to an already stunning outfit.

Accessories can have a lot of meaning to you as an individual, and they're excellent conversation starters that'll leave an impression on those you encounter.

Pick accessories with a message. A particular gemstone. Some beautiful beads. A different design. An exotic flair. A message or meaning related to your childhood or place of birth.

As you spread your wings and travel the world, hit up the local markets. They'll give you some unique accessories and some great stories to tell about it over drinks at the rooftop lounge or a dashing dinner date at the new spot downtown.

If your accessory is truly unique and special, do not spill the details easily. Let people guess. Make them wonder or work for it. If they can figure it out, it'll be a little Easter egg they'll remember for a long time and set you apart in their mind to build a special connection. They'll remember. Watch.

Lastly, it's hard to overdo it on the accessories unless you are pushing for plundering pirate or gypsy status. Keep it refined and broadly balanced, and you're good to go.

7. <u>BROAD BALANCE</u>

Your entire body is a canvas that needs to have the art spread out on. We spoke about how important a symmetrical physique is, but fashion plays by slightly different rules.

In fashion, pure symmetry is generic and bland. You want to mix things up a bit and flirt with a little dispersion. This is best done by the smaller elements of your look like planets circling the sun.

One style of accessories on one arm, and a different on another to a different degree. A little accent or design on one side to gently tip things in one direction. 3 rings on one hand and 1 on another.

Nevertheless, you don't want to be too top heavy or bottom heavy. You don't want to have too much weight on the left and not on the right. A touch can be trendy and tasteful, but too much is an eyesore. For example:

- Don't put 50 bracelets on one arm and then 0 on the other.
- Don't make your entire bottom half black and the top white.

The amount needed to bring balance into the look isn't as much as you'd think.

For the above examples, one or two bracelets on the other arm and shoes with a white accent or laces (or even some skin showing - think low cut shoes or rolled up pants) can be enough to bring some harmony back into the look.

8. BE BOLD

Fortune favors the bold, and the common and customary is left ignored.

All of the tips above are spot on and will contribute to a superb look, but always look to have a component of your look that's a little out there and rattles the cage.

This can be accomplished via the other principles, but sometimes it takes a little out of the box thinking. An unusual pattern or graphic. A unique accessory. A tattoo that's intriguing. All of these things are examples of ways to switch up the norm beyond normal convention.

Whatever it is, make it meaningful and special to you. Let it represent a strong component of who you are. You always want to have your calling card and that one special thing that separates you from the rest - and this isn't limited to just fashion, either.

No matter how you decide to carry this out, own it with unwavering confidence. No apologies. No remorse. This is you through and through.

9. SIMPLICITY

To wrap these all together, the last point is that of simplicity. Never lose sight of the bigger picture and allow things to get overcrowded. This will only confuse the eye, come off as too try-hard, and detract from the true prize, your physique.

Simplify and please the eye.

You want to create a clean, sharp look that comes off as normal and natural, not overly rehearsed. When in doubt, *less is more.*

A simple wardrobe will also allow you to mix and match easily and with more combinations. That means more versatility and potential for your creativity to shine.

It doesn't take much to have fashion that appeals to the eyes. Remember, your body is already lifting that heavy load. Fashion for a physique is just the simple things done RIGHT - just like most things in life.

10. VISUAL TEST

Equipped with these tips, you've got the fundamental principles you need to start piecing together a better wardrobe and a better look for that aesthetic physique, but there's one last thing...

The final boss must ALWAYS be the mirror.

These principles sound great in theory, but how does the outfit look in its totality when put into play? At the end of the day, THAT'S what it's all about. Each outfit is different and will ultimately be judged by mirror, mirror on the wall before hitting the world.

Over time, you'll see what works best with your look and personality within your wardrobe, and you'll develop a sixth sense for what to do when it's time to suit up and hit the streets.

AESTHETIC STYLE CHECKLIST

0. GET AESTHETIC
1. IT'S ALL IN THE FIT
2. MATCH YOU
3. MATCH THE REST
4. CONTRAST IS KING
5. HAVE A CENTERPIECE
6. ACCESSORIZE
7. BROAD BALANCE
8. BE BOLD
9. SIMPLICITY
10. VISUAL TEST

EXTRA TIPS:

- ❧ Get your grooming on point. Keep it well-maintained, and never head out less than proper and excellent.
- ❧ A splash of fragrance will work wonders. Alternate by occasion and season. Consider layering to develop your own signature scent. It'll be your calling card they'll never forget.
- ❧ Work to get the hairstyles that fit your face and look best.
- ❧ Whiten your smile and keep your breath minty fresh.
- ❧ Animate that style and physique with what you'll learn now:

42

BODY LANGUAGE

*I*S YOUR GOAL TO BE A STATUE ? Then skip past this section. If your goal is to *move* that aesthetic body you have created and work it in the real world to reap maximum success in all of your endeavors, then proceed.

You might have a great physique and dress for success, but the way in which you carry yourself just as important. Body language speaks more than words - both subconsciously to yourself and to others.

Even before you've achieved your goal physique, start implementing these tips today. There's no need to wait. Once you've determined something you want in your life, make those steps happen as soon as you can. By the time you've reached Olympus, it'll be ingrained in you and just another golden habit.

NATURAL AND FLOWING

Human aesthetics are demonstrated through flow - not rigid, stiff designs. The nectar of the eyes rests in organic, rounded shapes that sit gently and draw you near. Likewise, natural, flowing shapes in posing and body language demonstrate poise and ease in your environment.

Therefore, avoid fixed, rigid postures. You are not a robot or stick figure. If you are, hit the weights and bring your diet up to speed. This will demonstrate lack of control amongst your surroundings, nervousness, and timidity. Move with grace. Move without hesitation. Smooth.

Many find this difficult to do. They are too tense. The reason for this is simple: they feel the external pressure, and the weight of others looking at them is making it hard for them to move with flow.

To fix this, you've got to get to work on your mind because the mind is the source of reality and is holding you back.

Refine your meditations and let go of external judgment. The world is your playground, and no opinion can shake your steady soul.

CONTRAPPOSTO

Just like the ancient Greek figures frozen in marble, adopt the posture of contrapposto, where the angle of your hips and shoulders oppose each other.

To do this, you will put your weight on one leg and lean into it so that your hips tip up slightly. This naturally creates a relaxed posture of confidence and ease in your environment.

The hips are most important here:

- For women, the angle of the hips can be tipped off balance underneath a neutral shoulder posture. This is exudes sex appeal and femininity.
- Men need to avoid this altogether. For men, the hips must always be angled alongside a countered shoulder angle.

Try these in front of a full mirror and observe the rapid effects that take form. Practice them until it becomes second nature. You can slip into this as you stand in conversation or observation wherever you may roam.

TAKE YOUR TIME

Rushing and fumbling about communicates a lack of control and increases that same sensation in your own mind, leading to that anxious, hectic feeling within you.

- When you move, make your movements more deliberate and graceful.
- When you speak, don't be in a hurry to get it all out on one breath. Know your worth. They'll listen.

With everything you do, take your time.

You are in control of time and space; not the other way around.

Take that nugget of wisdom to heart because it speaks volumes.

You are not reactive. You demonstrate poise, control, and confidence in everything you do. The external world does not determine your internal state.

Make the conscious effort to slow things down in your day to day tasks. Even dip your toes in the waters of slowed down absurdity just so that you can experience what it feels like. It'll put you in the present moment and give you more enjoyment of everything you do through more mindfulness. You'll note how moving slower will give you that little oomph of confidence and surefootedness that cranks up your aura.

Walking from point A to point B is about the only thing you should be doing quickly. But with momentum, surefootedness, and purpose. This demonstrates power and confidence.

CONFIDENCE

Wherever you are, whatever you do: project unshakeable confidence.

Do not ever carry yourself like your existence is an apology. Carry yourself with pride and purpose. Chest up, shoulders back, and energy seemingly emanating off of you like a mirage of an oasis in the desert. Except yours is real. Your posture and results will thank you.

ALL IN THE EYES

The eyes are indeed the windows of the soul and can give away everything about your inner state.

Are you googly eyed quickly looking here, there, and everywhere? A shifty gaze indicates anxiety, insecurity, and weakness. Why are you looking around all over the place like the boogeyman is about to jump out from behind the corner at any moment?

Remember: <u>You are in control.</u>

Act as if you knew everything about everything and everyone in your vicinity and put them there on purpose. Why would you be nervous or paranoid?

When you walk or talk, keep a fixed gaze. When someone is in front of you, look them right in their eyes. Connect with them on a deep level. Don't let your eyes bounce around like they're in a pinball machine. When you decisively change where you look, don't be in any rush to do so.

NEUTRAL OR ABOVE

Whenever you look down – either with your eyes or your head – it shows sadness, lack of self-esteem, weakness, and other undesirable things. Stand up, walk down the hall, and try it for yourself.

In one instance, walk with your head held high, and in the other, walk with your head dipped downwards. In which one do you feel more confident, happy, and powerful?

To train yourself to do this, there's a very simple trick: Pretend like there's a block of wood attached to your neck right underneath your chin that physically prevents your head from dipping below neutral level.

Use this same idea with your eyes like you are the product of psycho surgery. Or that there were laser beams shooting out of your eyes and underneath neutral level there is an innocent child who will be blasted with flaming photons if you look down. Neutral or above. Never below.

Even when you text, hold your phone slightly out in front of you rather than straight down by your lap. Instant body language tune up. Better yet, stop texting so damn much at all. Life is happening all around you.

OPEN

A closed, minimized posture shows weakness and insecurity. It makes you appear fearful or uncomfortable in your surroundings. Always demonstrate an open posture. Uncross your arms, stand tall and never hunch over, and learn to lean back into your seat when you sit down.

This posture will show that you're at ease internally and have nothing to hide or be worried about. The more hectic or busy the surrounding environment is, the more power this has. You need to build up your forcefield like nothing can possibly affect you.

- Men, ensure that your openness takes up space and demonstrates dominance of your area – a symbol for the ability to dominate wherever you apply yourself
- Women, your openness is a delicate balance. You must appear completely open and confident, yet still mysterious and unable to be conquered. Too much openness is masculine, yet too much closure is timid. Find your sweet spot. Discover your enticing feminine charm.

LEARN FROM EXAMPLE

Those tips are golden, but body language is a far-reaching subject with much to learn that I couldn't possibly give you all here. You will constantly be finding ways to fine tune things and improve, so to help you do just that, I'm going to give you this simple homework assignment to fine tune your body language on your own.

Go out in your down time and at least once per week, fire up a good movie and relax.

Consciously observe the body language and mannerisms of the people. You will pick up on things from the actions of others and be able to then fine tune your behavior. Everything is an opportunity to learn and grow when you have an open mind.

Here we will focus on movies, as you have the opportunity to replay and dissect them with great ease:

1. OBSERVE

When you watch your favorite movies, observe how the actors move. Their facial expressions. The way they use their voice. Their body language. This is no accident. They dial this in to create a heightened effect on the audience, so it's an excellent learning tool for you.

2. ANALYZE

Don't just look at what they do. Pay attention to *how and why*. What's the context? What else is going on in the scene? The dialogue, the setting, and the reactions of the other characters will show you all that you need to know.

3. PRACTICE

Just like an actor or actress would, practice this in front of a mirror and videotape yourself. You can save clips of your favorite performances on screen and compare them side by side with how you do it to fine tune your movements.

4. INTERNALIZE

Practice until it becomes second nature. Put it in play at home and while you're out in the world. It may be awkward at first, but you're reprogramming your habits here. Stick with it. You can be whoever you want to be. All it takes is a little forethought and consistency.

Enjoyable, easy, and simple. Just how success should be.

In no time, you will renovate your movements and posture to a high degree of effectiveness and make the most out of all that hard work you've put in the weight room.

AFTER OLYMPUS

VENI, VIDI, VICI.
I CAME, I SAW, I CONQUERED.
Julius Caesar

MUCH TIME HAS PASSED since you set sail and departed from home to experience the journey of achieving aesthetics. You have gained the fundamental knowledge of training, nutrition, recovery, the mind, and much more that you can utilize to take yourself to your highest levels and the pinnacles you were destined to reach. And now your journey has come to a close.

Or has it?

For many, aesthetics are the end goal. There is nothing more than this. But the true architect of aesthetics recognizes that aesthetics are just the beginning. You learned how to lift. But have you learned how to live?

Before we part ways, I have one more lesson for you. The biggest.

THE 5 FACTORS OF HAPPINESS

What is the meaning of life..?

How many people have looked up in the sky and asked themselves this question...Different people will give you different answers, but everyone is just looking for one thing at the end of the day:

Happiness.

People chase this happiness in many different ways. Most of them are searching in the wrong places, but when all is said and done, everything comes down to this simple, yet complex thing. Happiness. But what is it?

The truth is, happiness isn't any *one* thing. Happiness is made up of a *variety* of factors that all support and lift each other. To achieve happiness and true success in life, you must aim to strike a balance in these 5 areas:

- ❧ WELL-BEING
- ❧ INNER PEACE
- ❧ FULFILLMENT
- ❧ GROWTH
- ❧ BENEFIT TO ALL

Architect, these are the pillars of your building of life. They've all got to be there to support it. If you knock one out, everything crumbles. Can such happiness ever be truly grasped in this life?

Perhaps not, but this is how you would do it.

WELL BEING

Many years ago, you saw the light of the world for the first time. Tears came streaming down your face, but you weren't sad. You were happy to be a part of what we call life.

As you grew up and took your first steps, you tried many other things for the first time. Delicious foods, the feeling of the warm water in the bath, and the cozy bed you rested your head in after a long day of play. These are your basic needs, and such simple things are life's greatest gifts.

Time passed by, and you discovered that out there in the world, there's much more to experience and explore. People, places, pleasures, and possessions.

Enjoy them all, but just like everything we've gone over so far that goes into building your work of art, it all has its sweet spot and limits.

Everything is there for you, but never let these things be the source of purpose in your life. You don't need much, and of the things you do need, you don't need much. Ambition is a virtue, but only when you apply it to the right things. Are you?

---

*A king or queen isn't made by their title or riches. It's **who you are** that makes the difference. The rest is just an accessory.*

Know your worth. Infinite.

BE MORE.

INNER PEACE

One Summer, you went to the beach and sat on the warm sand as you watched the waves of the ocean float in and out until the sun set and the fireflies flashed and disappeared into the night sky.

When you got older, you saw that life happens the same way.

Nothing lasts forever. Everything comes and goes. Everything is change. Yet there you are, watching it all pass by. You would be crazy to jump into the water and try to hold on to that wave forever. You would drown. So don't do the same in life.

Disconnect from your attachment to everything around you. Outcomes, people, possessions, and labels. Your value and state are distinct from them. You depend on nothing and no one. Instead, make *yourself* the source of your happiness and support in life.

KNOW YOURSELF
TRUST YOURSELF
LOVE YOURSELF

Only move forward if you're at peace with your path.

No matter what happens, you're still the captain. No matter what storms come, you will make it through and turn it into greatness.

How could you not? You are great yourself.

Until the day comes that your maker decides to take you, commit to the belief that there is nothing that can break you.

FULFILLMENT

Think of you and your life like a glass. It is built for a purpose and has great potential, but with nothing inside to fill it, it is nothing more than a simple object to look at.

How are you going to fill it up?

FULFILLMENT OF ACTION

There is nothing that can bring you greater joy and fulfillment than pursuing your passions and interests. Work is a thing of the past. You must find your beloved area to pour your life into.

If money was no issue at all, what would you do with your life?
If you could be anything you wanted, what would that be?
What would you do for nothing in return?

That is where you need to be. Get there, and everything else will come. Not the other way around. Chase nothing but your dreams. Be the eagle and soar. The entire sky is open for you to explore.

FULFILLMENT OF SELF

What does it mean to be human? Mind, body, and spirit in one. Live up to your potential and realize your capacity for great things.

Express yourself, create, think for yourself, experience, explore, discover, and act justly. Embrace who you are and hold yourself to a higher standard. Reject mediocrity. Abandon complacency. Be all that is worthy of a human being. You were born to live, not to survive. So live. True and you. Through and through. It's your right.

GROWTH

A seed isn't planted to be buried by dirt in the ground. Every day is an opportunity to learn, grow, and move forward in life to reach for the sun in the sky. Constantly think about how can you advance:

> ❧ YOURSELF

Your mind, body, and spirit. Your skillsets, virtues, and actions. You are the sculptor of all that is you. Who do you want to become?

> ❧ YOUR FIELD

The breadth of knowledge, the progression, and the advancements that will long outlive you. Be a part of something greater.

> ❧ THE WORLD

Your community, others, and the environment at large.

Every day of your life should be a good day and a day in which you moved forward - no matter how small. It all counts. This is the philosophy of kaizen - that is, continuous improvement.

Have firm goals that direct your actions. Aim high. Never settle. Having your sights set on progression will breathe new life into you. It's a never-ending journey of advancement to take you to another level. Progressive overload doesn't stop at the gym.

How can I be better today?

Start every morning with this question, and you will go far.

BENEFIT TO ALL

We live in a world full of competition. Me vs. you. Us vs. them. Only the strong shall survive. They've got it all wrong. There is no competition or enemy besides your own reflection.

What you do must not only be in your best interest, but it must also be in the best interest of *others*. No matter how tempted you may be, there is no reason to ever cause another person harm for your personal gain– physical or mental. You must be and do better.

You are ONE LIFE that may live for a good 70-80 years on this little blue marble in space if all works out well, but with that ONE life you have the ability to impact MILLIONS now and for generations to come through your actions. Even more immediately, you have the ability to impact *every individual* you come across every day.

They will look up to you now, but you must not look down on them. Every time someone comes into contact with you, you need to leave them better than you found them.

Young and old. Friend or foe. Black and white. Wrong or right. It doesn't matter.

You are in a privileged position of power, resources, knowledge, and understanding. Most others are not. Understand their position, have sympathy, and set the example. Lead them into victory.

Share your gifts, express what makes you who you are, and offer all the value you can to the world without expectation. There is nothing else for you to do. In return, it'll find its way to give you all that value back. And there is no greater feeling than that.

THE STRONGEST BUILDING

These factors all weave into and support one another. None alone are the solution, and when they are all at work together, each has new meaning and is carried out most effectively.

When looking at your life as a whole, reflect upon the extent to which all of these factors are at play. There are no contradictions between them, and if there are, it is a sign of improvement to be made on your part.

As I've shown you, specificity is paramount. You must know your goal and ensure that everything you do supports that goal.

Therefore, if these are the factors of true happiness, and your goal is to live a happy life, then you must always ask yourself whether what you are doing or experiencing is truly contributing to that goal and in line with the balance of these factors.

Chances are, you're far away from these, but don't let that discourage you. Just like the body has showed you thus far, *great things take time.* It's a constant journey, but remember: *your targets are everything.*

When you've got these 5 down, you will get a glimpse of what happiness really is. If the world is ever going to make it, it's going to be by these 5 factors. This is my life philosophy, and I wouldn't have it any other way.

Put these in play, and the throne will be yours someday.

TAKE FLIGHT

It is not death a man should fear, but he should fear never beginning to live.
Marcus Aurelius, Emperor of Rome

As I sit here writing my farewells, I'm overwhelmed to find that we're finally here. It's been one hell of a journey, and though I don't know you, by this point you know me, and so long as you can read these words, I'll be right there guiding you to greatness.

From my heart to yours, it's been a pleasure. Just as I made it home from those grueling runs years ago that changed my life, today *we all* made it home.

And this is where our story must come to a close...for now.

Go experience all that the world has to offer. Be a symbol for others. Set the example. Help lift them to their fullest potential just as I've lifted you. Go make yourself into the best version of yourself that you can possibly be.

Your life of aesthetics, personal growth, and happiness awaits you.

Now get out there and go live it.

I'll see you high in the sky.

ARCHITECT of AESTHETICS

A beautiful body perishes, but a work of art dies not.
Leonardo da Vinci

ABOUT THE AUTHOR

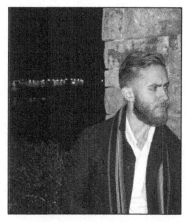

$\mathcal{J}$OSEPH MURCI is the author of *Architect of Aesthetics*, a book bringing together the art, science, and philosophy of building the ultimate physique.

From a young age, he has been obsessed with decoding the world around him and uses this passion to build better businesses, better people, and better lives for all across the globe. When he isn't training, writing, or exploring the world, you can catch him cruising the streets on his skateboard, creating music, lost in a book, or refining his skills in other areas.

For news, contact, coaching, and consultations, get in touch:

www.JOSEPHMURCI.com

THE 10 LAWS OF THE ARCHITECT OF AESTHETICS

I.   HONOR YOUR GOAL

II.   THE BODY OPERATES ON A SPECTRUM

III.   THE BODY OPERATES IN PHASES

IV.   THERE ARE NO HARD RULES. ONLY

       TECHNIQUES AND TOOLS

V.   CONSIDER ALL THE VARIABLES ON HAND

VI.   THE BODY IS MASTERFULLY BUILT TO SURVIVE

       AND ADAPT

VII.   SIMPLICITY IS THE SOLUTION

VIII.   MAKE GOLD OF WHAT IS GIVEN

IX.   STAY HUMBLE

X.   NEVER FORGET THE HUMAN BEING

THE MAXIMS OF AESTHETICS

I. The mind is the strongest muscle you have.

II. Success begins within. Before you can be it, first you must see it.

III. Learn from the greats - both in their victory and in their defeat.

IV. Chase not money nor fame. Chase your passion, and only then will the world remember your name.

V. A human being with no purpose is a human being with no pulse.

VI. Strive for balance above all...In lifting and in life.

VII. Too much given to one will cause all to topple.

VIII. Build upon your strengths and work with your weaknesses. Your only limitations are those you impose upon yourself.

IX. All is valid but not all is valuable.

X. Fitness is just the medium - not the mission.

XI. The people you surround yourself with are the predictors of your success.

XII. If you fail to plan, then you plan to fail.

XIII. You must be able to satisfactorily justify everything in your workout, diet program, and life.

XIV. If over time you aren't adding weight to the bar, over time you aren't going very far.

XV. Less is more. Push forward only when there is ground to gain.

XVI. Strive for excellence with every rep, just as you would strive for excellence with every day you live and everything that you do.

XVII. The numbers on the bar are not as important as the effects that lifting them correctly are.

XVIII. Focus on progression, not perfection.

XIX. Either your program or your results can be flashy, but rarely will you get both. And even if you do, there was probably a better way.

XX. When it's light, treat it like it's heavy. When it's heavy treat it like it's light.

XXI. Rest is just as important as routine

XXII. Your program should be enjoyable every day no matter what your current goal is.

XXIII. Working out is a privilege. Take care of your body so that it can take care of you.

XXIV. Track your progress or you are on the track to nowhere

XXV. Embrace the errors and pitfalls. They are the first step to further improvement

XXVI. The only negativity in your life should come from the eccentric portion of your lifts

REFERENCES

THE AESTHETIC PHYSIQUE

1. Zeki S, Ishizu T. Toward A Brain-Based Theory of Beauty. PLoS One. 2011; 6(7): e21852.
2. Wald C. Neuroscience: The aesthetic brain. Nature. 2015 Oct 8;526(7572):S2-3.
3. Zeki S. Clive Bell's "Significant Form" and the neurobiology of aesthetics. Front Hum Neurosci. 2013; 7:730.
4. Redies C. Combining universal beauty and cultural context in a unifying model of visual aesthetic experience. Front Hum Neurosci. 2015;9:218.
5. Bell C. (1914). Art. London: Chatto & Windus.
6. Kant I. (1790/1987). Critique of Judgment, trans. W. Pluhar. Indianapolis: Hackett Publishing Co, Inc.
7. Di Dio C, Macaluso E, Rizzolatti G. The golden beauty: brain response to classical and renaissance sculptures. Rustichini A, ed. *PLoS ONE*. 2007;2(11):e1201.
8. Tsukiura T, Cabeza R. Shared brain activity for aesthetic and moral judgments: implications for the beauty-is-good stereotype. Soc Cogn Affect Neurosci. 2011 Jan;6(1):138-48.
9. Wang T, Mo L, Mo C, Tan LH, Cant JS, Zhong L, Cupchik G. Is moral beauty different from facial beauty? Evidence from an fMRI study. Soc Cogn Affect Neurosci. 2015 Jun;10(6):814-23.
10. Chapman HA, Anderson AK. Things rank and gross in nature: a review and synthesis of moral disgust. Psychol Bull. 2013 Mar;139(2):300-27.
11. Olivera La Rosa A, Roselló Mir J. On the relationships between disgust and morality: a critical review. Psicothema. 2013;25(2):222-6.
12. Obermeier C, Menninghaus W, von Koppenfels M, et al. Aesthetic and emotional effects of meter and rhyme in poetry. Frontiers in Psychology. 2013;4:10.
13. Salimpoor VN, Benovoy M, Larcher K, Dagher A, Zatorre RJ. Anatomically distinct dopamine release during anticipation and experience of peak emotion to music. Nat Neurosci. 2011 Feb;14(2):257-62
14. Brattico P, Brattico E, Vuust P. Global sensory qualities and aesthetic experience in music. Front Neurosci. 2017 Apr 5;11:159.
15. Egermann H, Fernando N, Chuen L, McAdams S. Music induces universal emotion-related psychophysiological responses: comparing Canadian listeners to Congolese Pygmies. Front Psychol. 2015 Jan 7;5:1341.
16. Zeki S, Romaya JP, Benincasa DM, Atiyah MF. The experience of mathematical beauty and its neural correlates. Front Hum Neurosci. 2014 Feb 13;8:68.
17. Baumgartner T, Lutz K, Schmidt CF, Jäncke L. The emotional power of music: how music enhances the feeling of affective pictures. Brain Res. 2006 Feb 23;1075(1):151-64.
18. Rhodes G, Lee K, Palermo R, Weiss M, Yoshikawa S, Clissa P, Williams T, Peters M, Winkler C, Jeffery L. Attractiveness of own-race, other-race, and mixed-race faces. Perception. 2005;34(3):319-40.
19. Langlois JH, Kalakanis L, Rubenstein AJ, Larson A, Hallam M, Smoot M. Maxims or myths of beauty? A meta-analytic and theoretical review. Psychol Bull. 2000 May;126(3):390-423.
20. Wilson M, Daly M. Do pretty women inspire men to discount the future? Proc Biol Sci. 2004 May 7; 271(Suppl 4): S177-S179.

21. Lippa RA. The preferred traits of mates in a cross-national study of heterosexual and homosexual men and women: an examination of biological and cultural influences. Arch Sex Behav. 2007 Apr;36(2):193-208.
22. Kiire S. Effect of leg-to-body ratio on body shape attractiveness. Arch Sex Behav. 2016 May;45(4):901-10.
23. Grammer K, Sainani KL. Q&A: Karl Grammer. Innate attractions. Nature. 2015 Oct 8;526(7572):S11.
24. Singh D. Female mate value at a glance: relationship of waist-to-hip ratio to health, fecundity and attractiveness. Neuro Endocrinol Lett. 2002 Dec;23 Suppl 4:81-91.
25. Prum Ro. Aesthetic evolution by mate choice: Darwin's *really* dangerous idea. Philos Trans R Soc Lond B Biol Sci. 2012 Aug; 367(1600): 2253–2265.
26. Ramachandran VS, Hirstein W. The science of art: a neurological theory of aesthetic experience. Journal of Consciousness Studies. 1999; 6(6-7): 15-51
27. Carney DR, Cuddy AJ, Yap AJ. Power posing: brief nonverbal displays affect neuroendocrine levels and risk tolerance. Psychol Sci. 2010 Oct;21(10):1363-8.
28. Cuddy AJ, Wilmuth CA, Yap AJ, Carney DR. Preparatory power posing affects nonverbal presence and job interview performance. J Appl Psychol. 2015 Jul;100(4):1286-95.
29. Shariff A, Tracy JL, Markusoff JL. (Implicitly) judging a book by its cover: the power of pride and shame expressions in shaping judgments of social status. Psychol Bull. 2012 May; 38(9):1178-1193
30. Shafir T, Taylor SF, Atkinson AP, Langenecker SA, Zubieta JK. Emotion regulation through execution, observation, and imagery of emotional movements. Brain Cogn. 2013 Jul;82(2):219-27.
31. Shafir T, Tsachor RP, Welch KB. Emotion regulation through movement: unique sets of movement characteristics are associated with and enhance basic emotions. Front Psychol. 2016 Jan 11;6:2030.
32. Jakesch M, Leder H. Finding meaning in art: preferred levels of ambiguity in art appreciation. Q J Exp Psychol (Hove). 2009 Nov;62(11):2105-12.
33. Jakesch M, Goller J, Leder H. Positive fEMG Patterns with ambiguity in paintings. Frontiers in Psychology. 2017;8:785.
34. Jakesch M, Leder H, Forster M. Image ambiguity and fluency. PLoS One. 2013 Sep 5;8(9):e74084.
35. Millis K. Making meaning brings pleasure: the influence of titles on aesthetic experiences. Emotion. 2001 Sep;1(3):320-9.
36. Park SA, Yun K, Jeong J. Reappraising abstract paintings after exposure to background information. Solomon SG, ed. PLoS ONE. 2015;10(5):e0124159.

GENETICS

1. Bray MS, Hagberg JM, Pérusse L, Rankinen T, Roth SM, Wolfarth B, Bouchard C. The human gene map for performance and health-related fitness phenotypes: the 2006-2007 update. Med Sci Sports Exerc. 2009 Jan;41(1):35-73.
2. Bouchard C¹, Tremblay A, Després JP, Nadeau A, Lupien PJ, Thériault G, Dussault J, Moorjani S, Pinault S, Fournier G. The response to long-term overfeeding in identical twins. N Engl J Med. 1990 May 24;322(21):1477-82.
3. Bouchard C, Tremblay A. Genetic effects in human energy expenditure components. Int J Obes. 1990;14 Suppl 1:49-55; discussion 55-8.
4. Timmons JA. Variability in training-induced skeletal muscle adaptation. Journal of Applied Physiology. 2011;110(3):846-853.
5. Panizzon MS, Hauger R, Jacobson KC, Eaves LJ, York TP, Prom-Wormley E, Grant MD, Lyons MJ, McKenzie R, Mendoza SP, Xian H, Franz CE, Kremen WS. Genetic

and environmental influences of daily and intra-individual variation in
testosterone levels in middle-aged men. Psychoneuroendocrinology. 2013
Oct;38(10):2163-72.

LIFTING ACCESSORIES

1. Willms K, Wells R, Carnahan H. Glove attributes and their contribution to force
   decrement and increased effort in power grip. Hum Factors. 2009 Dec;51(6):797-
   812.
2. McGill SM, Norman RW, Sharratt MT. The effect of an abdominal belt on trunk
   muscle activity and intra-abdominal pressure during squat lifts. Ergonomics. 1990
   Feb;33(2):147-60.
3. Lee S, Kimmerly DS. Influence of music on maximal self-paced running
   performance and passive post-exercise recovery rate. J Sports Med Phys Fitness.
   2016 Jan-Feb;56(1-2):39-48.
4. Stork MJ, Kwan MY, Gibala MJ, Martin Ginis KA. Music enhances performance and
   perceived enjoyment of sprint interval exercise. Med Sci Sports Exerc. 2015
   May;47(5):1052-60.
5. Biagini MS, Brown LE, Coburn JW, Judelson DA, Statler TA, Bottaro M, Tran TT,
   Longo NA. Effects of self-selected music on strength, explosiveness, and mood. J
   Strength Cond Res. 2012 Jul;26(7):1934-8.
6. Bartolomei S, Di Michele R, Merni F. Effects of self-selected music on maximal
   bench press strength and strength endurance. Percept Mot Skills. 2015
   Jun;120(3):714-21.
7. Arazi H, Asadi A, Purabed M. Physiological and Psychophysical Responses to
   Listening to Music during Warm-Up and Circuit-Type Resistance Exercise in
   Strength Trained Men. J Sports Med (Hindawi Publ Corp). 2015;2015:389831.

OBJECTIVE OF TRAINING

1. Schoenfeld BJ. The mechanisms of muscle hypertrophy and their application to
   resistance training. J Strength Cond Res. 2010 Oct; 24(10): 2857-67
2. Schoenfeld BJ, Ogborn D, Krieger JW. Dose-response relationship between weekly
   resistance training volume and increases in muscle mass: A systematic review and
   meta-analysis. J Sports Sci. 2017 Jun;35(11):1073-1082.
3. Krieger J. Single vs. multiple sets of resistance exercise for muscle hypertrophy: a
   meta-analysis. Journal of Strength and Conditioning Research. 2010 Apr 24(4):1150-
   1159
4. Schoenfeld BJ, Ratamess NA, Peterson MD, Contreras B, Tiryaki-Sonmez G.
   Influence of resistance training frequency on muscular adaptations in well-trained
   men. J Strength Cond Res. 2015 Jul;29(7):1821-9.

INTENSITY

1. Schoenfeld BJ. Is there a minimum intensity threshold for resistance training-
   induced hypertrophic adaptations? Sports Med. 2013 Dec;43(12):1279-88.
2. Schoenfeld BJ, Wilson JM, Lowery RP, Krieger JW. Muscular adaptations in low-
   versus high-load resistance training: A meta-analysis. Eur J Sport Sci. 2016;16(1):1-
   10.

3. Schoenfeld BJ, Ratamess NA, Peterson MD, Contreras B, Sonmez GT, Alvar BA. Effects of different volume-equated resistance training loading strategies on muscular adaptations in well-trained men. J Strength Cond Res. 2014 Oct;28(10):2909-18

4. Schoenfeld, et al. Effects of low- vs. high-load resistance training on muscle strength and hypertrophy in well-trained men. Journal of Strength and Conditioning Research. 2015 Oct; 29(10):2954-2963

5. Schoenfeld BJ, et al. "Differential effects of heavy versus moderate loads on measures of strength and hypertrophy in resistance-trained men." Journal of Sports Science & Medicine 15.4 (2016): 715-722. Print.

6. Campos GE, et al. Muscular adaptations in response to three different resistance-training regimens: specificity of repetition maximum training zones. Eur J Appl Physiol. 2002 Nov;88(1-2):50-60.

7. Jenkins NDM, Miramonti AA, Hill EC, Smith CM, Cochrane-Snyman KC, Housh TJ, Cramer JT. Greater neural adaptations following high- vs. low-load resistance training. Front Physiol. 2017 May 29;8:331

8. Schoenfeld, et al. Muscle activation during low- versus high-load resistance training in well-trained men. European Journal of Applied Physiology December 2014, Volume 114, Issue 12, pp 2491-2497

9. Schoenfeld BJ, Contreras B, Ogborn D, Galpin A, Krieger J, Sonmez GT. Effects of varied versus constant loading zones on muscular adaptations in trained men. Int J Sports Med. 2016 Jun;37(6):442-7

10. Sanmy R. Nóbrega and Cleiton A. Libardi. Is resistance training to muscular failure necessary? Front Physiol. 2016; 7:10.

11. Sampson JA, Groeller H. Is repetition failure critical for the development of muscle hypertrophy and strength? Scand J Med Sci Sports. 2016 Apr;26(4):375-83.

12. Willardson JM. The application of training to failure in periodized multiple-set resistance exercise programs. J Strength Cond Res. 2007 May;21(2):628-31.

13. Davies T, Orr R, Halaki M, Hackett D. Effect of training leading to repetition failure on muscular strength: a systematic review and meta-analysis. Sports Med. 2016 Apr;46(4):487-502.

14. Martorelli S, Cadore EL, Izquierdo M, Celes R, Martorelli A, Cleto VA, Alvarenga JG, Bottaro M. Strength training with repetitions to failure does not provide additional strength and muscle hypertrophy gains in young women. Eur J Transl Myol. 2017 Jun;27(2):6339.

15. Helms ER, Cronin J, Storey A, Zourdos MC. "Application of the repetitions in reserve-based rating of perceived exertion scale for resistance training." Ed. Brad Schoenfeld. Strength and Conditioning Journal 2016; 38(4):42-49.

16. Fink J, Schoenfeld BJ, Kikuchi N, Nakazato K. Effects of drop set resistance training on acute stress indicators and long-term muscle hypertrophy and strength. J Sports Med Phys Fitness 2017 Apr

17. Henselmans M, Schoenfeld BJ. The effect of inter-set rest intervals on resistance exercise-induced muscle hypertrophy. Sports Medicine. 2014 Dec; 2012(14): 1635-1643

18. Schoenfeld et al. Longer interset rest periods enhance muscle strength and hypertrophy in resistance-trained men. Journal of Strength and Conditioning Research. 2016 Jul; 30(7):1805-1812

19. de Salles BF, Simão R, Miranda F, et al. Rest interval between sets in strength training. Sports Med. 2009;39(9):765-77.

20. Robins DW, et al. The effect of an upper-body agonist-antagonist resistance training protocol on volume load and efficiency. Journal of Strength and Conditioning Research. 2010 Oct; 24(10):2632-2640.

21. Maia MF, et al. Effects of different rest intervals between antagonist paired sets on repetition performance and muscle activation. Journal of Strength and Conditioning Research. 2014 Sep;28(9):2529-2535
22. Alcaraz PE, Sánchez-Lorente J, Blazevich AJ. Physical performance and cardiovascular responses to an acute bout of heavy resistance circuit training versus traditional strength training. J Strength Cond Res. 2008 May;22(3):667-71.
23. Eric Cressey and Mike Reinold, circa 2011. Ericcressey.com mikereinold.com

VOLUME

1. Klemp A, Dolan C, Quiles JM, Blanco R, Zoeller RF, Graves BS, Zourdos MC. Volume-equated high- and low-repetition daily undulating programming strategies produce similar hypertrophy and strength adaptations. Appl Physiol Nutr Metab. 2016 Jul;41(7):699-705.
2. Radaelli R, Fleck SJ, Leite T, Leite RD, Pinto RS, Fernandes L, Simão R. Dose-response of 1, 3, and 5 sets of resistance exercise on strength, local muscular endurance, and hypertrophy. J Strength Cond Res. 2015 May;29(5):1349-58.
3. Krieger J. Single vs. multiple sets of resistance exercise for muscle hypertrophy: a meta-analysis. Journal of Strength and Conditioning Research. 2010 Apr 24(4):1150-1159
4. Schoenfeld BJ, Ogborn D, Krieger JW. Dose-response relationship between weekly resistance training volume and increases in muscle mass: A systematic review and meta-analysis. J Sports Sci. 2017 Jun;35(11):1073-1082.
5. Burd NA, Holwerda AM, Selby KC, West DW, Staples AW, Cain NE, Cashaback JG, Potvin JR, Baker SK, Phillips SM. Resistance exercise volume affects myofibrillar protein synthesis and anabolic signalling molecule phosphorylation in young men. J Physiol. 2010 Aug 15;588(Pt 16):3119-30.
6. Wernbom M, Augustsson J, Thomeé R. The influence of frequency, intensity, volume and mode of strength training on whole muscle cross-sectional area in humans. Sports Med. 2007;37(3):225–64.
7. Stults-Kolehmainen MA, Bartholomew JB. Psychological stress impairs short-term muscular recovery from resistance exercise. Med Sci Sports Exerc. 2012 Nov;44(11):2220-7.
8. Bartholomew JB, Stults-Kolehmainen MA, Elrod CC, Todd JS. Strength gains after resistance training: the effect of stressful, negative life events. J Strength Cond Res. 2008 Jul;22(4):1215-21.

FREQUENCY

1. Burd NA, West DW, Moore DR, Atherton PJ, Staples AW, Prior T, Tang JE, Rennie MJ, Baker SK, Phillips SM. Enhanced amino acid sensitivity of myofibrillar protein synthesis persists for up to 24 h after resistance exercise in young men. J Nutr. 2011 Apr 1;141(4):568-73.
2. Tipton KD, Wolfe RR. Exercise, protein metabolism, and muscle growth. Int J Sport Nutr Exerc Metab. 2001 Mar;11(1):109-32.
3. MacDougall JD, Gibala MJ, Tarnopolsky MA, MacDonald JR, Interisano SA, Yarasheski KE. The time course for elevated muscle protein synthesis following heavy resistance exercise. Can J Appl Physiol. 1995 Dec;20(4):480-6.

4. Burd NA, Tang JE, Moore DR, Phillips SM. Exercise training and protein metabolism: influences of contraction, protein intake, and sex-based differences. Journal of Applied Physiology 2009 May. 106 (5): 1692-1701
5. Schoenfeld BJ, Ratamess NA, Peterson MD, Contreras B, Tiryaki-Sonmez G. Influence of resistance training frequency on muscular adaptations in well-trained men. J Strength Cond Res. 2015 Jul;29(7):1821-9.
6. Wernbom M, Augustsson J, Thomeé R. The influence of frequency, intensity, volume and mode of strength training on whole muscle cross-sectional area in humans. Sports Med. 2007;37(3):225-64.
7. Mclester Jr, Bishop E, Guilliams Me. Comparison of 1 day and 3 days per week of equal-volume resistance training in experienced subjects. Journal of Strength & Conditioning Research. 2000 Aug; 14(3)
8. Judge LW, Burke JR. The effect of recovery time on strength performance following a high-intensity bench press workout in males and females. Int J Sports Physiol Perform. 2010 Jun;5(2):184-96.
9. Hunter SK. Sex differences in human fatigability: mechanisms and insight to physiological responses. Acta Physiologica. 2014 Feb; 210(4):768-789
10. Maughan RJ, Harmon M, Leiper JB, Sale D, Delman A. Endurance capacity of untrained males and females in isometric and dynamic muscular contractions. European Journal of Applied Physiology and Occupational Physiology. 1986 Aug; 55(4): 395-400

EXERCISE SELECTION

1. de França HS, Branco PA, Guedes Junior DP, Gentil P, Steele J, Teixeira CV. The effects of adding single-joint exercises to a multi-joint exercise resistance training program on upper body muscle strength and size in trained men. Appl Physiol Nutr Metab. 2015 Aug;40(8):822-6.
2. Gentil P, Soares SR, Pereira MC, da Cunha RR, Martorelli SS, Martorelli AS, Bottaro M. Effect of adding single-joint exercises to a multi-joint exercise resistance-training program on strength and hypertrophy in untrained subjects. Appl Physiol Nutr Metab. 2013 Mar;38(3):341-4.
3. Fonseca RM, Roschel H, Tricoli V, de Souza EO, Wilson JM, Laurentino GC, Aihara AY, de Souza Leão AR, Ugrinowitsch C. Changes in exercises are more effective than in loading schemes to improve muscle strength. J Strength Cond Res. 2014 Nov;28(11):3085-92.
4. Antonio J. Nonuniform response of skeletal muscle to heavy resistance training: Can bodybuilders induce regional muscle hypertrophy? *J. Strength Cond. Res.* 2000;14(1):102-113.
5. Marcori, Alexandre & Moura, Túlio & Okazaki, Victor. Gastrocnemius muscle activation during plantar flexion with different feet positioning in physically active young men. Isokinetics and Exercise Science. 2016. 25. 1-5. 10.3233/IES-160654.
6. Assumpção CO, Tibana RA, Viana LC, Willardson JM, Prestes J. Influence of exercise order on upper body maximum and submaximal strength gains in trained men. Clin Physiol Funct Imaging. 2013 Sep;33(5):359-63.
7. Simão R, de Salles BF, Figueiredo T, Dias I, Willardson JM. Exercise order in resistance training. Sports Med. 2012 Mar 1;42(3):251-65.

FORM

1. Schoenfeld BJ, Ogborn D, Vigotsky AD, Franchi M, Krieger JW. Hypertrophic effects of concentric versus eccentric muscle actions: A systematic review and meta-analysis. J Strength Cond Res. 2017 May.
2. Schoenfeld BJ, Ogborn DI, Krieger JW. Effect of repetition duration during resistance training on muscle hypertrophy: a systematic review and meta-analysis. Sports Medicine. 2015 Apr; 45(4):577-585

MAKING GAINS

1. Medeiros HS Jr, Mello RS, Amorim MZ, Koch AJ, Machado M. Planned intensity reduction to maintain repetitions within recommended hypertrophy range. Int J Sports Physiol Perform. 2013 Jul;8(4):384-90.
2. Willardson JM, Simão R, Fontana FE. The effect of load reductions on repetition performance for commonly performed multijoint resistance exercises. J Strength Cond Res. 2012 Nov;26(11):2939-45.

PERIODIZATION

1. Rhea MR, Ball SD, Phillips WT, Burkett LN. A comparison of linear and daily undulating periodized programs with equated volume and intensity for strength. J Strength Cond Res. 2002 May;16(2):250-5.
2. Schoenfeld BJ, Contreras B, Ogborn D, Galpin A, Krieger J, Sonmez GT. Effects of varied versus constant loading zones on muscular adaptations in trained men. Int J Sports Med. 2016 Jun;37(6):442-7.
3. Fonseca RM, Roschel H, Tricoli V, de Souza EO, Wilson JM, Laurentino GC, Aihara AY, de Souza Leão AR, Ugrinowitsch C. Changes in exercises are more effective than in loading schemes to improve muscle strength. J Strength Cond Res. 2014 Nov;28(11):3085-92.
4. Antonio J. Nonuniform response of skeletal muscle to heavy resistance training: Can bodybuilders induce regional muscle hypertrophy? *J. Strength Cond. Res.* 2000;14(1):102-113.
5. McNamara JM, Stearne DJ. Flexible nonlinear periodization in a beginner college weight training class. J Strength Cond Res. 2010 Jan;24(1):17-22.

MAINTENANCE

1. Bickel CS, et al. Exercise dosing to retain resistance training adaptations in young and older adults. Med Sci Sports Exerc. 2011.

DELOADS

1. Ogasawara R, Yasuda T, Sakamaki M, Ozaki H, Abe T. Effects of periodic and continued resistance training on muscle CSA and strength in previously untrained men. Clin Physiol Funct Imaging. 2011 Sep;31(5):399-404.
2. Ogasawara R, Yasuda T, Ishii N, Abe T. Comparison of muscle hypertrophy following 6-month of continuous and periodic strength training. Eur J Appl Physiol. 2013 Apr;113(4):975-85.

3. Gentil P, Ferreira-Junior JB, Soares SR, Martorelli AS, Bottaro M, Cadore EL, Loenneke JP. Effects of periodic and continuous resistance training on muscle strength in detrained women. Percept Mot Skills. 2015 Dec;121(3):810-21.

BEFORE BATTLE

1. Schoenfeld BJ, Aragon A, Wilborn C, Urbina SL, Hayward SE, Krieger J. (2017) Pre-versus post-exercise protein intake has similar effects on muscular adaptations. PeerJ 5:e2825
2. Biagini MS, Brown LE, Coburn JW, Judelson DA, Statler TA, Bottaro M, Tran TT, Longo NA. Effects of self-selected music on strength, explosiveness, and mood. J Strength Cond Res. 2012 Jul;26(7):1934-8.
3. Tod D, Iredale F, Gill N. 'Psyching-up' and muscular force production. Sports Med. 2003;33(1):47-58.
4. Loizou G, Karageorghis CI. Effects of psychological priming, video, and music on anaerobic exercise performance. Scand J Med Sci Sports. 2015 Dec;25(6):909-20.

CARDIO

1. Wilson JM, Marin PJ, Rhea MR, Wilson SM, Loenneke JP, Anderson JC. Concurrent training: a meta-analysis examining interference of aerobic and resistance exercises. J Strength Cond Res. 2012 Aug;26(8):2293-307.
2. Baar K. Using molecular biology to maximize concurrent training. Sports Med. 2014 Nov;44 Suppl 2:S117-25.
3. Steele J, Fisher J, McGuff D, Bruce-Low S, Smith D. Resistance Training to Momentary Muscular Failure Improves Cardiovascular Fitness in Humans: A Review of Acute Physiological Responses and Chronic Physiological Adaptations. JEPonline 2012;15(3):53-80.
4. Alcaraz PE, Sánchez-Lorente J, Blazevich AJ. Physical performance and cardiovascular responses to an acute bout of heavy resistance circuit training versus traditional strength training. J Strength Cond Res. 2008 May;22(3):667-71.
5. Helms ER, Fitschen PJ, Aragon AA, Cronin J, Schoenfeld BJ. Recommendations for natural bodybuilding contest preparation: resistance and cardiovascular training. J Sports Med Phys Fitness. 2015 Mar;55(3):164-78.
6. Schoenfeld BJ, Aragon AA, Wilborn CD, Krieger JW, Sonmez GT. Body composition changes associated with fasted versus non-fasted aerobic exercise. Journal of the International Society of Sports Nutrition. 2014;11:54.

CALORIES

1. Levine JA, Eberhardt NL, Jensen MD. Role of nonexercise activity thermogenesis in resistance to fat gain in humans. Science. 1999 Jan 8;283(5399):212-4.
2. Aragon AA, Schoenfeld BJ, Wildman R, Kleiner S, VanDusseldorp T, Taylor L, Earnest CP, Arciero PJ, Wilborn C, Kalman DS, Stout JR, Willoughby DS, Campbell B, Arent SM, Bannock L, Smith-Ryan AE, Antonio J. International society of sports nutrition position stand: diets and body composition. J Int Soc Sports Nutr. 2017 Jun;14:16.
3. Rozenek R, Ward P, Long S, Garhammer J. Effects of high-calorie supplements on body composition and muscular strength following resistance training. J Sports Med Phys Fitness. 2002 Sep;42(3):340-7.

4. Garthe I, Raastad T, Refsnes PE, Koivisto A, Sundgot-Borgen J.Effect of two different weight-loss rates on body composition and strength and power-related performance in elite athletes.Int J Sport Nutr Exerc Metab. 2011 Apr;21(2):97-104.
5. Helms ER, Aragon AA, Fitschen PJ. Evidence-based recommendations for natural bodybuilding contest preparation: nutrition and supplementation. Journal of the International Society of Sports Nutrition 2014;11:20
6. First learned this from Lyle McDonald, a great thinker of the field many years ago. You can read more of his work at www.bodyrecomposition.com

MACRONUTRIENTS

1. Morton RW, Murphy KT, McKellar SR, et al. A systematic review, meta-analysis and meta-regression of the effect of protein supplementation on resistance training-induced gains in muscle mass and strength in healthy adults. Br J Sports Med. 2017 Jul.
2. Jäger R, Kerksick CM, Campbell BI, Cribb PJ, Wells SD, Skwiat TM, Purpura M, et al. International Society of Sports Nutrition Position Stand: protein and exercise. J Int Soc Sports Nutr. 2017 Jun 20;14:20.
3. Helms ER, Zinn C, Rowlands DS, Brown SR. A systematic review of dietary protein during caloric restriction in resistance trained lean athletes: a case for higher intakes. Int J Sport Nutr Exerc Metab. 2014 Apr;24(2):127-38.
4. Antonio J, Ellerbroek A, Silver T, Vargas L, Tamayo A, Buehn R, Peacock CA. A high protein diet has no harmful effects: a one-year crossover study in resistance-trained males. J Nutr Metab. 2016;2016:9104792. Epub 2016 Oct 11.
5. Antonio J, Peacock CA, Ellerbroek A, Fromhoff B, Silver T. The effects of consuming a high protein diet (4.4 g/kg/d) on body composition in resistance-trained individuals. J Int Soc Sports Nutr. 2014 May 12;11:19.

MEAL TIMING

1. Bellisle F, McDevitt R, Prentice, AM. Meal frequency and energy balance. British Journal of Nutrition. 1997 Apr;77(1)57-70
2. Schoenfeld BJ, Aragon AA, Krieger JW. Effects of meal frequency on weight loss and body composition: a meta-analysis. Nutr Rev. 2015;73(2): 69-82.
3. Cameron JD, Cyr MJ, Doucet E. Increased meal frequency does not promote greater weight loss in subjects who were prescribed an 8-week equi-energetic energy-restricted diet. Br J Nutr. 2010 Apr;103(8):1098-101.
4. Leidy HJ, Armstrong CL, Tang M, Mattes RD, Campbell WW. The influence of higher protein intake and greater eating frequency on appetite control in overweight and obese men. Obesity (Silver Spring). 2010 Sep;18(9):1725-32.
5. Tinsley GM, Forsse JS, Butler NK, Paoli A, Bane AA, La Bounty PM, Morgan GB, Grandjean PW. Time-restricted feeding in young men performing resistance training: A randomized controlled trial. Eur J Sport Sci. 2017 Mar;17(2):200-207.
6. Moro T, Tinsley G, Bianco A, Marcolin G, Pacelli QF, Battaglia G, Palma A, Gentil P, Neri M, Paoli A. Effects of eight weeks of time-restricted feeding (16/8) on basal metabolism, maximal strength, body composition, inflammation, and cardiovascular risk factors in resistance-trained males. J Transl Med. 2016 Oct 13;14(1):290.
7. The credit for popularizing this approach must go to Martin Berkhan, circa 2010. You can read more of his work at ww.leangains.com

8.   Schoenfeld BJ, Aragon A, Wilborn C, Urbina SL, Hayward SE, Krieger J. (2017) Pre-versus post-exercise protein intake has similar effects on muscular adaptations. PeerJ 5:e2825
9.   Capaldo B, Gastaldelli A, Antoniello S, Auletta M, Pardo F, Ciociaro D, Guida R, Ferrannini E, Saccà L Splanchnic and leg substrate exchange after ingestion of a natural mixed meal in humans. Diabetes. 1999 May;48(5):958-66.

FOOD CHOICES

1.   Hoefkens C, Sioen I, Baert K, De Meulenaer B, De Henauw S, Vandekinderen I, Devlieghere F, Opsomer A, Verbeke W, Van Camp J. Consuming organic versus conventional vegetables: the effect on nutrient and contaminant intakes. Food Chem Toxicol. 2010 Nov;48(11):3058-66.
2.   Magkos F, Arvaniti F, Zampelas A. Putting the safety of organic food into perspective. Nutr Res Rev. 2003 Dec;16(2):211-22.
3.   Dangour AD, Dodhia SK, Hayter A, Allen E, Lock K, Uauy R. Nutritional quality of organic foods: a systematic review. Am J Clin Nutr. 2009 Sep;90(3):680-5.
4.   Surwit RS, et al. Metabolic and behavioral effects of a high-sucrose diet during weight loss. Am J Clin Nutr. 1997 Apr;65(4):908-15.

MEAL TIME

1.   Arch JJ, Brown KW, Goodman RJ, Della Porta MD, Kiken LG, Tillman S. Enjoying food without caloric cost: The impact of brief mindfulness on laboratory eating outcomes.Behav Res Ther. 2016 Apr;79:23-34.
2.   Beshara M, Hutchinson AD, Wilson C. Does mindfulness matter? Everyday mindfulness, mindful eating and self-reported serving size of energy dense foods among a sample of South Australian adults. Appetite. 2013 Aug;67:25-9.
3.   O'Reilly GA, Cook L, Spruijt-Metz D, Black DS. Mindfulness-based interventions for obesity-related eating behaviours: a literature review.Obes Rev. 2014 Jun;15(6):453-61.

SUPPLEMENTS

1.   Kreider RB, Wilborn CD, Taylor L, et al. ISSN exercise & sport nutrition review: research & recommendations. Journal of the International Society of Sports Nutrition. 2010;7:7.
2.   Simopoulos AP. Omega-3 fatty acids and athletics. Curr Sports Med Rep. 2007 Jul;6(4):230-6.
3.   Kreider RB, Kalman DS, Antonio J, Ziegenfuss TN, Wildman R, Collins R, Candow DG, Kleiner SM, Almada AL, Lopez HL. International Society of Sports Nutrition position stand: safety and efficacy of creatine supplementation in exercise, sport, and medicine. J Int Soc Sports Nutr. 2017 Jun;14:18.
4.   Da Silva VL, Messias FR, Zanchi NE, Gerlinger-Romero F, Duncan MJ, Guimarães-Ferreira L. Effects of acute caffeine ingestion on resistance training performance and perceptual responses during repeated sets to failure. J Sports Med Phys Fitness. 2015 May;55(5):383-9.

5. Duncan MJ, Stanley M, Parkhouse N, Cook K, Smith M. Acute caffeine ingestion enhances strength performance and reduces perceived exertion and muscle pain perception during resistance exercise. Eur J Sport Sci. 2013;13(4):392-9.
6. Evans SM, Griffiths RR. Caffeine tolerance and choice in humans. Psychopharmacology (Berl). 1992;108(1-2):51-9.

ALCOHOL

1. Koziris LP, et al. Effect of acute postexercise ethanol intoxication on the neuroendocrine response to resistance exercise. J Appl Physiol. 2000 Jan;88(1):165-72.
2. Sierksma A, et al. Effect of moderate alcohol consumption on plasma dehydroepiandrosterone sulfate, testosterone, and estradiol levels in middle-aged men and postmenopausal women: a diet-controlled intervention study. Alcohol Clin Exp Res. 2004 May;28(5):780-5.
3. Parr EB, Camera DM, Areta JL, Burke LM, Phillips SM, Hawley JA, Coffey VG. Alcohol ingestion impairs maximal post-exercise rates of myofibrillar protein synthesis following a single bout of concurrent training. PLoS One. 2014 Feb 12;9(2):e88384
4. Gaziano JM, Gaziano TA, Glynn RJ, Sesso HD, Ajani UA, Stampfer MJ, Manson JE, Hennekens CH, Buring JE. Light-to-moderate alcohol consumption and mortality in the Physicians' Health Study enrollment cohort. J Am Coll Cardiol. 2000 Jan;35(1):96-105.
5. Sesso HD, Stampfer MJ, Rosner B, Hennekens CH, Manson JE, Gaziano JM. Seven-year changes in alcohol consumption and subsequent risk of cardiovascular disease in men. Arch Intern Med. 2000 Sep 25;160(17):2605-12.
6. Camargo CA Jr, Hennekens CH, Gaziano JM, Glynn RJ, Manson JE, Stampfer MJ. Prospective study of moderate alcohol consumption and mortality in US male physicians. Arch Intern Med. 1997 Jan 13;157(1):79-85.
7. Kato I, Kiyohara Y, Kubo M, Tanizaki Y, Arima H, Iwamoto H, Shinohara N, Nakayama K, Fujishima M. Insulin-mediated effects of alcohol intake on serum lipid levels in a general population: the Hisayama Study. J Clin Epidemiol. 2003 Feb;56(2):196-204.
8. Holahan CJ, Schutte KK, Brennan PL, et al. Wine Consumption and 20-Year Mortality Among Late-Life Moderate Drinkers. Journal of Studies on Alcohol and Drugs. 2012;73(1):80-88.
9. Mitchell MC, Teigen EL, Ramchandani VA. Absorption and Peak Blood Alcohol Concentration After Drinking Beer, Wine, or Spirits. Alcoholism, Clinical and Experimental Research. 2014;38(5):1200-1204.
10. Jones AW, Jönsson KA, Kechagias S. Effect of high-fat, high-protein, and high-carbohydrate meals on the pharmacokinetics of a small dose of ethanol. Br J Clin Pharmacol. 1997 Dec;44(6):521-6.
11. Rose AK, Hardman CA, Christiansen P. The effects of a priming dose of alcohol and drinking environment on snack food intake. Appetite. 2015 Dec;95:341-8.

SLEEP

1. Brandt R, Bevilacqua GG, Andrade A. Perceived Sleep Quality, Mood States, and Their Relationship With Performance Among Brazilian Elite Athletes During a Competitive Period.J Strength Cond Res. 2017 Apr;31(4):1033-1039.
2. Copenhaver EA, Diamond AB. The Value of Sleep on Athletic Performance, Injury, and Recovery in the Young Athlete. Pediatr Ann. 2017 Mar 1;46(3):e106-e111.

3. Rae DE, Chin T, Dikgomo K, Hill L, McKune AJ, Kohn TA, Roden LC. One night of partial sleep deprivation impairs recovery from a single exercise training session. Eur J Appl Physiol. 2017 Apr;117(4):699-712.

4. Lentino CV, Purvis DL, Murphy KJ, Deuster PA. Sleep as a component of the performance triad: the importance of sleep in a military population. US Army Med Dep J. 2013 Oct-Dec:98-108.

5. Loprinzi PD, Loenneke JP. Engagement in muscular strengthening activities is associated with better sleep. Prev Med Rep. 2015 Oct 31;2:927-9.

6. Alley JR, Mazzochi JW, Smith CJ, Morris DM, Collier SR. Effects of resistance exercise timing on sleep architecture and nocturnal blood pressure. J Strength Cond Res. 2015 May;29(5):1378-85.

7. Chang AM, Aeschbach D, Duffy JF, Czeisler CA. Evening use of light-emitting eReaders negatively affects sleep, circadian timing, and next-morning alertness. Proc Natl Acad Sci U S A. 2015 Jan 27;112(4):1232-7.

8. Cajochen C, Frey S, Anders D, Späti J, Bues M, Pross A, Mager R, Wirz-Justice A, Stefani O. Evening exposure to a light-emitting diodes (LED)-backlit computer screen affects circadian physiology and cognitive performance. J Appl Physiol (1985). 2011 May;110(5):1432-8.

9. van der Lely S, Frey S, Garbazza C, Wirz-Justice A, Jenni OG, Steiner R, Wolf S, Cajochen C, Bromundt V, Schmidt C. Blue blocker glasses as a countermeasure for alerting effects of evening light-emitting diode screen exposure in male teenagers. J Adolesc Health. 2015 Jan;56(1):113-9.

SOFT TISSUE WORK/FOAM ROLLING

1. Peacock CA, Krein DD, Silver TA, Sanders GJ, VON Carlowitz KA. An Acute Bout of Self-Myofascial Release in the Form of Foam Rolling Improves Performance Testing. Int J Exerc Sci. 2014 Jul 1;7(3):202-211.

2. Cheatham SW, Kolber MJ, Cain M, Lee M. The effects of self-myofascial release using a foam roll or roller massager on joint range of motion, muscle recovery, and performance: a systematic review. Int J Sports Phys Ther. 2015 Nov;10(6):827-38.

3. Schroeder AN, Best TM. Is self myofascial release an effective preexercise and recovery strategy? A literature review. Curr Sports Med Rep. 2015 May-Jun;14(3):200-8.

4. Beardsley C, Škarabot J. Effects of self-myofascial release: A systematic review. J Bodyw Mov Ther. 2015 Oct;19(4):747-58.

5. Mohr AR, Long BC, Goad CL. Effect of foam rolling and static stretching on passive hip-flexion range of motion. J Sport Rehabil. 2014 Nov;23(4):296-9.

6. Su H, Chang NJ, Wu WL, Guo LY, Chu IH. Acute Effects of Foam Rolling, Static Stretching, and Dynamic Stretching During Warm-Ups on Muscular Flexibility and Strength in Young Adults. J Sport Rehabil. 2016 Oct 13:1-24.

7. Pearcey GE, Bradbury-Squires DJ, Kawamoto JE, Drinkwater EJ, Behm DG, Button DC. Foam rolling for delayed-onset muscle soreness and recovery of dynamic performance measures. J Athl Train. 2015 Jan;50(1):5-13.

8. Macdonald GZ, Button DC, Drinkwater EJ, Behm DG. Foam rolling as a recovery tool after an intense bout of physical activity. Med Sci Sports Exerc. 2014 Jan;46(1):131-42.

CUTTING PLATEAUS

1. Keys A, Brozek J, Henschel A, Mickelsen O, Taylor HL. The biology of human starvation. Minneapolis (MN): The University of Minnesota Press; 1950.
2. Müller MJ, Enderle J, Pourhassan M, Braun W, Eggeling B, Lagerpusch M, Glüer CC, Kehayias JJ, Kiosz D, Bosy-Westphal A. Metabolic adaptation to caloric restriction and subsequent refeeding: the Minnesota Starvation Experiment revisited. Am J Clin Nutr. 2015 Oct;102(4):807-19.
3. Swartz AM, Squires L, Strath SJ. Energy expenditure of interruptions to sedentary behavior. Int J Behav Nutr Phys Act. 2011 Jun 27;8:69.

PROGRESS PITFALLS

1. Lowery RP, Joy JM, Loenneke JP, de Souza EO, Machado M, Dudeck JE, Wilson JM. Practical blood flow restriction training increases muscle hypertrophy during a periodized resistance training programme. Clin Physiol Funct Imaging. 2014 Jul;34(4):317-21.
2. Scott BR, Loenneke JP, Slattery KM, Dascombe BJ. Blood flow restricted exercise for athletes: A review of available evidence. J Sci Med Sport. 2016 May;19(5):360-7.
3. Loenneke JP, Wilson JM, Marín PJ, Zourdos MC, Bemben MG. Low intensity blood flow restriction training: a meta-analysis. Eur J Appl Physiol. 2012 May;112(5):1849-59.
4. Shaw G, Lee-Barthel A, Ross ML, Wang B, Baar K. Vitamin C-enriched gelatin supplementation before intermittent activity augments collagen synthesis. Am J Clin Nutr. 2017 Jan;105(1):136-143.
5. Ogasawara R, Yasuda T, Sakamaki M, Ozaki H, Abe T. Effects of periodic and continued resistance training on muscle CSA and strength in previously untrained men. Clin Physiol Funct Imaging. 2011 Sep;31(5):399-404.
6. Ogasawara R, Yasuda T, Ishii N, Abe T. Comparison of muscle hypertrophy following 6-month of continuous and periodic strength training. Eur J Appl Physiol. 2013 Apr;113(4):975-85.
7. Gentil P, Ferreira-Junior JB, Soares SR, Martorelli AS, Bottaro M, Cadore EL, Loenneke JP. Effects of periodic and continuous resistance training on muscle strength in detrained women. Percept Mot Skills. 2015 Dec;121(3):810-21.
8. Bickel CS, et al. Exercise dosing to retain resistance training adaptations in young and older adults. Med Sci Sports Exerc. 2011.

MIND OVER MUSCLE

1. Goldfield GS. Body image, disordered eating and anabolic steroid use in female bodybuilders. Eat Disord. 2009 May-Jun;17(3):200-10.
2. Mangweth B, Pope HG Jr, Kemmler G, Ebenbichler C, Hausmann A, De Col C, Kreutner B, Kinzl J, Biebl W. Body image and psychopathology in male bodybuilders. Psychother Psychosom. 2001 Jan-Feb;70(1):38-43.
3. Goldfield GS, Blouin AG, Woodside DB. Body image, binge eating, and bulimia nervosa in male bodybuilders. Can J Psychiatry. 2006 Mar;51(3):160-8.
4. Blouin AG, Goldfield GS. Body image and steroid use in male bodybuilders. Int J Eat Disord. 1995 Sep;18(2):159-65.
5. Aspa. "Home." Home | MentalHealth.gov, Department of Health and Human Services, 31 July 2012, www.mentalhealth.gov/.

6. "Mental Disorders." World Health Organization, World Health Organization, www.who.int/mental_health/management/en/.

7. Petterson H, Olson BL. Effects of Mindfulness-Based Interventions in High School and College Athletes for Reducing Stress and Injury, and Improving Quality of Life. J Sport Rehabil. 2016 Aug 24:1-18.

8. Bühlmayer L, Birrer D, Röthlin P, Faude O, Donath L. Effects of Mindfulness Practice on Performance-Relevant Parameters and Performance Outcomes in Sports: A Meta-Analytical Review. Sports Med. 2017 Jun 29. [Epub ahead of print]

9. Haase L, May AC, Falahpour M, Isakovic , Simmons AN, Hickman SD, Liu TT, Paulus MP. A pilot study investigating changes in neural processing after mindfulness training in elite athletes. Front Behav Neurosci. 2015 Aug 27;9:229.

10. Scott-Hamilton J, Schutte NS, Brown RF. Effects of a Mindfulness Intervention on Sports-Anxiety, Pessimism, and Flow in Competitive Cyclists.Appl Psychol Health Well Being. 2016 Mar;8(1):85-103.

11. Spijkerman MP, Pots WT, Bohlmeijer ET. Effectiveness of online mindfulness-based interventions in improving mental health: A review and meta-analysis of randomised controlled trials. Clin Psychol Rev. 2016 Apr;45:102-14.

12. Sharma M, Rush SE. Mindfulness-based stress reduction as a stress management intervention for healthy individuals: a systematic review. J Evid Based Complementary Altern Med. 2014 Oct;19(4):271-86.

13. Marchand WR. Mindfulness-based stress reduction, mindfulness-based cognitive therapy, and Zen meditation for depression, anxiety, pain, and psychological distress. J Psychiatr Pract. 2012 Jul;18(4):233-52.

14. Shonin E, Van Gordon W, Griffiths MD. Mindfulness-based interventions: towards mindful clinical integration. Frontiers in Psychology. 2013;4:194.

15. Kabat-Zinn J, Massion AO, Kristeller J, Peterson LG, Fletcher KE, Pbert L, Lenderking WR, Santorelli SF.Effectiveness of a meditation-based stress reduction program in the treatment of anxiety disorders. Am J Psychiatry. 1992 Jul;149(7):936-43.

16. Feicht T, Wittmann M, Jose G, Mock A, von Hirschhausen E, Esch T. Evaluation of a seven-week web-based happiness training to improve psychological well-being, reduce stress, and enhance mindfulness and flourishing: a randomized controlled occupational health study. Evidence-based Complementary and Alternative Medicine : eCAM. 2013;2013:676953.

17. Brand S, Holsboer-Trachsler E, Naranjo JR, Schmidt S. Influence of mindfulness practice on cortisol and sleep in long-term and short-term meditators. Neuropsychobiology. 2012;65(3):109-18.

18. Dalen J, Smith BW, Shelley BM, Sloan AL, Leahigh L, Begay D. Pilot study: Mindful Eating and Living (MEAL): weight, eating behavior, and psychological outcomes associated with a mindfulness-based intervention for people with obesity. Complement Ther Med. 2010 Dec;18(6):260-4.

19. Katterman SN, Kleinman BM, Hood MM, Nackers LM, Corsica JA. Mindfulness meditation as an intervention for binge eating, emotional eating, and weight loss: a systematic review. Eat Behav. 2014 Apr;15(2):197-204.

20. Mantzios M, Wilson JC. Mindfulness, eating behaviours, and obesity: a review and reflection on current findings. Curr Obes Rep. 2015 Mar;4(1):141-6.

21. Skanavi S, Laqueille X, Aubin HJ. Mindfulness based interventions for addictive disorders: a review.Encephale. 2011 Oct;37(5):379-87.

22. Montero-Marin J, Puebla-Guedea M, Herrera-Mercadal P, Cebolla A Soler J, Demarzo M, Vazquez C, Rodríguez-Bornaetxea F, Garcia-Campayo J. Psychological Effects of a 1-Month Meditation Retreat on Experienced Meditators: The Role of Non-attachment. Front Psychol. 2016 Dec 12;7:1935

23. M G R, B S, E S, S Rai K. Efficacy of rajayoga meditation on positive thinking: an index for self-satisfaction and happiness in life. J Clin Diagn Res. 2013 Oct;7(10):2265-7.

24. Barnes S, Brown KW, Krusemark E, Campbell WK, Rogge RD. The role of mindfulness in romantic relationship satisfaction and responses to relationship stress. J Marital Fam Ther. 2007 Oct;33(4):482-500.

25. Sun S, Yao Z, Wei J, Yu R. Calm and smart? A selective review of meditation effects on decision making. Front Psychol. 2015 Jul 24;6:1059.

26. Grant JA, Rainville P. Pain sensitivity and analgesic effects of mindful states in Zen meditators: a cross-sectional study. Psychosom Med. 2009 Jan;71(1):106-14.

27. Zeidan F, Gordon NS, Merchant J, Goolkasian P. The effects of brief mindfulness meditation training on experimentally induced pain. J Pain. 2010 Mar;11(3):199-209.

28. Fjorback LO. Mindfulness and bodily distress. Dan Med J. 2012 Nov;59(11):B4547.

29. Mrazek MD, Franklin MS, Phillips DT, Baird B, Schooler JW. Mindfulness training improves working memory capacity and GRE performance while reducing mind wandering. Psychol Sci. 2013 May;24(5):776-81.

30. Chiesa A, Calati R, Serretti A. Does mindfulness training improve cognitive abilities? A systematic review of neuropsychological findings. Clin Psychol Rev. 2011 Apr;31(3):449-64.

Made in the USA
Coppell, TX
15 July 2020

30889079R00350